Lymphadenectomy in Urologic Oncology: Indications, Controversies and Complications

Guest Editor

REZA GHAVAMIAN, MD

UROLOGIC CLINICS
OF NORTH AMERICA

www.urologic.theclinics.com

November 2011 • Volume 38 • Number 4

SAUNDERS an imprint of ELSEVIER, Inc.

W.B. SAUNDERS COMPANY
A Division of Elsevier Inc.

1600 John F. Kennedy Blvd. ● Suite 1800 ● Philadelphia, PA 19103-2899

http://www.theclinics.com

UROLOGIC CLINICS OF NORTH AMERICA Volume 38, Number 4
November 2011 ISSN 0094-0143, ISBN-13: 978-1-4557-1048-5

Editor: Stephanie Donley
Developmental Editor: Teia Stone

Urologic Clinics of North America (ISSN 0094-0143) is published quarterly by Elsevier Inc., 360 Park Avenue South, New York, NY 10010-1710. Months of issue are February, May, August, and November. Business and Editorial Offices: 1600 John F. Kennedy Blvd., Suite 1800, Philadelphia, PA 19103-2899. Periodicals postage paid at New York, NY and additional mailing offices. Subscription prices are $311.00 per year (US individuals), $519.00 per year (US institutions), $363.00 per year (Canadian individuals), $636.00 per year (Canadian institutions), $451.00 per year (foreign individuals), and $636.00 per year (foreign institutions). Foreign air speed delivery is included in all *Clinics* subscription prices. All prices are subject to change without notice. **POSTMASTER:** Send address changes to *Urologic Clinics of North America*, Elsevier Health Sciences Division, Subscription Customer Service, 3251 Riverport Lane, Maryland Heights, MO 63043. Customer Service: 1-800-654-2452 (US). From outside the United States, call 1-314-447-8871. Fax: 1-314-447-8029. E-mail: JournalsCustomerServiceusa@elsevier.com (for print support) and JournalsOnlineSupport-usa@elsevier.com (for online support).

Reprints. For copies of 100 or more, of articles in this publication, please contact the Commercial Reprints Department, Elsevier Inc., 360 Park Avenue South, New York, New York 10010-1710. Tel.: 212-633-3813; Fax: 212-462-1935; E-mail: reprints@elsevier.com.

Urologic Clinics of North America is covered in MEDLINE/PubMed (*Index Medicus*), *Excerpta Medica, Current Contents/ Clinical Medicine, Science Citation Index,* and *ISI/BIOMED.*

Printed in the United States of America.

Contributors

GUEST EDITOR

REZA GHAVAMIAN, MD
Professor of Clinical Urology; Director of
Urologic Oncology Program, Department
of Urology, Montefiore Medical Center,
Albert Einstein College of Medicine, Bronx,
New York

AUTHORS

RILEY E. ALEXANDER, MD, MBA
Department of Pathology and Laboratory
Medicine, Indiana University School of
Medicine, Indianapolis, Indiana

CHRISTOPHER L. AMLING, MD
Division of Urology, Oregon Health and
Science University, Portland, Oregon

FIONA C. BURKHARD, MD
Associated Professor, Department of Urology,
University Hospital Bern, Bern, Switzerland

BRETT CARVER, MD
Assistant Attending, Assistant Member,
Memorial Sloan-Kettering Cancer Center,
New York, New York

BRIAN F. CHAPIN, MD
Department of Urology, University of Texas MD
Anderson Cancer Center, Houston, Texas

LIANG CHENG, MD
Departments of Pathology and Laboratory
Medicine and Urology, Indiana University
School of Medicine, Indianapolis, Indiana

VICTORIA CHERNYAK, MD
Assistant Professor of Radiology of Albert
Einstein College of Medicine, Department of
Radiology, Montefiore Medical Center, Bronx,
New York

SCOTT E. DELACROIX Jr, MD
Department of Urology, University of Texas MD
Anderson Cancer Center, Houston, Texas

BRIAN D. DUTY, MD
Attending Physician, Department of Urology,
North Shore Long Island Jewish Health
System, The Smith Institute for Urology,
New Hyde Park, New York

MATHEW T. GETTMAN, MD
Professor of Urology, Department of Urology,
Mayo Clinic, Rochester, Minnesota

REZA GHAVAMIAN, MD
Professor of Clinical Urology; Director of
Urologic Oncology Program, Department of
Urology, Montefiore Medical Center, Albert
Einstein College of Medicine, Bronx,
New York

A. ARI HAKIMI, MD
Department of Urology, Montefiore Medical
Center, Albert Einstein College of Medicine,
Bronx, New York

SIMON HORENBLAS, MD, PhD
Professor of Urology, Head of Department
of Urology, The Netherlands Cancer
Institute–Antoni van Leeuwenhoek Hospital,
Amsterdam, The Netherlands

LOUIS R. KAVOUSSI, MD, MBA
Professor and Chair, Department of Urology,
North Shore Long Island Jewish Health
System, The Smith Institute for Urology,
New Hyde Park, New York

JEFFREY C. LA ROCHELLE, MD
Division of Urology, Oregon Health and Science University, Portland, Oregon

ANDREW K. LEE, MD
Associate Professor, Division of Radiation Oncology, The University of Texas MD Anderson Cancer Center, Houston, Texas

DANIEL J. LEWINSHTEIN, MD
Suo Fellow in Urologic Oncology, Division of Urology, Virginia Mason Medical Center, Seattle, Washington

CHRISTOPHER R. PORTER, MD
Director of Urologic Oncology, Division of Urology, Virginia Mason Medical Center, Seattle, Washington

THOMAS J. PUGH, MD
Assistant Professor, Division of Radiation Oncology, The University of Texas MD Anderson Cancer Center, Houston, Texas

FARHANG RABBANI, MD
Department of Urology, Albert Einstein College of Medicine; Associate Professor, Montefiore Medical Center, Bronx, New York

BEAT ROTH, MD
Department of Urology, University Hospital Bern, Bern, Switzerland

ORNOB P. ROY, MD, MBA
Department of Urology, North Shore Long Island Jewish Health System, The Smith Institute for Urology, New Hyde Park, New York

JOEL SHEINFELD, MD
Deputy Chief, Urology Service; William G. Cahan Chair in Surgery, Memorial Sloan-Kettering Cancer Center, New York, New York

URS E. STUDER, MD
Professor, Department of Urology, University Hospital Bern, Bern, Switzerland

MING-TSE SUNG, MD
Departments of Pathology and Laboratory Medicine, Kaohsiung Chang Gung Memorial Hospital and Chang Gung University College of Medicine, Niao Sung District, Kaohsiung, Taiwan

TATUM TARIN, MD
Urologic Oncology Fellow, Memorial Sloan-Kettering Cancer Center, New York, New York

CHRISTOPHER J. WEIGHT, MD
Department of Urology, Mayo Clinic, Rochester, Minnesota

STEVE K. WILLIAMS, MD
Department of Urology, Albert Einstein College of Medicine, Bronx, New York

CHRISTOPHER G. WOOD, MD
Professor and Deputy Chairman, Department of Urology, University of Texas MD Anderson Cancer Center, Houston, Texas

PASCAL ZEHNDER, MD
Department of Urology, University Hospital Bern, Bern, Switzerland

Contents

> The history of urologic lymphadenectomy is rich and diverse. Our current under-
> standing of its use and benefits is a product of the hard work of numerous physicians
> and scientists from many nations. Standard dissection templates for the various
> urologic malignancies are based on a complete understanding of the anatomy of
> the lymphatic system, which has developed immensely since Hippocrates first
> described the white blood of the lymphatic system while performing an axillary dis-
> section. It is hoped that the next 100 years will bring even greater comprehension of
> its value and utility.

> Pelvic lymph node dissection is the only reliable technique to detect low-volume
> lymph node involvement in prostate cancer. Extended lymph node dissections
> that include the internal iliac chain in addition to the external iliac and obturator
> packets have shown a significantly higher proportion of patients to have lymphatic
> involvement than previously recognized. The improved staging afforded by a more
> extended dissection raises several questions. Addressing these questions is the
> focus of this review.

> Pelvic lymph node dissection (PLND) at the time of cystectomy remains the most ac-
> curate method of staging and can have a positive impact on cancer control, and
> there is general agreement as to its necessity at the time of surgery. There is, how-
> ever, a lack of consensus regarding the terminology of PLND and controversy con-
> cerning the optimal extent of lymph node dissection, especially because recent
> investigations have suggested a survival benefit with extended PLND.

> With the rapid and widespread adoption of minimally invasive procedures (laparo-
> scopic and robotic) for the treatment of prostate and bladder cancers in the last
> decade, concerns have been raised regarding whether the technique can emulate
> the time-tested gold standard open procedures. This article briefly reviews the indi-
> cations for lymph node dissection for bladder and prostate cancer, and reviews the
> role of extended lymphadenectomy in each procedure. Much of the focus of this
> review is on minimally invasive approaches and the technical aspects of the proce-
> dures, the feasibility of the robotic technique, and early oncologic outcomes.

node involvement. It focuses on the indications of surgical management of the regional nodes, the extent of the surgery, and its complications. Also, neoadjuvant therapy is covered.

Accurate lymph node staging in genitourinary (GU) malignancies is important for planning an appropriate treatment and establishing an accurate prognosis. This article discusses the novel imaging techniques for detection of metastases in various GU malignancies, including prostate, bladder, penile, and testicular cancers. Discussion includes nuclear medicine techniques of ^{18}F-fluorodeoxyglucose positron emission tomography/computed tomography (PET/CT), ^{11}C-choline and ^{18}F-choline PET/CT, and ProstaScint scanning, as well as sentinel lymph node mapping. Magnetic resonance (MR) techniques include lymphotropic nanoparticle-enhanced MR imaging and diffusion-weighted MR imaging.

Lymphadenectomy (LAD) is an important staging and treatment modality of oncologic surgery. LAD in genitourinary malignancies presents inherent difficulties to the urologist and pathologist because of the differences in anatomic sites and primary histologic type. This review focuses on pathologic evaluation and how communication between urologist and pathologist is necessary to provide optimal care. Recommendations covering general specimen submission and processing are discussed, as well as more specific recommendations concerning the kidney, upper urinary tract, urinary bladder, prostate, testes, and penis. Emerging areas of prognostic significance and the impact that improved molecular techniques are contributing to diagnostic interpretation are highlighted.

Radiation therapy (RT) represents an important therapeutic component in the management of genitourinary (GU) malignancies. RT is used to treat patients with proven involvement of the regional lymph nodes or delivered electively to patients at risk for occult regional lymph node metastases. Advances in treatment planning and delivery of various types of RT provide the technology to precisely plan, target, and deliver RT with the goal of optimizing the radiation dose to the target while sparing normal tissue. This article provides an overview of the modalities, indications, and techniques of RT for treatment of the lymphatic basins in GU malignancies.

Lymphadenectomy in urologic surgery provides accurate staging and may be therapeutic in some patients with lymph node metastases. In addition to the associated cost, pelvic lymph node dissection (PLND) has the potential for morbidity. This article focuses on the complications associated with PLND, including lymphocele, thromboembolic events, ureteral injury, nerve injury, vascular injury, and lymphedema. With improvements in surgical technique and perioperative care, the morbidity associated with lymphadenectomy may be minimized.

GOAL STATEMENT

The goal of *Urologic Clinics of North America* is to keep practicing urologists and urology residents up to date with current clinical practice in urology by providing timely articles reviewing the state of the art in patient care.

ACCREDITATION

The *Urologic Clinics of North America* is planned and implemented in accordance with the Essential Areas and Policies of the Accreditation Council for Continuing Medical Education (ACCME) through the joint sponsorship of the University of Virginia School of Medicine and Elsevier. The University of Virginia School of Medicine is accredited by the ACCME to provide continuing medical education for physicians.

The University of Virginia School of Medicine designates this enduring material activity for a maximum of 15 *AMA PRA Category 1 Credit*(s)™ for each issue, 60 credits per year. Physicians should claim only the credit commensurate with the extent of their participation in the activity.

The American Medical Association has determined that physicians not licensed in the US who participate in this CME enduring material activity are eligible for a maximum of 15 *AMA PRA Category 1 Credit*(s)™ for each issue, 60 credits per year.

Credit can be earned by reading the text material, taking the CME examination online at http://www.theclinics.com/home/cme, and completing the evaluation. After taking the test, you will be required to review any and all incorrect answers. Following completion of the test and evaluation, your credit will be awarded and you may print your certificate.

FACULTY DISCLOSURE/CONFLICT OF INTEREST

The University of Virginia School of Medicine, as an ACCME accredited provider, endorses and strives to comply with the Accreditation Council for Continuing Medical Education (ACCME) Standards of Commercial Support, Commonwealth of Virginia statutes, University of Virginia policies and procedures, and associated federal and private regulations and guidelines on the need for disclosure and monitoring of proprietary and financial interests that may affect the scientific integrity and balance of content delivered in continuing medical education activities under our auspices.

The University of Virginia School of Medicine requires that all CME activities accredited through this institution be developed independently and be scientifically rigorous, balanced and objective in the presentation/discussion of its content, theories and practices.

All authors/editors participating in an accredited CME activity are expected to disclose to the readers relevant financial relationships with commercial entities occurring within the past 12 months (such as grants or research support, employee, consultant, stock holder, member of speakers bureau, etc.). The University of Virginia School of Medicine will employ appropriate mechanisms to resolve potential conflicts of interest to maintain the standards of fair and balanced education to the reader. Questions about specific strategies can be directed to the Office of Continuing Medical Education, University of Virginia School of Medicine, Charlottesville, Virginia.

The faculty and staff of the University of Virginia Office of Continuing Medical Education have no financial affiliations to disclose.

The authors/editors listed below have identified no professional or financial affiliations for themselves or their spouse/partner:
Riley E. Alexander, MD, MBA; Christopher L. Amling, MD; Fiona C. Burkhard, MD; Brett Carver, MD; Brian F. Chapin, MD; Liang Cheng, MD; Scott E. Delacroix, Jr, MD; Stephanie Donley, (Acquisitions Editor); Mathew T. Gettman, MD; Simon Horenblas, MD, PhD; Jeffrey C. La Rochelle, MD; Daniel J. Lewinshtein, MD; Thomas J. Pugh, MD; Farhang Rabbani, MD; Beat Roth, MD; Joel Sheinfeld, MD; Urs E. Studer, MD; Ming-Tse Sung, MD; Tatum Tarin, MD; Christopher J. Weight, MD; Steve K. Williams, MD; Christopher G. Wood, MD; and Pascal Zehnder, MD.

The authors/editors listed below identified the following professional or financial affiliations for themselves or their spouse/partner:
Victoria Chernyak, MD is on the Speakers' Bureau for Lantheus Medical Imaging.
Andrew K. Lee, MD is employed by M.D. Anderson.
Christopher R. Porter, MD is employed by Virginia Mason Medical Center.
William Steers, MD (Test Author) is employed by the American Urologic Association, is a reviewer and consultant for NIH, and is an investigator for Allergan.

Disclosure of Discussion of Non-FDA Approved Uses for Pharmaceutical Products and/or Medical Devices
The University of Virginia School of Medicine, as an ACCME provider, requires that all faculty presenters identify and disclose any off-label uses for pharmaceutical and medical device products. The University of Virginia School of Medicine recommends that each physician fully review all the available data on new products or procedures prior to clinical use.

TO ENROLL

To enroll in the Urologic Clinics of North America Continuing Medical Education program, call customer service at 1-800-654-2452 or visit us online at www.theclinics.com/home/cme. The CME program is available to subscribers for an additional fee of $207.00.

Urologic Clinics of North America

THE CLINICS ARE NOW AVAILABLE ONLINE!

Access your subscription at:
www.theclinics.com

Preface

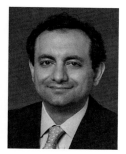

Reza Ghavamian, MD
Guest Editor

The practice of urologic oncology continues to evolve. The last two decades have witnessed a wide expansion of the literature pertaining to urologic malignancies. More recently, there have been surgical advances, notably adoption of minimally invasive methods for many urologic oncologic procedures. Much of the focus has always been on the surgical treatment of local disease. Yet, patterns of spread, dissemination, and metastasis are important considerations in urologic malignancies and have also deservedly been the focus of recent study. Cancer dissemination can occur by one of two route: hematogenously or by the lymphatic system. Lymphatic spread, by many accounts and for many urologic cancers, is considered the first step in systemic dissemination. For the most part, contrary to hematogenous spread and with some distinct exceptions as discussed in this issue of the *Urologic Clinics*, lymphatic spread occurs along a reasonably predicted route for each organ afflicted.

It is therefore not surprising that lymphadenectomy is an important component of oncologic surgery in most disciplines regardless of the organ in question. Its potential value and role in most urologic malignancies are no different. It can provide important information with regards to the regional extent of the disease. This information can then be utilized to formulate adjuvant treatment strategies and provide prognostic information for patients. With recent advances in radiation therapy and development of effective targeted and chemotherapeutic therapies, potential adjuvant therapies now exist. In addition, recent advances in imaging have led to a better predictive capability in the clinical diagnosis of lymph node involvement and hence the clinical staging of urologic malignancies prior to possible surgical intervention. Imaging also plays a crucial role in

the follow-up of the primary tumor and its nodal drainage system. The surgical and medical treatment of the primary tumor can thus be tailored for the individual patient.

The lymphatic drainage system and the importance of the management of the lymph nodes in the curative management of the primary malignancy are understood and established for some urologic cancers more than others. For example, the role and extent of lymphadenectomy and the pattern of lymphatic spread in testicular cancer and to a large extent in penile cancer is established. However, the role of lymphadenectomy and extent of lymphadenectomy are subject to recent debate and some controversy in prostate and bladder cancer. There is less information in the role of lymphadenectomy in renal cell carcinoma, with regards to both the need for lymphadenectomy and its extent. In this era of targeted therapy for renal cell carcinoma, understanding the patterns of lymphatic involvement in this particular malignancy can lead to better selection of patients for adjuvant systemic treatment.

With all the recent attention, publications, and known controversies in the management of the lymph nodes in urologic malignancies, a comprehensive issue focused on lymphadenectomy is long overdue. In this issue of the *Urologic Clinics*, an attempt is made to address the importance of lymphadenectomy in the management of urologic malignancies in the form of an up-to-date single resource. This is done by organizing a comprehensive compilation of original articles addressing important facets of this topic for all urologic malignancies. To achieve this, I have enlisted the help of colleagues, all of whom are recognized experts in the subject matter of their respective articles. The first article is interesting in that it addresses

Urol Clin N Am 38 (2011) xi–xii
doi:10.1016/j.ucl.2011.07.014
0094-0143/11/$ – see front matter © 2011 Elsevier Inc. All rights reserved.

urologic.theclinics.com

anatomy, and most importantly, the history and evolution of lymphadenectomy for all urologic cancers. Articles focusing on recent advances in imaging, pathologic assessment and handling, and the role of radiation therapy for the treatment for lymph node involvement in urologic malignancies are included. There is an article addressing minimally invasive lymphadenectomy for prostate and bladder cancer in which a defined and equivalent role for this technology does exist. A separate provocative article on laparoscopic lymphadenectomy for testicular cancer is also included. Finally, a separate article on complications of lymphadenectomy is presented.

It is my hope that this issue of the *Urologic Clinics* provides the reader with insightful, comprehensive, and up-to-date information about the role of lymphadenectomy in the management of common urologic malignancies. I wanted to thank originally Kerry Holland and subsequently Stephanie Donley from Elsevier for their cooperation and aid in bringing this project to fruition.

Reza Ghavamian, MD
Department of Urology
Montefiore Medical Center
Albert Einstein College of Medicine
3400 Bainbridge Avenue
Bronx, NY 10467, USA

E-mail address:
rghavami@montefiore.org

The History and Anatomy of Urologic Lymphadenectomy

Daniel J. Lewinshtein, MD[a], Christopher R. Porter, MD[b],*

KEYWORDS
- History • Anatomy • Lymphadenectomy • Kidney cancer
- Bladder cancer • Prostate cancer • Testes cancer
- Penile cancer

HISTORY OF THE LYMPHATIC SYSTEM

The history of the lymphatic system dates back to the biblical era. There are many references in both the early Hebrew and Greek literature to severe swelling of the lower extremities. Unknowingly, these authors described afflictions of the lymphatic system that would only be comprehended millennia later. Hippocrates (460–370 BC) was the first to actually describe the lymphatic system itself. After performing axillary lymph node dissections he commented on the "white blood" contained within them.[1] Aristotle (384–322 BC) went on to describe "fibers which course between blood vessels and nerves and contain clear liquid."[2] Celsus (30 BC to 50 AD) was the first person to name a symptom complex associated with lymphatic dysfunction and is credited with the term elephantiasis, which he used to describe persons with extreme edema of the lower extremities because it resembled the hide of an elephant.[3] The first to describe lymphatics associated with an organ system was Erasistratus (310–250 BC), a respected anatomist of Alexandria, who described "white arteries" of the small bowel.[4] Surprisingly, Vesalius, who is considered the founder of modern anatomy and who described the vascular system in detail, made no mention of the lymphatic system.[5] It was not until 1622 that an anatomist had accurately dissected and surmised the function of the lymphatics. Aselli, an anatomist and surgeon in Milan, performed a vivisection on a dog to demonstrate its nerves to colleagues.[6] In addition, he sought to analyze the function of the diaphragm and swept the bowel downwards. To his amazement, he observed multiple white chords over the bowel and mesentery, which he opened and reported white fluid emanating from them. The next day he had wanted to reproduce the same dissection on another dog, but to his disappointment, he did not observe the white chords. He hypothesized that their presence was related to the time of feeding, and he reperformed the experiment on a recently fed dog, and to his delight, he observed the white chords again. He named these chords *venae albae et lactae* and suggested that chyle was absorbed from the intestines via these chords and transported to the liver because, at the time, it was erroneously considered the origin of blood.

Pecquet (1622–1674), an anatomist at Montpellier, made the next major discovery. In 1651, he published a report on experiments he had performed as a medical student on the thoracic cavities of dogs. He noted that white fluid emanated from a stump in the superior vena cava and thought this was an abscess. However, upon pressing the abdomen, the flow increased. He went on to describe the cisterna chili, the thoracic duct, and its insertion point at the confluence of the left jugular and subclavian veins.[7]

In 1643, Bartholin confirmed Pecquet's findings in humans. Moreover, he demonstrated that these vessels also flow from the liver, and are, thus, not confined to the intestines. He published *Vasa*

The authors have nothing to disclose.
a Division of Urology, Virginia Mason Medical Center, Seattle, WA, USA
b Division of Urology, Virginia Mason Medical Center, C7-URO, 1100 9th Avenue, Seattle, WA 98101, USA
* Corresponding author.
E-mail address: Christopher.porter@vmmc.org

Urol Clin N Am 38 (2011) 375–386
doi:10.1016/j.ucl.2011.07.007

Lymphatica, and his name for these newly discovered vessels has been retained to this day.[8] In 1935, Drinker demonstrated that one of the most important functions of the lymphatic system was to absorb protein from the interstitium and return it to the venous system to maintain blood volume.[9] These aforementioned persons made the key discoveries regarding the anatomy and function of the lymphatic system.

EMBRYOLOGY OF THE LYMPHATIC SYSTEM

Although a large body of work exists on the function of the lymphatic system, its genesis is not completely elucidated. However, it is recognized that initially the primordial lymphatic system derives from 2 paired and 2 unpaired endothelial sacs that arise as outgrowths from the primitive venous system during the fifth gestational week.[2] First, 2 paired sacs appear at the junction of the subclavian and jugular veins; these outpouchings create the lymphatic sacs of the upper limbs (**Fig. 1**). Subsequently, 2 more unpaired sacs arise, one in the retroperitoneal space at the root of the mesentery and another dorsal to the mesentery; the latter becomes the cisterna chili. Finally, 2 paired sacs, the iliac lymphatics, emanate from the junction between the sciatic and the femoral veins. Several endothelial channels link these primordial lymphatic sacs by the ninth gestational week to form a complex network. Around this time, mesenchymal cells invade the lymphatic sacs; once encapsulated, the lymphatic sacs become

true lymph nodes. True lymphatic function derives from the invasion of the sacs by lymphocytes.

The upper and the lower lymphatic system are connected by the thoracic duct. Originally, the jugular lymphatic sacs are connected to the cisterna chili by 2 thoracic ducts that have an anastomotic channel between them.[10] Regression occurs such that the final thoracic duct is formed from the caudal right duct, the anastomotic channel, and the proximal left duct.

HISTORY OF SURGICAL LYMPHADENECTOMY

The importance of the lymphatic system with respect to malignant spread was first recognized in breast cancer. Ambrose Pare (1510–1590), a French battlefield surgeon, was probably the first surgeon to observe that the axillary lymph nodes may be involved in breast cancer.[10] In the same era, Michael Servetus (1511–1553), a Spanish scientist, suggested that these nodes be removed as part of a radical mastectomy.[10] Their thoughts were largely ignored and axillary dissection was only revisited 100 years later when Henri Le Dran and Jean Petit, 2 eminent French surgeons, suggested that axillary dissection may have a therapeutic benefit.[11]

In 1844, Joseph Pancoast authored the first published report describing lymphadenectomy (LND), which described axillary dissection.[12] However, the technique only become widely accepted and disseminated through the surgical community when, in 1895, Halsted published his report on axillary dissection (**Fig. 2**). He advocated a systematic and sequential dissection and argued for the removal of the nodes en bloc with the primary cancer.[13] Rapidly, surgeons from other organ systems recognized the importance of LND in cancer surgery. Moynihan, a contemporary of Halsted, referring to rectal surgery, exclaimed: "the surgery of malignant disease is not the surgery of organs; it is the anatomy of the lymphatic system."[14] In fact, the most accepted theory of cancer dissemination at the time was the lymphatic dominant spread postulated by the Handley and popularized by Halsted, which stated that cancer spread to lymph nodes first and secondarily via lymphatic channels from the lymph nodes to visceral organs. It was thought that the cancer cells became trapped in the lymph nodes, and there was a window period within which distant metastases could be avoided despite nodal involvement.[15] This theory was challenged as early as 1913 when Tyzzer reported on several patients with distant metastases in the absence of regional nodal involvement.[16] The theory was further challenged by Fisher who reported in

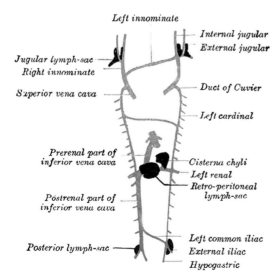

Fig. 1. The 6 primordial lymphatic sacs. (*From* Lewis WJ. Gray's anatomy of the human body. 20th edition. Philadelphia: Lea and Febiger; 1918.)

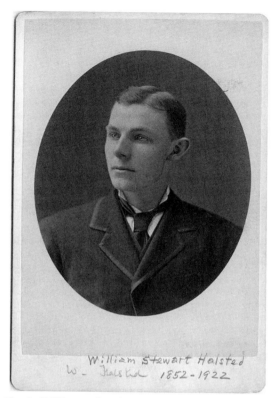

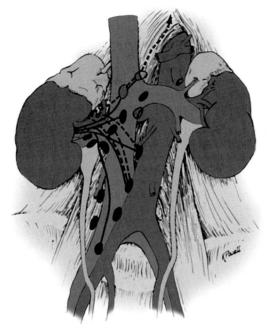

Fig. 2. William Halsted circa 1874. (*Courtesy of* Yale University Manuscripts & Archives Digital Images Database, New Haven, CT.)

Fig. 3. Regional lymphatic drainage of the right kidney. The lower line is the upper limit of a standard node dissection and the upper line is the upper limit of an extended node dissection. (*From* Wein AJ. Campbell-Walsh urology. 9th edition. Philadelphia: Saunders; 2007. Figure 1–35; with permission.)

1964 that LND did not decrease the appearance of distant metastases and hypothesized that the cancer was a systemic disease from the outset whereby cancer cells escape into both the systemic circulation and lymphatic system in all patients.[17] It is now apparent that cancer spreads via both pathways. However, it is recognized that the Halstedian principle is sound in asserting that cancer is a local disease that becomes systemic if left untreated and, thus, cure is possible if the disease remains local or locoregional.[18]

THE ANATOMY AND HISTORY OF LYMPHADENECTOMY FOR SPECIFIC UROLOGIC MALIGNANCIES
Kidney

The lymphatic drainage of the 2 kidneys varies. The left kidney drains primarily into the para-aortic nodes, which are bordered cranially by the diaphragm and caudally by the inferior mesenteric artery.[19] Rarely, the left kidney may drain into the retrocrural nodes or directly into the thoracic duct. The right kidney drains primarily into the para-caval, precaval, and interaortocaval nodes (**Fig. 3**).[20]

Classically, renal cancer presented with a triad of flank pain, hematuria, and a palpable flank mass. However, with the advent of modern imaging, less than 10% of contemporary patients will present with this constellation.[21] Moreover, less than 5% of contemporary patients will exhibit lymphadenopathy on preoperative imaging.[22] However, this was not the case in 1948 when Mortensen first described the modern radical nephrectomy, which included removing all contents within the Gerota fascia, including the kidney, adrenal, and perirenal fat.[23] It was not until 1963 that Robson reported that 22.5% of patients in his case series had renal-hilar lymph node involvement and, thus, he suggested performing a regional LND along with radical nephrectomy.[24] When he updated his series in 1969, he demonstrated a significant survival advantage in patients who had received a regional LND, even after adjustment for tumor size.[25] The template for renal LND has not really changed since that time, and although several retrospective series have demonstrated survival benefit in those undergoing LND,[26,27] the only randomized trial published did not corroborate those earlier findings.[22] Moreover, since the advent of laparoscopic nephrectomy and because of its extensive use, the performance of a renal LND has decreased substantially.[28]

Bladder

The lymphatic drainage of the bladder is complex and dependent on bladder location. The wall itself has lymphatics in the submucosa, detrusor, and the perivesical fat. The nodes of the base, neck, and trigone terminate in the internal, external, and sacral nodes. The anterior wall nodes primarily feed the external iliac. The posterior wall drains into the hypogastric nodes.[29] The second echelon of drainage is the common iliac and distal aorto-caval nodes.[30] Regional lymph node mapping has identified the external iliac (65%) and obturator (74%) to be the 2 most commonly involved sites of metastases.[31]

At the time of cystectomy for muscle invasive disease, nearly 25% of patients will have pathologic lymph node metastases.[32] Although LND has become a standard component of the contemporary radical cystectomy, this was not always the case. Despite the Halstedian view that primary cancers with solely lymph node involvement were amenable to surgical treatment,[13] the prevailing view in the bladder cancer community flanking the turn of the century was that grossly palpable nodes indicated uniformly fatal disease. The first study to challenge this dogma was reported by Colston and Leadbetter[33] in 1936, who performed

autopsies on 98 patients with bladder cancer. They observed a significant number of patients that had solely nodal metastases and, therefore, hypothesized that these patients were potentially curable with surgery. Ten years later, Jewett and Strong[34] confirmed these findings in 1946 in a similar autopsy study that included patients with extravesical disease. Moreover, they demonstrated a correlation between the depth of the bladder tumor and nodal metastatic burden. Their findings became the basis for the Marshall-Jewett system, the first staging system for bladder cancer.[34,35]

It was not until 1950 that data emerged suggesting a clinical benefit from pelvic LND. Colby and Kerr[36] reported on 2 patients with nodal disease that experienced long-term survival. Moreover, the investigators reported a high number of local recurrences, and, thus, suggested 2 technical improvements: wide bladder excision and inclusion of a pelvic LND (PLND), both of which have stood the test of time. That same year (1950), Leadbetter and Cooper were the first to describe a detailed technical template for performing LND for bladder cancer. Based on the established bladder lymphatic drainage patterns, their limits were the distal aorta proximally, the genitofemoral nerve laterally, and both the circumflex iliac vein and the node of Cloquet distally.[30] This template essentially represents a contemporary extended pelvic LND (ePLND) (**Fig. 4**).[37] The survival benefit of ePLND for patients with nodal disease was later validated by reports from both Whitmore[38] and Leadbetter[39] himself describing nodal positive

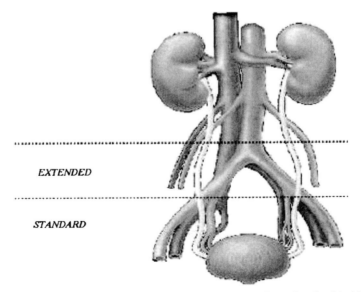

EXTENDED

STANDARD

Fig. 4. Proximal extent of standard versus extended pelvic lymph node dissection for bladder cancer at time of radical cystectomy. (*From* Raj GV, Bochner BH. Radical cystectomy and lymphadenectomy for invasive bladder cancer: towards the evolution of an optimal surgical standard. Sem Oncol 2007;34:110–21; with permission.)

patients with long-term survival. Moreover, the latter study concluded that ePLND was not associated with increased morbidity. In 1982, Skinner[40] published his first series on the contemporary use of an ePLND and demonstrated 30% long-term survival in patients who were node positive.

The utility of the template described by Leadbetter and championed by Skinner remained unchallenged for almost 40 years. However, in 1987, a study by Wishnow[41] suggested that LND above the bifurcation could be safely avoided proximal to the iliac bifurcation in those patients with no gross pelvic nodal disease. This limited template became known as the standard or limited PLND even though his results were based on only 18 patients who were node positive (see **Fig. 3**). More recent data from Stein,[32] at the University of Southern California, and other large cohort studies refute this hypothesis,[42] and an ePLND is the template that has emerged as the standard of care in centers of excellence today.[37]

Prostate

The first radical prostatectomy was described by Kucher[43] in 1866 and was completed via the perineal approach. However, the technique only became widely accepted after Hugh Hampton Young[44] reported on his initial series of patients in 1905, with a more anatomic and practical description. In 1945, Millin described the retropubic prostatectomy for benign disease,[45] which was later modified by Whitmore to treat malignant disease and, thus, included LND in some patients.[46] However, the procedure was not widely practiced because of the significant morbidity associated with the procedure.[47] Thus, the transperineal approach, precluding formal PLND, became the procedure of choice for clinically localized prostate malignancy until reports in the late 1970s suggested that PLND had increased sensitivity for detecting occult lymph node involvement (LNI) compared with preoperative imaging techniques and, thus, added important staging information.[48] Around the same time, in 1982, Walsh[49] described the anatomic retropubic radical prostatectomy (RRP), which benefited from enhanced understanding of the dorsal venous complex, and, thus, blood loss and consequent morbidity could be reduced. Moreover, reports from Walsh detailing enhanced understanding of the urinary sphincter and the neurovascular bundles provided for superior continence and sexual function outcomes.[50] Thus, RRP with concomitant PLND became a standard of care for all patients with locally resectable prostate cancer until the Partin tables were published, which accurately quantified the risk of occult lymph node involvement.[51]

With the advancement in urologic laparoscopy around the early 1990s, laparoscopic pelvic LND developed into a useful tool for detecting occult lymph node metastases in patients in whom external beam radiotherapy[52] was planned or in patients who were undergoing perineal prostatectomy.[53] Formal pelvic LND is still widely practiced in men undergoing both open and laparoscopic RRP and remains the most accurate modality for identifying pelvic metastases.[54]

Although LND was thought to confer staging information and enhance prognostication,[48] the therapeutic benefit in men with prostate cancer remained controversial even in patients with clinically unapparent LNI (stage D1).[55] In fact, Walsh surmised in 1987 that: "It is unlikely that radical surgery will cure any patient with Stage D1 adenocarcinoma of the prostate."[56] However, in that same year, data emerged supporting a therapeutic benefit for PLND. Golimbu and colleagues,[57] in a study of 42 patients, demonstrated enhanced survival in patients with minimal LNI detected after PLND compared with a matched cohort that had not undergone PLND. Although no randomized controlled trials have been performed to support curative PLND, multiple case series support moderate cancer-specific survival outcomes for patients with LNI.[58,59] Moreover, in 2006, Masterson and Joslyn demonstrated improved survival outcomes in patients that had undergone ePLND compared with standard PLND in patients who were node negative[60] and node positive,[61] respectively.

Standard PLND for prostate cancer, which is now considered a limited dissection, extends proximally from the iliac bifurcation to the circumflex iliac vein distally and medially from the obturator nerve to the external iliac vein laterally (**Fig. 5**).[62] In 2002, Heidenreich[63] reported that performing an ePLND, including external, internal, and common iliac; obturator; and presacral, increased the detection of lymph node metastases from 12% to 27% (see **Fig. 5**). Moreover, there were patients that had solely positive hypogastric nodes, which laid doubt to the dogma that the obturator and external iliac nodes were the primary prostate drainage sites.[63] Others have reported similar findings.[64,65] Most recently, Mattei and colleagues,[66] using intraprostatic technetium injection and fused single-photon emission computed tomography (SPECT) combined with either computed tomography (CT) or magnetic resonance imaging (MRI), demonstrated that more than 35% of the prostate landing zones are proximal to the iliac bifurcation and that more than 20% of the primary echelon nodes may be proximal to the ureteric crossing of the iliac vessels (**Fig. 6**).

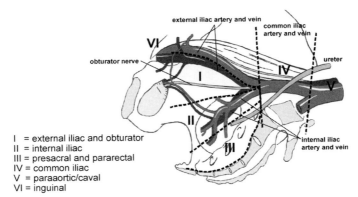

I   = external iliac and obturator
II = internal iliac
III = presacral and pararectal
IV = common iliac
V   = paraaortic/caval
VI = inguinal

Fig. 5. The various lymphatic drainage regions of the prostate. Region I defines the standard PLND where nodes from the obturator fossa and the external iliac vein are removed. Regions I to III define an extended PLND for prostate cancer that adds the hypogastric and presacral nodes. (*From* Mattei A, Fuechsel FG, Bhatta Dhar N, et al. The template of the primary lymphatic landing sites of the prostate should be revisited: results of a multimodality mapping study. Eur Urol 2008;53:118–25; with permission.)

Testes

The human urogenital ridge is undifferentiated at 8 weeks of gestation and lies near the developing kidney attached dorsally via the cranial suspensory ligament and ventrally by the progenitor of the gubernaculum.[67] After differentiation, testicular descent begins and the testes arrive at their pelvic location by the third gestational month. The testes enter the inguinal canal by 21 weeks and usually arrive at their scrotal location by 28 weeks.[68] The vascular and lymphatic supply of the testes is, therefore, derived from the upper retroperitoneum.

Although testicular descent was first described by John Hunter,[29] it was not until the early 1900s that lymphatic drainage was described independently by Jamiesen,[69] Most,[70] and Cuneo.[71] Moreover, Cuneo[71] and one of his contemporaries,

Chevassu,[72] suggested performing resection of retroperitoneal masses in conjunction with orchiectomy in the treatment of testis cancer. Before this era, the association between testis cancer and retroperitoneal masses was observed because Kocker, Potts, and Von Bergman all performed unsuccessful resections of these masses in the 1800s.[73]

In 1914, Hinman[74] published the first case series of patients who had undergone retroperitoneal lymph node dissection (RPLND). One of those cases, performed by Cuneo, had long-term survival despite a node positive for teratoma and is likely the first successful example of a curative RPLND. Hinman, in the same article, reported on 4 other long-term survivors with node-positive disease operated on at Johns Hopkins, which was the initial spark in developing interest in the surgical treatment of stage II disease.

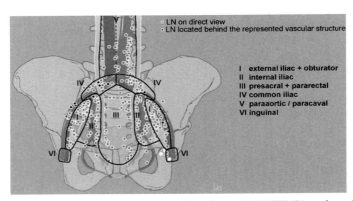

○ LN on direct view
• LN located behind the represented vascular structure

I   external iliac + obturator
II internal iliac
III presacral + pararectal
IV common iliac
V   paraaortic / paracaval
VI inguinal

Fig. 6. Primary lymphatic landing sites of the prostate based on SPECT/CT/MRI and confirmed by surgery in patients with prostate cancer. Regions of various proposed primary landing sites are identified by roman numerals. Landing sites anterior to vessels are green and those posterior to vessels are yellow. (*From* Mattei A, Fuechsel FG, Bhatta Dhar N, et al. The template of the primary lymphatic landing sites of the prostate should be revisited: results of a multimodality mapping study. Eur Urol 2008;53:118–25; with permission.)

Patton, an Army surgeon at Walter Reed Medical Center, was the first to demonstrate the enhanced efficacy of surgery over radiotherapy for stage II nonseminomatous germ cell tumors in a large cohort.[75] In his series, no patient with node positive disease treated with adjuvant radiotherapy achieved long-term survival, whereas 47% of those treated with orchiectomy and RPLND achieved cure.

Staubitz[76] and Whitmore[77] later published reports demonstrating greater than 60% survival in patients with pathologic stage II disease, which solidified interest in surgery for stage II disease.

The thoracoabdominal approach, first described by Cooper and colleagues[78] and later popularized by Skinner[79] and Fraley,[80] was borrowed from esophageal surgeons in the 1950s because of its enhanced access to upper abdominal anatomy.[81]

Donohue[82] first described the extended bilateral suprarenal RPLND in 1977. This template was bordered by the diaphragm superiorly and included the suprarenal and the retrocrural space, the ureters laterally, and the bifurcation of the common iliac inferiorly. This extensive template was a function of both the inadequate imaging techniques and the ineffective chemotherapy of that era.

Serendipitously, lymphangiographic studies of testicular lymphatic drainage performed in the 1960s by Sayegh[83] and others demonstrating retroperitoneal crossover spurred urologists to more accurately characterize side-specific drainage patterns based upon actual RPLND specimens. Performing positive node distribution analysis, Whitmore,[84] Weissbach,[85] and Donohue[86] all demonstrated that metastases had a predilection for unilateral involvement and that unifocal pathologic stage IIa disease was not seen in the suprahilar region (Fig. 7). It was also clearly demonstrated that the primary landing zone of the right testes was the interaortocaval region, whereas the left drained primarily to the para-aortic and preaortic region. Taken together, these results suggested that suprahilar dissection may be safely omitted and that unilateral templates could be implemented with minimal risk for missed disease in patients with clinical stage I disease.

In 1977, Einhorn[87] reported on the use of platinum-based chemotherapy for advanced testis cancer, which revolutionized the care and prognosis of these patients.[87] This breakthrough introduced a new term in testis cancer: "post-chemotherapy RPLND"[81] Systemic therapy allowed surgeons to resect masses that were previously unresectable even with extensive vascular mobilization and control[82] and to simplify difficult resections. To

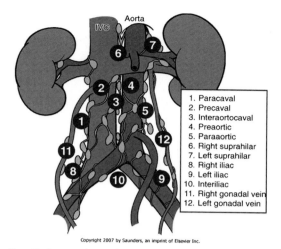

Fig. 7. Anatomic nodal regions of the retroperitoneum. The right and left testes drain primarily to the interaortocaval and para-aortic regions, respectively. IVC, inferior vena cava. (*From* Wein AJ. Campbell-Walsh urology. 9th edition. Philadelphia: Saunders; 2007. Figure 30–3; with permission.)

date, several investigators have reported successful curative outcomes in the setting of postchemotherapy RPLND in patients with both teratoma and non-teratomatous disease.[88–90]

The next major breakthrough in RPLND was improving fertility postoperatively via implementing novel surgical dissection. Urologists understood that the connection between the postganglionic sympathetic fibers and the hypogastric plexus in the para-aortic region was critical for ejaculation (Fig. 8). Narayan was the first to report on improved fertility rates after RPLND with meticulous dissection,[91] and in the late 1980s both Jewett[92] and Colleselli[93] published detailed prospective templates for preserving the para-aortic sympathetic nerves, which allowed for preservation of ejaculation postoperatively.

In summary, RPLND has evolved significantly over the last 100 years and is now a vital treatment of all stages of testis cancer treatment.

Penis

The primary drainage of the penis is the inguinal nodes. The inguinal nodes are confined to the femoral triangle, which is bordered by the inguinal ligament superiorly, the sartorius laterally, and the adductor longus medially.[94] The floor of the triangle is made from the iliopsoas laterally and the pectineus medially. The drainage pattern, proven to be bilateral with lymphoscintigraphy studies,[95] has been well described by several

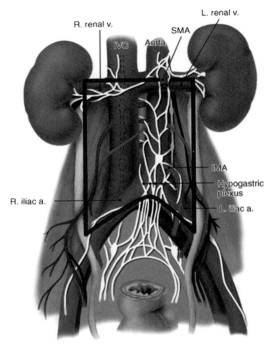

Fig. 8. Surgical template for a bilateral RPLND with identification of the postganglionic sympathetic fibers. IMA, inferior mesenteric artery; IVC, inferior vena cava; SMA, superior mesenteric artery. (*From* Wein AJ. Campbell-Walsh urology. 9th edition. Philadelphia: Saunders; 2007. Figure 30–4; with permission.)

investigators.[96,97] The inguinal nodes are separated into the deep and the superficial group by the fascia lata. The superficial nodes lie deep to the Scarpa fascia and generally number between 8 and 25. The deep nodes are fewer and lie deep to the fascia lata and congregate around the fossa ovalis, which is the opening of the fascia lata where the saphenous vein enters to join the femoral vein. The node of Cloquet is the most cephalad of the deep nodes and is located between the femoral vein and the lacunar ligament. It also is the communicating point to the next echelon of drainage: the pelvic nodes.

According to Das,[98] the surgical extirpation of malignancies of the penis was first advocated by Celsus in the first century AD. Thiersch, in 1875, published the first detailed description of radical surgery to cure localized penile cancer.[47] Only 11 years later, based on lymphatic drainage patterns, MacCormack suggested performing total penectomy with bilateral inguinal lymphadenectomy for cure.[47] Daseler, in 1948, studied 450 cadavers and published a more detailed description of

penile lymphatic drainage than previously understood.[99] He described 5 groups of superficial nodes: (1) central nodes around the saphenofemoral junction, (2) superolateral nodes around the superficial circumflex vein, (3) inferolateral nodes around the lateral femoral cutaneous and superficial circumflex veins, (4) superomedial nodes around the superficial external pudendal and superficial epigastric veins, and (5) inferomedial nodes around the greater saphenous vein. Again in 1948, Buonofsky described the transposition of the Sartorius to prevent femoral vessel erosion after groin dissection.[47]

John Spratt, a pioneer in groin dissection for multiple malignancies in Missouri in the 1960s, first published the standard groin dissection, which is used in patients with penile carcinoma to this day. He described a quadrilateral template for dissection of the superficial nodes with the corners being the anterior superior iliac spine (ASIS), a point on the outer thigh 20 cm caudal from the ASIS, a point 2 cm cephalad from the pubic tubercle, and the fourth point on the inner thigh at the same level as the point on the outer thigh (**Fig. 9**).[100]

In 1977, Cabanas reported on his seminal work with sentinel node biopsy, and he advocated inguinal dissection be omitted in those with a negative sentinel node.[101] He based his recommendations on static lymphangiographic studies and suggested that the primary drainage of the penis was always a node near the superficial epigastric vein. However, this technique has largely fallen out of favor since many other groups have found a significant number of patients harboring metastatic disease despite a negative sentinel node.[102,103]

Although groin dissection was considered standard of care for patients with palpable disease, its benefit in patients with high-risk primary features but clinically negative nodes was unclear until the early 1980s. However, in 1984, Johnson reported a survival benefit in those patients that had nonpalpable inguinal nodes that had undergone prophylactic groin dissection.[104] Since that time, other reports have drawn similar conclusions,[105–107] and prophylactic groin dissection in patients with high-risk features in the primary lesion has become the standard of care for patients with penile cancer.[108]

With the introduction of prophylactic groin dissection,[104] the morbidity of the standard template was examined[109] and centers of excellence explored technical variations to mitigate morbidity. In 1988, Catalona[110] published a report on modified inguinal LND that targeted the medial inguinal nodes in patients with clinically negative

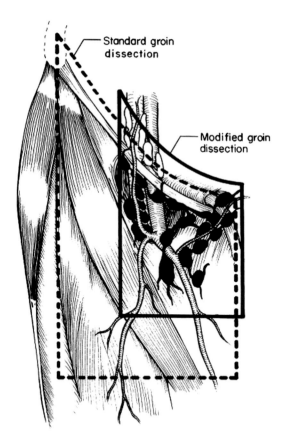

Standard groin dissection

Modified groin dissection

Fig. 9. Comparison of the limits of dissection of the modified Catalona compared with a standard groin dissection. (*From* Colberg JW, Andriole GL, Catalona WJ. Long-term follow-up of men undergoing modified inguinal lymphadenectomy for carcinoma of the penis. BJU 1997;79:54–7; with permission.)

inguinal nodes (see **Fig. 9**). The major modifications were: (1) a shorter incision, (2) preservation of tissue superficial to the Scarpa fascia, (3) dissection of tissue only medial to the femoral vessels, (4) preservation of the saphenous vein, and (5) omitting transposition of the sartorius.

REFERENCES

1. Hippocrates. The genuine books of Hippocrates. Translation by Francis Adams. London: Sydenham Society; 1849.
2. Skandalakis JE. Skandalakis' surgical anatomy: the embryologic and anatomic basis of modern surgery, vols. 1 & 2. Athens (Greece): Paschalidis Medical Publications; 2004.
3. Hajdu SI. A note from history: the first two laboratory scientists. Ann Clin Lab Sci 2002;32(4):438–40.
4. Fulton J. The early history of lymphatics. Bull Hennepin Co Med Soc 1938;9:5–10.
5. Vesalius A. On the fabric of the human body. Translated by W. F. Richardson and J. B. Carman. San Francisco (CA): Norman Publishing; 1998–2009.
6. Aselli G. De lactibus sine lacteis venis, quatro vasorum mesaraicorum genere, novo invento. Disertatis qua senteniae anatomicae multae uel parum perceptae illustrtur. Milan (Italy): JB Bidellum; 1627 [in Latin].
7. Pecquet J. Experimenta nova anatomica quibus incoguitum hactemus chyli receptaculum, et ab eo per thoracem in ramos usque sub claibious vasa lactae detegunter. Paris: Craimosy & Gab Cramoisy; 1651 [in Latin].
8. Bartholin T. Vasa Lymphatica, nuper Hafniae in animantibus inventa et hepatis exsequiae. Copenhagen (Denmark): Petri hakii; 1653 [in Latin].
9. Drinker CK. Lymphatic, lymph, and tissue fluid. Baltimore (MD): The Williams and Wilkins Co; 1933.
10. Robinson JO. Treatment of breast cancer through the ages. Am J Surg 1986;151(3):317–33.
11. Syme J. Principles of surgery. London: H Balliere; 1842.
12. Cooper W. The history of radical mastectomy. Ann Med Hist 1941;3:36–54.
13. Halsted WS. The results of operations for the cure of cancer of the breast performed at the Johns Hopkins Hospital from June, 1889, to January, 1894. Ann Surg 1894;20:497–555.
14. Moynihan GA. The surgical treatment of cancer of the sigmoid flexure and rectum. Surg Gynecol Obstet 1908;6:463–6.
15. Natarajan S, Taneja C, Cady B. Evolution of lymphadenectomy in surgical oncology. Surg Oncol Clin N Am 2005;14(3):447–59, v.
16. Tyzzer EE. Factors in the production and growth of tumor metastases. J Med Res 1913;28(2):309–32, 301.
17. Fisher B, Fisher ER. Biologic aspects of cancer-cell spread. Proc Natl Cancer Conf 1964;5:105–22.
18. Koscielny S, Tubiana M, Le MG, et al. Breast cancer: relationship between the size of the primary tumour and the probability of metastatic dissemination. Br J Cancer 1984;49(6):709–15.
19. Anderson K, Kabalin J, Caddedu J. Chapter 1 – Surgical anatomy of the retroperitoneum, adrenals, kidneys, and ureters. In: Wein AJ, Kavoussi LR, Novick AC, et al, editors. Campbell-Walsh urology. Philadelphia: Saunders; 2007. p. 3–37.
20. Wein AJ. Campbell-Walsh urology. Philadelphia: Saunders Elsevier; 2007.
21. Jayson M, Sanders H. Increased incidence of serendipitously discovered renal cell carcinoma. Urology 1998;51(2):203–5.
22. Blom JH, van Poppel H, Marechal JM, et al. Radical nephrectomy with and without lymph-node dissection: final results of European Organization for Research and Treatment of Cancer

(EORTC) randomized phase 3 trial 30881. Eur Urol 2009;55(1):28–34.

23. Mortensen H. Transthoracic nephrectomy. J Urol 1948;60(6):855–8.

24. Robson CJ. Radical nephrectomy for renal cell carcinoma. J Urol 1963;89:37–42.

25. Robson CJ, Churchill BM, Anderson W. The results of radical nephrectomy for renal cell carcinoma. J Urol 1969;101(3):297–301.

26. Pantuck AJ, Zisman A, Dorey F, et al. Renal cell carcinoma with retroperitoneal lymph nodes: role of lymph node dissection. J Urol 2003;169(6): 2076–83.

27. Canfield SE, Kamat AM, Sanchez-Ortiz RF, et al. Renal cell carcinoma with nodal metastases in the absence of distant metastatic disease (clinical stage TxN1-2M0): the impact of aggressive surgical resection on patient outcome. J Urol 2006;175(3 Pt 1):864–9.

28. Bhayani SB, Clayman RV, Sundaram CP, et al. Surgical treatment of renal neoplasia: evolving toward a laparoscopic standard of care. Urology 2003;62(5):821–6.

29. Skandalakis JE. Surgical anatomy: the embryologic and anatomic basis of modern surgery. Vol chapter 25. New York: McGraw Hill; 2004.

30. Leadbetter WF, Cooper JF. Regional gland dissection for carcinoma of the bladder; a technique for one-stage cystectomy, gland dissection, and bilateral uretero-enterostomy. J Urol 1950;63(2):242–60.

31. Smith JA Jr, Whitmore WF Jr. Regional lymph node metastasis from bladder cancer. J Urol 1981; 126(5):591–3.

32. Stein JP, Lieskovsky G, Cote R, et al. Radical cystectomy in the treatment of invasive bladder cancer: long-term results in 1,054 patients. J Clin Oncol 2001;19(3):666–75.

33. Colston JA, Leadbetter WF. Infiltrating carcinoma of the bladder. J Urol 1936;36:669–89.

34. Jewett HJ, Strong GH. Infiltrating carcinoma of the bladder; relation of depth of penetration of the bladder wall to incidence of local extension and metastases. J Urol 1946;55:366–72.

35. Marshall VF. The relation of the preoperative estimate to the pathologic demonstration of the extent of vesical neoplasms. J Urol 1952;68(4): 714–23.

36. Kerr WS, Colby FH. Pelvic lymph node dissection and total cystectomy in the treatment of carcinoma of the bladder. J Urol 1950;63:842–51.

37. Sanderson KM, Stein JP, Skinner DG. The evolving role of pelvic lymphadenectomy in the treatment of bladder cancer. Urol Oncol 2004;22(3):205–11 [discussion: 212–3].

38. Whitmore WF Jr, Marshall VF. Radical total cystectomy for cancer of the bladder: 230 consecutive cases five years later. J Urol 1962;87:853–68.

39. Dretler SP, Ragsdale BD, Leadbetter WF. The value of pelvic lymphadenectomy in the surgical treatment of bladder cancer. J Urol 1973;109(3): 414–6.

40. Skinner DG. Management of invasive bladder cancer: a meticulous pelvic node dissection can make a difference. J Urol 1982;128(1):34–6.

41. Wishnow KI, Johnson DE, Ro JY, et al. Incidence, extent and location of unsuspected pelvic lymph node metastasis in patients undergoing radical cystectomy for bladder cancer. J Urol 1987;137(3): 408–10.

42. Leissner J, Ghoneim MA, Abol-Enein H, et al. Extended radical lymphadenectomy in patients with urothelial bladder cancer: results of a prospective multicenter study. J Urol 2004;171(1): 139–44.

43. Kuchler H. Uber prostataver-Grosserungen. Deutsch Klin 1866;18:458.

44. Young HH. The early diagnosis and radical cure of carcinoma of the prostate: being a study of 40 cases and presentation of a radical operation which was carried out in four cases. Johns Hopkins Hosp Bull 1905;16:315–21.

45. Denmeade SR, Isaacs JT. Development of prostate cancer treatment: the good news. Prostate 2004; 58(3):211–24.

46. Whitmore WF Jr, Mackenzie AR. Experience with various operative procedures for the total excision of prostate cancer. Cancer 1959;12:396–405.

47. Garrett JE, Rowland RG. Evolution of radical procedures for urologic cancer. Surg Oncol Clin N Am 2005;14(3):553–68, vii.

48. McLaughlin AP, Saltzstein SL, McCullough DL, et al. Prostatic carcinoma: incidence and location of unsuspected lymphatic metastases. J Urol 1976;115(1):89–94.

49. Reiner WG, Walsh PC. An anatomical approach to the surgical management of the dorsal vein and Santorini's plexus during radical retropubic surgery. J Urol 1979;121(2):198–200.

50. Walsh PC, Lepor H, Eggleston JC. Radical prostatectomy with preservation of sexual function: anatomical and pathological considerations. Prostate 1983;4(5):473–85.

51. Partin AW, Kattan MW, Subong EN, et al. Combination of prostate-specific antigen, clinical stage, and Gleason score to predict pathological stage of localized prostate cancer. A multi-institutional update. JAMA 1997;277(18):1445–51.

52. Prout GR Jr, Griffin PP, Daly JJ, et al. Nodal involvement as prognostic indicator in prostatic carcinoma. Urology 1981;17(Suppl 3):72–9.

53. Levy DA, Resnick MI. Laparoscopic pelvic lymphadenectomy and radical perineal prostatectomy: a viable alternative to radical retropubic prostatectomy. J Urol 1994;151(4):905–8.

54. Parker CC, Husband J, Dearnaley DP. Lymph node staging in clinically localized prostate cancer. Prostate Cancer Prostatic Dis 1999;2(4): 191–9.

55. Donohue RE, Mani JH, Whitesel JA, et al. Stage D1 adenocarcinoma of prostate. Urology 1984;23(2): 118–21.

56. Walsh PC, Lepor H. The role of radical prostatectomy in the management of prostatic cancer. Cancer 1987;60(Suppl 3):526–37.

57. Golimbu M, Provet J, Al-Askari S, et al. Radical prostatectomy for stage D1 prostate cancer. Prognostic variables and results of treatment. Urology 1987;30(5):427–35.

58. Daneshmand S, Quek ML, Stein JP, et al. Prognosis of patients with lymph node positive prostate cancer following radical prostatectomy: long-term results. J Urol 2004;172(6 Pt 1):2252–5.

59. Briganti A, Karnes JR, Da Pozzo LF, et al. Two positive nodes represent a significant cut-off value for cancer specific survival in patients with node positive prostate cancer. A new proposal based on a two-institution experience on 703 consecutive N+ patients treated with radical prostatectomy, extended pelvic lymph node dissection and adjuvant therapy. Eur Urol 2009;55(2):261–70.

60. Masterson TA, Bianco FJ Jr, Vickers AJ, et al. The association between total and positive lymph node counts, and disease progression in clinically localized prostate cancer. J Urol 2006;175(4): 1320–4 [discussion: 1324–5].

61. Joslyn SA, Konety BR. Impact of extent of lymphadenectomy on survival after radical prostatectomy for prostate cancer. Urology 2006;68(1):121–5.

62. Thurairaja R, Studer UE, Burkhard FC. Indications, extent, and benefits of pelvic lymph node dissection for patients with bladder and prostate cancer. Oncologist 2009;14(1):40–51.

63. Heidenreich A, Varga Z, Von Knobloch R. Extended pelvic lymphadenectomy in patients undergoing radical prostatectomy: high incidence of lymph node metastasis. J Urol 2002;167(4):1681–6.

64. Allaf ME, Palapattu GS, Trock BJ, et al. Anatomical extent of lymph node dissection: impact on men with clinically localized prostate cancer. J Urol 2004;172(5 Pt 1):1840–4.

65. Clark T, Parekh DJ, Cookson MS, et al. Randomized prospective evaluation of extended versus limited lymph node dissection in patients with clinically localized prostate cancer. J Urol 2003;169(1): 145–7 [discussion: 147–8].

66. Mattei A, Fuechsel FG, Bhatta Dhar N, et al. The template of the primary lymphatic landing sites of the prostate should be revisited: results of a multimodality mapping study. Eur Urol 2008;53(1):118–25.

67. van der Schoot P. The name cranial ovarian suspensory ligaments in mammalian anatomy should be used only to indicate the structures derived from the foetal cranial mesonephric and gonadal ligaments. Anat Rec 1993;237(3):434–8.

68. Wyndham NR. A morphological study of testicular descent. J Anat 1943;77(Pt 2):179–88, 173.

69. Jamieson JK, Dobson JF. The lymphatics of the testicle. Lancet 1910;1:493.

70. Most A. Uber die lymphgefässe und lymphdrüssen des hodens. Arch f Anat u Entweckingsgesh 1899; 113:387–93 [in German].

71. Cuneo B. Note sur les lymphatiques du testicule. Bull et Mem Soc Anat de Paris 1901;76:105 [in French].

72. Chevassu M. Deux cas d'epitheliome du testicule traite par castration et l'ablation des ganglions lumboaortique. Bull et Mem Soc de Chir Paris 1910;36: 236–62 [in French].

73. Kober G. Teratoma testis, 114 cases. Am J Med Sci 1899;CX-VII:535.

74. Hinman F. The operative treatment of tumors of the testicle. JAMA 1914;58:2009–15.

75. Patton JF, Hewitt CB, Mallis N. Diagnosis and treatment of tumors of the testis. J Am Med Assoc 1959; 171:2194–8.

76. Staubitz WJ, Early KS, Magoss IV, et al. Surgical management of testes tumor. J Urol 1974;111:205–9.

77. Whitmore W. Retroperitoneal lymphadenectomy for testicular cancer. Contemp Surg 1975;6:486–96.

78. Cooper J, Leadbetter W, Chute R. The thoracoabdominal approach for retroperitoneal gland dissection: its application to testis tumors. Surg Gynecol Obstet 1950;90:486.

79. Skinner DG. Advances in the management of nonseminomatous germinal tumours of the testis. Br J Urol 1977;49(6):553–60.

80. Fraley EE, Markland C, Lange PH. Surgical treatment of stage I and stage II nonseminomatous testicular cancer in adults. Urol Clin North Am 1977;4(3):453–63.

81. Donohue JP. Evolution of retroperitoneal lymphadenectomy (RPLND) in the management of nonseminomatous testicular cancer (NSGCT). Urol Oncol 2003;21(2):129–32.

82. Donohue JP. Retroperitoneal lymphadenectomy: the anterior approach including bilateral suprarenal-hilar dissection. Urol Clin North Am 1977;4(3):509–21.

83. Busch FM, Sayegh ES. Roentgenographic visualization of human testicular lymphatics: a preliminary report. J Urol 1963;89:106–10.

84. Ray B, Hajdu SI, Whitmore WF Jr. Proceedings: distribution of retroperitoneal lymph node metastases in testicular germinal tumors. Cancer 1974; 33(2):340–8.

85. Weisbach L, Boedefeld E. Localization of solitary and multiple metastasis in stage II non seminomatous testis tumors as a basis for a modified staging lymph node dissection in stage I. J Urol 1982;138:77–82.

86. Donohue J, Zachary J, Maynard S. Distribution of nodal metastases in non-seminomatous testicular cancer. J Urol 1982;128:315–20.

87. Einhorn L, Donohue J. Cis-diamminedichloroplatinum, vinblastine and bleomycin chemotherapy in disseminated testicular cancer. Ann Intern Med 1977;87:293–8.

88. Murphy B, Breeden E, Donohue J, et al. Surgical salvage of chemorefractory germ cell tumors. J Clin Oncol 1993;11:324–9.

89. Donohue J, Thornhill J, Foster R, et al. Vascular considerations in post chemotherapy RPLND. Part I-vena cava: part II-aorta. World J Urol 1994;12: 182–9.

90. Nash P, Liebovitch I, Foster R, et al. En bloc nephrectomy in patients undergoing post chemotherapy RPLND for advanced NSGCT: indications, implications and outcomes. J Urol 1998;159:707–10.

91. Narayan P, Lange P, Fraley E. Ejaculation and fertility after extended retro-peritoneal lymph node dissection for testicular cancer. World J Urol 1982;127:685.

92. Jewett M, Kong Y, Goldberg J. Retroperitoneal lymphadenectomy for testicular tumor with preservation of ejaculation. J Urol 1988;139:1220–4.

93. Colleselli K, Poisel S, Schachtner W, et al. Nerve sparing bilateral retroperitoneal lymphadenectomy anatomical study and operative approach. J Urol 1990;144:293–7.

94. Spratt J. Groin dissection. J Surg Oncol 2000; 73(4):243–62.

95. Valdes Olmos RA, Tanis PJ, Hoefnagel CA, et al. Penile lymphoscintigraphy for sentinel node identification. Eur J Nucl Med 2001;28(5):581–5.

96. Cabanas RM. Anatomy and biopsy of sentinel lymph nodes. Urol Clin North Am 1992;19(2):267–76.

97. Dewire D, Lepor H. Anatomic considerations of the penis and its lymphatic drainage. Urol Clin North Am 1992;19(2):211–9.

98. Das S. Penile amputations for the management of primary carcinoma of the penis. Urol Clin North Am 1992;19:277–82.

99. Daseler E, Barry J, Reimann A. Radical excision of the inguinal and iliac lymph glands (a study based upon 450 anatomical dissections and upon supportive clinical observation). Surg Gynecol Obstet 1948;87.

100. Spratt J, Shiber W, Dillard B. Groin dissection. In: Spratt J, Shiber W, Dillard B, editors. "Anatomy and surgical technique of groin dissection". St Louis (MO): CV Mosby Company; 1965. p. 1–97.

101. Cabanas RM. An approach for the treatment of penile carcinoma. Cancer 1977;39(2):456–66.

102. Perinetti E, Crane DB, Catalona WJ. Unreliability of sentinel lymph node biopsy for staging penile carcinoma. J Urol 1980;124(5):734–5.

103. Fowler JE Jr. Sentinel lymph node biopsy for staging penile cancer. Urology 1984;23(4):352–3.

104. Johnson DE, Lo RK. Management of regional lymph nodes in penile carcinoma. Five-year results following therapeutic groin dissections. Urology 1984;24(4):308–11.

105. McDougal WS, Kirchner FK Jr, Edwards RH, et al. Treatment of carcinoma of the penis: the case for primary lymphadenectomy. J Urol 1986;136(1): 38–41.

106. Kroon BK, Horenblas S, Lont AP, et al. Patients with penile carcinoma benefit from immediate resection of clinically occult lymph node metastases. J Urol 2005;173(3):816–9.

107. Leijte JA, Kirrander P, Antonini N, et al. Recurrence patterns of squamous cell carcinoma of the penis: recommendations for follow-up based on a two-centre analysis of 700 patients. Eur Urol 2008; 54(1):161–8.

108. Margulis V, Sagalowsky AI. Penile cancer: management of regional lymphatic drainage. Urol Clin North Am 2010;37(3):411–9.

109. Ravi R. Morbidity following groin dissection for penile carcinoma. Br J Urol 1993;72(6):941–5.

110. Catalona WJ. Modified inguinal lymphadenectomy for carcinoma of the penis with preservation of saphenous veins: technique and preliminary results. J Urol 1988;140(2):306–10.

Role of Lymphadenectomy for Prostate Cancer: Indications and Controversies

Jeffrey C. La Rochelle, MD, Christopher L. Amling, MD*

KEYWORDS
- Lymphadenectomy • Prostate cancer
- Lymph node dissection • Staging

As a staging modality, pelvic lymph node dissection remains an important component of radical prostatectomy (RP) due, in part, to the low sensitivity of preoperative imaging studies. CT and MRI are able to detect approximately only 40% of cases with low-volume nodal involvement.[1] Ferumoxtran, an MRI-based intravenous lymph node imaging agent, has been used to demonstrate microscopic nodal deposits with impressive results,[2] but it remains unapproved by the US Food and Drug Administration. Additionally, examining the images of each lymph node for the small filling defects that indicate a metastatic deposit is time consuming. Fluorocholine-based positron emission tomography has shown some potential[3] but it is still an experimental technique with questionable sensitivity.[4] Thus, for the foreseeable future, pelvic node dissection remains the most reliable technique for the detection of low-volume nodal involvement in prostate cancer.

The last article in *Urologic Clinics of North America* to discuss the indications of pelvic lymph node dissection for prostate cancer was in 2001.[5] The focus of that review and most relevant urologic literature at that time was on the effort to identify patients at very low risk for lymph node metastasis who could be spared a node dissection with its additional operative time and morbidity. Given that a node dissection was considered primarily a staging method rather than a therapeutic one, it was generally believed that the staging accuracy afforded by the preoperative clinical variables of prostate-specific antigen (PSA), biopsy Gleason score, and clinical tumor stage (ie, Partin tables) was often adequate for low-risk patients. Accumulating data since that review has challenged previous beliefs. Extended lymph node dissections that include the internal iliac chain in addition to the external iliac and obturator packets (**Fig. 1**) have shown a significantly higher proportion of patients to have lymphatic involvement than previously recognized.

There is now little doubt that an extended node dissection detects more patients with lymph node involvement (LNI) compared with a limited dissection. The improved staging afforded by a more extended dissection raises several questions. First, are there still patients at very low risk for LNI who can be spared a lymph node dissection? Second, is there a therapeutic benefit to an extended dissection? Third, what are the drawbacks of doing an extended lymph node dissection? Fourth, should patients with nodal involvement on an extended dissection be treated the same as patients with nodal disease on a limited dissection (ie, Should they be excluded from adjuvant radiation and/or be offered immediate androgen-deprivation therapy)? Lastly, what are the current

Division of Urology, Oregon Health & Science University, 3303 Southwest Bond Avenue, CH10U, Portland, OR 97239, USA
* Corresponding author.
E-mail address: amling@ohsu.edu

Urol Clin N Am 38 (2011) 387–395
doi:10.1016/j.ucl.2011.07.009
0094-0143/11/$ – see front matter © 2011 Published by Elsevier Inc.

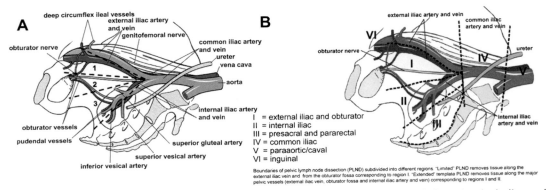

Fig. 1. (*A*) Template for an ePLND, which includes zones 1–3, compared with a limited dissection including only zones 1 and 2. (*B*) Potential landing zones for prostate cancer lymph node metastases, with a proposed modified PLND template, including zones I, II, and IV. ([*A*] *From* Bader P, Burkhard FC, Markwalder R, et al. Disease progression and survival of patients with positive lymph nodes after radical prostatectomy. Is there a chance of cure? J Urol 2003;169:849–54; with permission; and [*B*] *From* Mattei A, Fuechsel FG, Bhatta Dhar N, et al. The template of the primary lymphatic landing sites of the prostate should be revisited: results of a multimodality mapping study. Eur Urol 2008;53:118–25; with permission.)

recommendations from the American Urological Association (AUA), the European Association of Urology (EAU), and the National Comprehensive Cancer Network (NCCN) regarding patient selection and extent of dissection? Addressing these questions is the focus of this review, although some cannot be definitively answered given the current limitations of the literature.

EVIDENCE FOR IMPROVED STAGING BY EXTENDED LYMPH NODE DISSECTION

There has been a growing appreciation over the past 10 years that a limited pelvic lymph node dissection (limPLND) at the time of RP, which removes nodes from only the external iliac and obturator locations, can miss a significant percentage of potentially cancer-bearing nodal tissue.[6–9] A mapping study by Mattei and colleagues[7] using a radiolabeled tracer injected into the prostate followed by single-photon emission CT scanning,

intraoperative lymphatic mapping with a gamma probe, and a superextended lymph node dissection extending above the aortic bifurcation demonstrated that the primary lymphatic landing sites of the prostate can also include presacral, pararectal, paracaval, para-aortic, and even inguinal lymph nodes (**Fig. 2**). The investigators calculated that a limPLND includes only 38% of prostate-draining nodes and that an extended pelvic lymph node dissection (ePLND), including the tissue along the internal and distal common iliac vessels, would remove 75%. This study did not report on the distribution of patients with exclusive drainage to basins outside the limited and extended dissection templates who might therefore be understaged by the different pelvic lymph node dissection (PLND) schema. A report by Schumacher and colleagues[10] of 122 node-positive patients described the likelihood of having positive lymph nodes outside the limPLND template, exclusively or in combination with other sites.

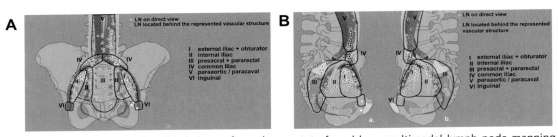

Fig. 2. (*A, B*) Distribution of nodal drainage from the prostate found by a multimodal lymph node mapping study. (*From* Mattei A, Fuechsel FG, Bhatta Dhar N, et al. The template of the primary lymphatic landing sites of the prostate should be revisited: results of a multimodality mapping study. Eur Urol 2008;53:118–25; with permission.)

Overall, 70% had positive nodes in the internal iliac basin, and 21% were positive only in this area. This compared with 9% positive only in the external iliac distribution and 16% positive only in the obturator fossa. It is not surprising that Heidenreich and colleagues[6] reported a significantly higher rate of positive lymph nodes in 103 patients undergoing RP with ePLND compared with 100 patients undergoing RP with limPLND (26% vs 12%) who were otherwise well matched for Gleason score, clinical tumor stage, and PSA. Likewise, Touijer and colleagues[11] reported a hazard ratio of 7.15 for positive nodes in patients undergoing an ePLND compared with those undergoing only an external iliac dissection in a group with a greater than 1% risk for nodal involvement based on the Partin tables.

IS THERE STILL A LOW-RISK POPULATION THAT CAN BE SPARED A LYMPH NODE DISSECTION?

It is well established that an ePLND demonstrates a higher rate of LNI compared with a limPLND. Does this finding extend, however, to patients previously considered low-risk for LNI based on preoperative variables? In a large series of men from Johns Hopkins treated with RP over the past 30 years, the rate of positive lymph nodes decreased from 11% in 1982 through 1991 to 1% in 2000 through 2005.[12] The decline was due in part to migration toward lower stages because of increasing use of PSA screening, but there also were decreasing rates of positive lymph nodes within the predefined risk categories based on PSA, Gleason score, and clinical tumor stage. This led to questions about the utility of a lymph node dissection in the large segment of men undergoing surgery for low-risk disease. Cagiannos and colleagues[13] developed a nomogram using standard preoperative variables with the goal of identifying men at very low risk of nodal involvement who could be spared a PLND, and community-based data from the Cancer of the Prostate Strategic Urologic Research Endeavor (CaPSURE) demonstrated decreasing rates of PLND at the time of RP.[14]

With the awareness that removing more nodes can lead to increased detection of nodal metastases,[6,10,11,15] is there still a substantial segment of men who are still at very low risk for LNI at ePLND, or is the prevalence of occult positive nodes in men with prostate cancer high enough that nearly all patients should undergo an ePLND? This question cannot be answered in an absolute sense because the underlying characteristics of a patient population determine how often LNI would be found on ePLND. Additionally, patients' and practitioners' tolerance for the risk of understaging is potentially variable. Using a reasonable population estimate of the incidence of LNI at RP with ePLND, however, along with an acceptable arbitrary cutoff for the risk of LNI in an individual patient that should trigger an ePLND, it can begin to be determined which and how many patients could safely have an ePLND omitted with low risk of understaging. Godoy and colleagues[16] from Memorial Sloan-Kettering Cancer Center did just this using a recalibrated nomogram based on findings from 3721 patients undergoing RP with ePLND. Given an overall 7% incidence of LNI, along with an individual cutoff of greater than or equal to 2% (ie, patients with nomogram-calculated risk of positive nodes greater than or equal to 2% would undergo ePLND), the investigators estimated that approximately 35% of patients could be spared an ePLND by using their nomogram. In their study population, which had an actual 5.2% incidence of LNI, 53% of patients were categorized as low risk and less than 1% of that group had positive nodes at ePLND. Briganti and colleagues[17] developed a similar nomogram based on 602 patients undergoing RP with ePLND. One aspect that potentially makes it difficult to use this nomogram is that their absolute lowest measurable probability of LNI was 2%, which is likely due to the higher rate of LNI (11%) in their study. This higher LNI rate is attributable either to a difference in populations or to the fact that the mean number of nodes removed in their report was 17 compared with 11 in the study by Godoy and colleagues.

There has been concern that using preoperative variables may underestimate the true risk of LNI at the time of ePLND. Studies that demonstrated higher than expected LNI in patients with PSA less than or equal to 10 or a biopsy Gleason score less than or equal to 6 used methods that are difficult to compare with current practice.[18,19] Biopsy templates were not reported, and fine-needle aspiration was used in one study. In the report by Weckermann and colleagues[18] of higher than expected LNI in patients with Gleason score less than or equal to 6 and PSA less than or equal to 10 (5.4%–11.3%), there was a substantial rate of upgrading and/or upstaging at surgery (46%–80%). In a report by Burkhard and colleagues,[19] 23% of patients with pathologic Gleason score of 5 and 25% with Gleason score of 6 prostate cancer had LNI. The median PSAs of these groups, however, were 11 and 13, respectively. An updated report from this group found that among patients with both pathologic Gleason score of 5 or 6 and PSA less than or equal to 10, the rate of LNI was 4.5%.[20] No clinical tumor stage was given for these patients. Therefore, it seems that in ostensibly low-risk patients with LNI, there are often other clinical risk factors present that would remove many, but not all, from the low-risk category.

In conclusion, it seems that in spite of a higher rate of LNI at RP than was previously recognized, there is still a significant number of men who would not be understaged by omission of a PLND. That number is smaller than previously appreciated, however. For men with a higher risk of LNI, an ePLND is a significantly better method of staging, although the cutoff risk level that should trigger an ePLND is somewhat arbitrary. Nomograms or risk categories that predict the probability of LNI found with limPLND underestimate the actual risk of LNI, and ePLND-based prediction tools are preferable.

IS AN EXTENDED LYMPH NODE DISSECTION POTENTIALLY THERAPEUTIC?

The question looming over much of the discussion surrounding ePLND is whether finding and removing limited metastatic deposits in pelvic lymph nodes can potentially cure patients or at least measurably delay progression. Prostate cancer does not follow a routine progression to the regional lymph nodes before systemic dissemination, as is evidenced by the surprising rate of PSA-positive epithelial cells in bone marrow aspirates of patients with otherwise pathologically organ-confined disease.[21] Patients with a negative PLND have a better prognosis than those with LNI, but node-negative status is not associated with durable recurrence-free survival to the same extent as in urothelial, germ cell, or penile tumors. There are no prospective, randomized trials that have compared the outcome of patients with or without PLND. Nevertheless, there is some indirect evidence that patients with limited LNI or with negative nodes may get a therapeutic benefit from a node dissection. These data, however, must be interpreted with caution. A report from Josyln and Konety describing results from the Surveillance, Epidemiology and End Results (SEER) database is often cited by proponents of the therapeutic benefit of PLND.[22] In that report, the authors demonstrated a survival advantage for both node-negative and node-positive patients when greater than 4 nodes were removed compared with those having fewer nodes removed. A key point that should not be overlooked is that this survival benefit can potentially be attributed to the so-called Will Rogers effect, which can occur when comparing outcomes in patients who have been staged differently.[23,24] Patients remaining in the node-negative group

after having a more extensive node dissection are more likely to be truly node negative and therefore have a better outcome compared with those included in the node-negative category after a limited dissection, some of whom are likely harboring occult LNI. The same holds true for the node-positive group, whereby those included in the node-positive group after an extensive node dissection may have less overall disease and therefore a better prognosis than patients found to have nodal metastases after a limited dissection who likely have more extensive disease. The paradoxic effect of this phenomenon is that by transferring patients with limited LNI out of the node-negative group and into the node-positive group through better identification (more extensive PLND), both node-negative and node-positive patients seem to do better than historical controls, in spite of there having been no change in overall or individual outcomes. In that same report, node-negative patients with more than 10 nodes removed also had a cancer-specific survival (CSS) advantage, which was attributed to the possibility that micrometastases were removed.[22] This could also be explained, however, by the Will Rogers effect. Likewise, a retrospective study by Masterson and colleagues[25] that found improved recurrence-free survival in node-negative patients with higher number of removed nodes could similarly be explained.

Several investigators have retrospectively reported on large single-institution experiences with the aim of elucidating a possible therapeutic benefit for PLND. Weight and colleagues[26] updated the Cleveland Clinic experience with Kaplan-Meier 10-year estimated biochemical relapse (BCR)-free survival in favorable risk patients with (n = 140) and without (n = 196) a limPLND. No difference was detected (88% vs 84%, P = .33). The investigators admitted they could not specifically comment on the value of an ePLND and that their study may have been underpowered to detect a small benefit to PLND. DiMarco and colleagues[27] described the Mayo Clinic experience with 7036 node-negative patients undergoing RP with PLND between 1987 and 1999. The average number of lymph nodes removed steadily declined during that time period, from 14 in 1987 to 5 in 1999. A multivariate analysis of outcome based on grade, clinical stage, PSA, year of surgery, and number of nodes removed failed to show any BCR-free survival benefit in any risk category for increased number of nodes removed at PLND. Presumably, removing fewer nodes would leave more residual occult positive nodes and lead to higher rates of progression, particularly in higher risk disease, but this was not seen. Lastly, Allaf and colleagues[15] from Johns Hopkins reported on BCR-free survival in patients with LNI found at RP by two high-volume surgeons, one who routinely performed a limPLND and one who performed an ePLND. There was a trend toward improved BCR-free survival in patients with LNI undergoing ePLND (n = 71) versus limPLND (n = 22) (34.4% vs 16.5%, P = .07). A significant difference in BCR-free survival was reached in the subgroup with LNI but less than 15% of nodes involved (42.9% vs 10%, P = .01). The number of nodes removed by each surgeon was not significantly different in this subgroup (15.9 vs 15.1) in spite of the difference in extent of dissection. Even though this report is encouraging with respect to the possibility of a therapeutic effect, there is still a distinct chance that the Will Rogers effect is at work here. More patients in the ePLND group may truly have had limited LNI due to a wider sampling compared with the group with limited LNI based on a limPLND, many of whom may have had a higher actual burden of LNI.

Although there is no conclusive evidence that a PLND results in improved prostate cancer outcomes, a significant percentage of men with LNI across several studies consistently have prolonged BCR-free survival without adjuvant therapy, even men undergoing limPLND.[10,28–31] Five-year to-10-year BCR-free rates range from 4% to 40% in these reports, with patients with fewer positive nodes consistently having a better prognosis. It is difficult to imagine an explanation for this outcome other than a low but significant percentage of men with low-volume LNI can be cured of their disease or at least have a long-term delay in progression. Extensive lymph node dissection in bladder cancer, a more aggressive pelvic cancer with an overlapping lymphatic drainage pattern, can also cure some patients with limited LNI. It should, therefore, not be surprising that the same seems true in prostate cancer, although admittedly an ePLND in prostate cancer is not as extensive as the typical dissection in bladder cancer.

Without a prospective randomized trial of ePLND versus limited or no PLND, it is impossible to unequivocally answer the question of whether an ePLND results in a measurable therapeutic benefit. Until such data exist, retrospective analyses, with all of their inherent selection bias, must be relied on. Most reports consistently show a reasonable percentage of men with LNI with long-term recurrence-free survival, however, which should at least prompt strong consideration of a PLND. Given that an ePLND is more likely to remove cancer-bearing nodes in patients at higher risk of LNI, it is likely that any possible therapeutic advantage to PLND will be greater in an ePLND.

WHAT ARE THE DRAWBACKS OF AN EXTENDED LYMPH NODE DISSECTION?

With its definite staging advantage and possible therapeutic benefit, is there any reason to not perform an ePLND? The predominant risk of a PLND is lymphocele, which happens when lymphatic fluid accumulates in the extraperitoneal pelvic compartment. The definition of lymphocele varies, with some defining it as prolonged elevated drain output and others reserving the term for fluid collections after drain removal that are found incidentally or due to the onset of symptoms. Postoperative management algorithms determining how long a drain stays in place can influence the incidence of lymphocele, depending on the definition. Deep vein thrombosis (DVT) is also a risk of PLND, and it may occur as a result of vascular compression or injury during PLND or secondarily due to compression by a lymphocele. Heparin given to lessen the risk of DVT can increase lymphatic flow and the risk of lymphocele.[32] Administering heparin in the upper arm rather than the leg may reduce this risk.[33] Lymphedema is another possible, although infrequent, consequence of PLND. Other complications, such as ureteral or obturator nerve injury, happen on occasion but are generally rare.

A study performed by Clark and colleagues[34] prospectively recorded complications in 123 patients undergoing an ePLND on one side and a limPLND on the other, thereby eliminating the surgeon as a variable. Three of 4 lymphoceles, 2 of 2 DVTs, and 3 of 5 cases of lower-extremity edema occurred on the side of ePLND. Musch and colleagues[35] retrospectively analyzed complications in 867 limPLNDs and 434 ePLNDs. They found the odds ratio for lymphocele in ePLND to be 3 compared with limPLND (9.4% vs 3.3%). The incidence of DVT was associated with the development of a lymphocele. There was a total of 8 ureteral and 2 obturator nerve injuries across both groups. Briganti and colleagues[36] compared 767 ePLNDs with 196 limPLNDs and found a 10.3% rate of lymphocele in the ePLND group versus 4.6% in the limPLND cases. They used a definition of greater than 50 mL/day for over 7 days as their definition of lymphocele. They did not find a higher rate of DVT in the ePLND group, perhaps because the length of time the drains were left in prevented fluid accumulation and vein compression. They did not report any cases of ureteral injury.

An effort to lessen risks of ePLND by only performing an ePLND on the side of the dominant prostate tumor based on biopsy is ill advised. A mapping study by Tokuda and colleagues[37] showed that positive nodes can occur on the contralateral side from the dominant tumor in 30% to 40% of cases with LNI. It is possible that robotic assisted laparoscopic prostatectomy (RALP) will demonstrate a lower rate of lymphocele because the transperitoneal approach allows drainage of lymphatic fluid into the peritoneal space where it can be resorbed. A report by Zorn and colleagues[38] showed a 2% rate of lymphocele in 296 patients undergoing RALP with PLND, a rate somewhat lower than large open series. In an analysis of 773 patients undergoing laparoscopic RP, however, the risk of DVT was higher in the patients undergoing PLND than those in whom it was omitted (1.5% vs 0%, $P = .047$) in spite of no patients experiencing a symptomatic lymphocele.[39] Early ambulation and sequential compression devices were used in lieu of pharmacologic prophylaxis.

The benefits of ePLND come at a cost, primarily in the increased risk of lymphocele and perhaps DVT. Patients undergoing an ePLND may need to have longer postoperative drainage to avoid symptomatic lymphoceles with their associated risk of DVT if undergoing a retropubic approach. The role of drainage in patients undergoing RALP with ePLND remains undefined, although DVT prophylaxis seems warranted in this group.

SHOULD PATIENTS WITH LNI FOUND AT ePLND BE EXCLUDED FROM ADJUVANT RADIATION FOR pT3 DISEASE OR POSITIVE MARGINS, AND SHOULD THEY BE STARTED ON ADJUVANT ANDROGEN DEPRIVATION THERAPY?

Adjuvant radiation to the prostate fossa in men with locally advanced prostate cancer has been shown to result in improved CSS in a prospective randomized trial.[40] The study that demonstrated this benefit excluded men with LNI or who were at higher risk for LNI but did not undergo a PLND. Given that the men without LNI in this study had high-risk disease and most probably underwent a limPLND, it seems likely that a substantial number of men in this study had some degree of occult LNI. It is possible that the survival benefit in this study was concentrated in the men who were free of occult metastases, and if this were the case, an ePLND would be a more effective method of selecting appropriate candidates for adjuvant radiation. A report by Da Pozza and colleagues[41] suggests that patients with LNI may benefit from the addition of adjuvant radiation treatment (RT). In a retrospective analysis of 250 patients with LNI on ePLND with a mean of 2.5 nodes involved and a median follow-up of 7.5 years, the group that received AR (with 75%

receiving whole-pelvic irradiation) in combination with adjuvant androgen deprivation therapy (ADT) seemed to have improved outcomes relative to the group that received ADT alone. At 10 years, a trend was seen toward improved BCR-free survival after RT and ADT versus ADT alone (51% vs 41%, $P = .11$), in spite of a higher proportion with poor-risk features in the RT group. Multivariate analysis for BCR-free and CSS did show a highly significant advantage for RT plus ADT (BCR-free survival hazard ratio 0.49, $P<.01$; CSS hazard ratio 0.38, $P<.01$). Although far from conclusive, this provocative study suggests that patients with limited LNI after ePLND may benefit from adjuvant RT, although whole-pelvic irradiation and ADT may be necessary components of this treatment.

The nomogram developed by Stephenson and colleagues[42] used to predict the probability of response to salvage RT for a rising PSA also lends indirect support for the consideration of RT in patients with LNI. Depending on the presence of other adverse prognostic factors, LNI reduces the chance of response by 15% to 25%, but it does not seem to preclude the possibility of benefit. Only 3% (48 patients) included in the analysis had LNI, but the majority probably had a limPLND at most. Given that all patients in the study had PSA failure after RP, it seems likely that a significant fraction had occult LNI. Although speculative, it seems distinctly possible that if the analysis could have incorporated the true LNI status based on ePLND, the nomogram-calculated decrement in the probability of responding to salvage RT due to LNI might be less.

Adjuvant ADT after RP in patients with LNI is supported by a prospective randomized trial of 100 patients that demonstrated a survival benefit for adjuvant use versus initiation at the time of clinical progression.[38] The median number of nodes assessed was between 11 and 14, and the median number of positive nodes was 2. It is currently unknown whether all patients with LNI would benefit from the use of adjuvant ADT, in particular those with limited LNI based on an ePLND. As discussed previously, several reports have demonstrated that a proportion of men with LNI have prolonged BCR-fee survival without the use of adjuvant therapy. Initiation of ADT constitutes overtreatment in at least 15% of these men. Each of those reports found that the number of nodes involved was one of the most important variables, and 2 of them specifically found the ratio of positive nodes to the number of nodes removed ($\leq$15%–20%) to be particularly informative.[30,31] A recent analysis found that patients with less than or equal to 2 nodes positive on ePLND had a significantly better prognosis than those with a higher burden of LNI.[43] All patients in that analysis received adjuvant ADT, so no determination of whether adjuvant ADT can be avoided in patients with limited LNI can be made based on those data. They do show, however, that patients with limited LNI do not all have the dismal prognosis previously associated with node-positive prostate cancer.

Adjuvant ADT is beneficial in many, if not most, patients with LNI. A subset of these men, however, does not progress, in particular those with limited LNI. ePLND is better able than limPLND to identify which men have higher and lower burdens of LNI and, therefore, which men are at higher and lower risk for prostate cancer progression. Patients with limited LNI on ePLND may be good candidates for a watchful waiting approach, whereby ADT could be initiated at the time of PSA progression rather than immediately after surgery. Likewise, men with limited LNI may still be reasonable candidates for adjuvant or salvage radiation if other indications are present.

WHAT ARE THE CURRENT RECOMMENDATIONS FOR PATIENT SELECTION AND EXTENT OF PLND?

Currently, the AUA, the EAU, and the NCCN each has different recommendations regarding PLND. The AUA 2009 Best Practice Statement for PSA states that the possible staging and therapeutic benefits of an ePLND must be balanced against the increased morbidity.[44] The statement adds that a PLND can be appropriately omitted in patients with Gleason score less than or equal to 6 and PSA less than or equal to 10. The EAU, however, is explicit about when a PLND should be done and how extensive it should be, according to 2010 guidelines.[45] They recommend that a PLND be done when the risk of LNI is greater than or equal to 7%, although they do not specify which prediction tool should be used. Furthermore, they state that an ePLND should always be the technique used, which should cover the external iliac vessels, the obturator fossa, and nodes medial and lateral to the internal iliac artery. They mention, but do not specifically advocate, that the common iliac nodes can be removed distal to the ureteric crossing. The NCCN, in its prostate cancer guidelines, version 1.2011, states that an ePLND has the chance to cure some men with micrometastatic LNI and is, therefore, preferred to a limPLND.[46] They recommend that an ePLND be done when the risk of LNI is greater than or equal to 2%, without a specific prediction tool specified. They state the ePLND should

include the nodes within the area demarcated by the external iliac vein anteriorly, the pelvic sidewall laterally, the bladder wall medially, the floor of the pelvis posteriorly, Cooper ligament distally, and the internal iliac artery proximally. If the NCCN guidelines were followed and then the Briganti nomogram used to predict the likelihood of LNI (1 of only 2 currently based on ePLND results), an ePLND would be indicated for every patient undergoing RP.[17]

SUMMARY

PLND is still the only reliable technique to detect low-volume LNI in prostate cancer, which is present to a much greater degree than previously appreciated. An ePLND covering the internal iliac artery in addition to the traditional external iliac/obturator fossa dissection is significantly more sensitive in detecting nodal involvement, at the cost of a modestly higher rate of lymphocele formation. Patients with a limited burden of nodal involvement do not usually have the dismal prognosis previously associated with node-positive prostate cancer, and a small but significant percentage of these men may be cured surgically. The role of adjuvant radiation and adjuvant ADT in this group is still being defined, but these patients may be reasonable candidates for adjuvant or salvage radiation and for deferred ADT. Current recommendations vary, but 2 of the 3 main guideline-issuing organizations state a preference for an extended dissection rather than a limited one, with lymph node dissection only omitted when the risk of LNI is low (2%–7%).

REFERENCES

1. Hovels AM, Heesakkers RA, Adang EM, et al. The diagnostic accuracy of CT and MRI in the staging of pelvic lymph nodes in patients with prostate cancer: a meta-analysis. Clin Radiol 2008;63: 387–95.

2. Heesakkers RA, Hovels AM, Jager GJ, et al. MRI with a lymph-node-specific contrast agent as an alternative to CT scan and lymph-node dissection in patients with prostate cancer: a prospective multi-cohort study. Lancet Oncol 2008;9:850–6.

3. Poulsen MH, Bouchelouche K, Gerke O, et al. [18F]-fluorocholine positron-emission/computed tomography for lymph node staging of patients with prostate cancer: preliminary results of a prospective study. BJU Int 2010;106:639–43.

4. Hacker A, Jeschke S, Leeb K, et al. Detection of pelvic lymph node metastases in patients with clinically localized prostate cancer: comparison of [18F] fluoro-choline positron emission tomography-computerized

tomography and laparoscopic radioisotope guided sentinel lymph node dissection. J Urol 2006;176: 2018–9.

5. Link RE, Morton RA. Indications for pelvic lymphadenectomy in prostate cancer. Urol Clin North Am 2001;28:491–8.

6. Heidenreich A, Varga Z, von Knobloch R. Extended pelvic lymphadenectomy in patients undergoing radical prostatectomy: high incidence of lymph node metstasis. J Urol 2002;167:1681–6.

7. Mattei A, Fuechsel FG, Bhatta Dhar N, et al. The template of the primary lymphatic landing sites of the prostate should be revisited: results of a multimodality mapping study. Eur Urol 2008;53:118–25.

8. Bader P, Burkhard FC, Markwalder R, et al. Disease progression and survival of patients with positive lymph nodes after radical prostatectomy. Is there a chance of cure? J Urol 2003;169:849–54.

9. Murray SK, Breau RH, Guha AK, et al. Spread of prostate carcinoma to the perirectal lymph node basin. Am J Surg Pathol 2004;28:1154–62.

10. Schumacher MC, Burkhard FC, Thalmann GN, et al. Good outcome for patients with few lymph node metastases after radical retropubic prostatectomy. Eur Urol 2008;54:344–52.

11. Toujier K, Rabbani F, Otero JR, et al. Standard versus limited pelvic lymph node dissection for prostate cancer in patients with a predicted probability of nodal metastasis greater than 1%. J Urol 2007;178:120–4.

12. Makarov DV, Trock BJ, Humphreys EB, et al. Updated nomogram to predict pathologic stage of prostate cancer given prostate-specific antigen level, clinical stage, and biopsy Gleason score (Partin Tables) based on cases from 2000 to 2005. Urology 2007;69:1095–101.

13. Cagiannos I, Karakiewicz P, Eastham JA, et al. A preoperative nomogram identifying decreased risk of positive pelvic lymph nodes in patients with prostate cancer. J Urol 2003;170:1798–803.

14. Kawakami J, Meng MV, Sadetsky N, et al. Changing patterns of pelvic lymphadenectomy for prostate cancerL: results from CaPSURE. J Urol 2006;176: 1382–6.

15. Allaf ME, Palapattu GS, Trock BJ, et al. Anatomical extent of lymph node dissection: impact on men with clinically localized prostate cancer. J Urol 2004;172:1840–4.

16. Godoy G, Chong KT, Cronin A et al. Extent of pelvic lymph node dissection and the impact of standard template dissection on nomogram prediction of lymph node involvement. Eur Urol 2011;60:195–201.

17. Briganti A, Chun FKH, Salanoia A, et al. Validation of a nomogram predicting the probability of lymph node invasion among patients undergoing radical prostatectomy and an extended pelvic lymphadenectomy. Eur Urol 2006;49:1019–27.

18. Weckermann D, Goppelt M, Dorn R, et al. Incidence of positive pelvic lymph nodes in patients with prostate cancer, a prostate-specific antigen (PSA) level of <10 ng/ml and biopsy Gleason score of < 6, and their infuence on PSA progression-free survival after radical prostatectomy. BJU Int 2006;97:1173–8.

19. Burkhard FC, Pader P, Schneider E, et al. Reliability of preoperative values to determine the need for lymphadenectomy in patients with prostate cancer and meticulous lymph node dissection. Eur Urol 2002;42:84–92.

20. Schumacher MC, Burkhard FC, Thalmann GN, et al. Is pelvic lymph node dissection necessary in patients with a serum PSA, 10ng/ml undergoing radical prostatectomy for prostate cancer? Eur Urol 2006;50:272–9.

21. Morgan TM, Lange PH, Porter MP, et al. Disseminated tumor cells in prostate cancer patients after radical prostatectomy and without evidence of disease predicts biochemical recurrence. Clin Cancer Res 2009;15:677–83.

22. Joslyn SA, Konety BR. Impact of extent of lymphadenectomy on survival after radical prostatectomy for prostate cancer. Urology 2006;68:121–5.

23. Albertsen PC, Hanley JA, Barrows GH, et al. Prostate cancer and the Will Rogers phenomenon. J Natl Cancer Inst 2005;17:1248–53.

24. Gofrit ON, Zorn KC, Steinberg GD, et al. The Will Rogers phenomenon in urological oncology. J Urol 2008;179:28–33.

25. Masterson TA, Bianco FJ, Vickers AJ, et al. The association between total and positive lymph node counts, and disease progression in clinically localized prostate cancer. J Urol 2006;175:1320–5.

26. Weight CJ, Reuther AM, Gunn PW, et al. Limited pelvic lymph node dissection does not improve survival at 10 years after radical prostatectomy in patients with low-risk prostate cancer. Urology 2008;71:141–5.

27. DiMarco DS, Zincke H, Sebo TJ, et al. The extent of lymphadenectomy for pTXN0 prostate cancer does not affect prostate cancer outcome in the prostate specific antigen era. J Urol 2005;173:1121–5.

28. Messing EM, Manola J, Yao J, et al. Immediate versus deferred androgen deprivation treatment in patients with node-positive prostate cancer after radical prostatectomy and pelvic lymphadenectomy. Lancet Oncol 2006;7:472–9.

29. Boorjian SA, Thompson RH, Siddiqui S, et al. Long-term outcome afetr radical prostatectomy for patients with lymph node positive prostate cancer in the prostate specific antigen era. J Urol 2007; 178:864–71.

30. Daneshmand S, Quek ML, Stein JP, et al. Prognosis of patients with lymph node positive prostate cancer following radical prostatectomy: long-term results. J Urol 2004;172:2252–5.

31. Palapattu GS, Allaf ME, Trock BJ, et al. Prostate specifc antigen progression in men with lymph node metastases following radical prostatectomy: results of long-term follow-up. J Urol 2004;172: 1860–4.

32. Bigg SW, Catalona WJ. Prophylactic mini-dose heparin in patients undergoing radical retropubic prostatectomy. A prospective trial. Urology 1992; 39:309–13.

33. Kropfl D, Krause R, Hartung R, et al. Subcutaneous heparin injection in the upper arm as a method of avoiding lymphoceles after lymphadenectomies in the lower part of the body. Urol Int 1987;42:416–23.

34. Clark T, Parekh DJ, Cookson MS, et al. Randomized prospective evaluation of extended versus limited lymph node dissection in patients with clinically localized prostate cancer. J Urol 2003;169:145–8.

35. Musch M, Klevecka V, Roggenbuck U, et al. Complications of pelvic lymphadenectomy in 1,380 patients undergoing radical retropubic prostatectomy between 1993 and 2006. J Urol 2008;179:923–9.

36. Briganti A, Chun FK, Salonia A, et al. Complications and other surgical outcomes associated with extended pelvic lymphadenectomy in men with localized prostate cancer. Eur Urol 2006;50:1006–13.

37. Tokuda Y, Carlino LJ, Gopalan A, et al. Prostate cancer topography and patterns pf lymph node metastasis. Am J Surg Pathol 2010;34:1862–7.

38. Zorn KC, Katz MH, Bernstein A, et al. Pelvic lymphadenectomy during robot-assisted radical prostatectomy: assessing nodal yield, perioperative outcomes, and complications. Urology 2009;74:296–304.

39. Eifler JB, Levinson AW, Hyndman ME, et al. Pelvic lymph node dissection is associated with symptomatic venous thromboembolism during laparoscopic radical prostatectomy. J Urol 2011;185: 1661–6.

40. Thompson IM, Tangen CM, Paradelo J, et al. Adjuvant radiotherapy for pathological T3N0M0 prostate cancer significantly reduces risk of metastases and improves survival: long-term followup of a randomized clinical trial. J Urol 2009;181:956–62.

41. Da Pozza LF, Cozzarini C, Briganti A, et al. Long-term follow-up of patients with prostate cancer and nodal metastases treated by pelvic lymphadenopathy and radical prostatectomy: the positive impact of adjuvant radiotherapy. Eur Urol 2009;55:1003–11.

42. Stephenson AJ, Scardino PT, Kattan MW, et al. Predicting the outcome of salvage radiation therapy for recurrent prostate cancer after radical prostatectomy. J Clin Oncol 2007;25:2035–41.

43. Briganti A, Karnes JR, Da Pazzo LF, et al. Two positive nodes represent a significant cut-off value for cancer-specific survival in patients with node positive prostate cancer. A new proposal based on a two-institution experience on 703 consecutive N+ patients treated with radical prostatectomy, extended pelvic lymph node dissection and adjuvant therapy. Eur Urol 2009;55:261–70.

44. American Urological Association Prostate-Specific Antigen Best Practice Statement: 2009 Update. Available at: auanet.org. Accessed March 3, 2011.

45. European Association of Urology 2010 Guidelines on Prostate Cancer. Available at: uroweb.org. Accessed March 3, 2011.

46. National Comprehensive Cancer Network Guidelines Version 1.2011 Prostate Cancer. Available at: nccn.org. Accessed January 3, 2011.

Lymphadenectomy for Bladder Cancer: Indications and Controversies

Fiona C. Burkhard, MD, Beat Roth, MD, Pascal Zehnder, MD, Urs E. Studer, MD*

KEYWORDS

- Pelvic lymph node dissection • Cystectomy
- Invasive bladder cancer • Template • Outcome

Pelvic lymph node dissection (PLND) at the time of cystectomy remains the most accurate method of staging and can have a positive impact on cancer control, and there is general agreement as to its necessity at the time of surgery. There is, however, a lack of consensus regarding the terminology of PLND and controversy concerning the optimal extent of lymph node (LN) dissection, especially because recent investigations have suggested a survival benefit with extended PLND.

INDICATIONS

Twenty percent to 40% of patients with bladder cancer present with muscle invasive disease and approximately 25% are found to have LN metastases at the time of cystectomy.[1–6] PLND remains the only way to achieve accurate staging because the available imaging studies are limited either by having to base their identification of pathology on LN size[7] or by their unacceptably low sensitivity rates.[8]

The incidence of LN positivity increases with increasing tumor stage, from approximately 2% to 5% in pT1 tumors to 16% to 22% in pT2, 34% to 51% in pT3, and 41% to 50% in pT4 tumors.[1,2,4,9–11] Shariat and colleagues[12] and Palapattu and colleagues[13] showed that even patients with carcinoma in situ only or pT0 after transurethral resection of Tis, T1, T2, or T3 disease at the time of cystectomy had a 3% rate of LN metastases with

5-year bladder cancer-specific survival estimates of 95% and 91%, respectively. Patient selection is an unquantifiable factor and, therefore, the results must be interpreted with caution. Nevertheless, although the risk of LN metastases is assumed low in patients with nonmuscle invasive bladder cancer requiring cystectomy, these results have demonstrated a potential benefit of PLND even in these low-risk patients. In summary, if cystectomy is indicated, then PLND should be performed.

CONTROVERSIES
Terminology

There is a certain degree of confusion surrounding the definitions of PLND in bladder cancer. Historically, a standard PLND included the removal of all lymphatic tissue between the bladder and pelvic sidewall and along the external and internal iliac vessels proximally up to the midportion of the common iliac vessels, including tissue from the fossa of Marcille.[14] Distally the limits were defined by the crossing of the circumflex iliac vein over the external iliac artery and the LN of Cloquet. Today, limited PLND is generally restricted to removal of the lymphatic tissue in the obturator fossa, in some cases with a dissection along the external iliac vessels. In contrast, an extended PLND includes all lymphatic tissue up to the boundaries of the aortic bifurcation. Some centers also include the LNs surrounding the distal aorta and inferior

Department of Urology, University Hospital Bern, 3010 Bern, Switzerland
* Corresponding author.
E-mail address: Urs.Studer@insel.ch

Urol Clin N Am 38 (2011) 397–405
doi:10.1016/j.ucl.2011.07.011

urologic.theclinics.com

vena cava up to the level of the takeoff of the inferior mesenteric artery (IMA).[2,10,15]

To avoid confusion with the terminology, the authors propose subdividing the current terminology into 3 groups (**Fig. 1**). Limited PLND refers to tissue along the external iliac vein and from the obturator fossa. The limits of an extended PLND are laterally, the genitofemoral nerve; medially, the bladder wall; distally, the inguinal ligament and the pelvic floor; dorsally, the hypogastric vessels, including both the medial (considered presacral by some) and the lateral sides; and proximally, along either side of the common iliac vessels up to where the retracted ureter crosses them (ie, approximately between the proximal and middle third of the common iliac vessels). Also included is the tissue in the fossa of Marcille, dorsolateral to the bifurcation of the common iliac vessels and dorsal to the external iliac vein (considered presciatic by some). For a superextended PLND, the proximal border is extended up to the level of the origin of the IMA. The true presacral nodes, which lie dorsal to the bladder and rectum and are few in number, are, to the authors' knowledge, hardly ever included in a PLND for bladder cancer.

What Can Be Considered an Adequate Template for PLND?

The lymphatic drainage pattern of a malignant tumor determines the field of LN dissection. The available data on lymphatic tumor spread have been gained by using surgical specimens to identify the location of LN metastases.[1,10,15,16] Leissner and colleagues[10] examined LNs at 12 different anatomic sites in 290 patients who underwent radical cystectomy and a superextended PLND. Sixteen percent of LN metastases were found above the aortic bifurcation but only in patients with 2 or more LN metastases. None of the 29 single LN metastases was located above the aortic bifurcation. In this setting, a limited PLND would have missed 27% and extending the PLND to the iliac bifurcation, 10% of positive LNs in patients with a single positive node, respectively.[10] This is in line with the report of Dangle and colleagues,[16] who demonstrated that a limited PLND fails to identify positive nodes in 25% and a standard PLND (up to the iliac bifurcation) in 11% of patients. Vazina and colleagues[1] evaluated 176 patients undergoing radical cystectomy and superextended PLND. Of those with pT3 or pT4 disease stage, 16% had LN metastases along

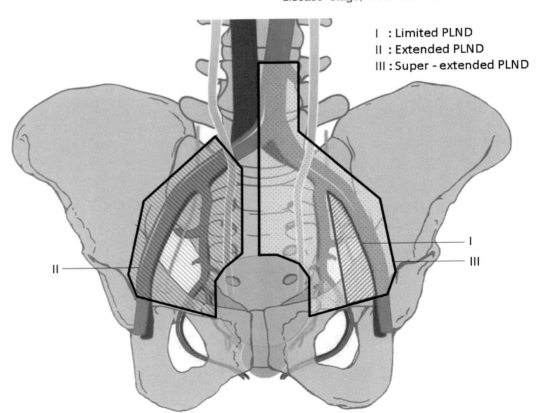

I : Limited PLND
II : Extended PLND
III : Super - extended PLND

Fig. 1. Depicts the boundaries of a limited (I), extended (II), and superextended (III) PLND.

the common iliac artery and at or above the aortic bifurcation but always combined with other LN metastases inside the small pelvis. In a prospective mapping study of 200 patients, Ghoneim's group evaluated the probability of disease (node-positive) clearance with increasingly wider fields of LN dissection. After removal of all LNs in the pelvis (extended dissection), 65% of all positive nodes were identified. By extending the dissection to the level of the aortic bifurcation, this proportion increased to 79%. Again, no metastatic lesions located solely outside of the small pelvis (skip lesions) were found.[15] Of the 48 LN-positive patients, 39% presented with bilateral LN involvement, leading to a recommendation of bilateral resection. These findings imply that a solitary LN metastasis outside the pelvis is rare and that exposing patients to the risk of including the nodes up to the IMA may be of limited benefit. LN metastases can be found at the level of the aortic bifurcation and IMA. They are generally associated, however, with multiple affected LNs with a correspondingly poor prognosis.

Certain problems are inherent to all mapping studies. The location to which the tissue is assigned may vary. For example, tissue from the common iliac bifurcation can be considered external, internal, common iliac, or from the obturator fossa, depending on the institutional standards. Another issue is that information is only gained on the nodes that were removed and not on the nodes that were possibly missed. If no nodes were retrieved at the aortic level, then the conclusion is that there are no positive nodes to be found at that location.

A recently published study identifying the true lymphatic drainage pattern of the bladder, however, is less limited by these problems. By applying new imaging techniques to accurately define the bladder's primary lymphatic landing sites, for the first time, further insight into the lymphatic drainage pattern of the bladder was gained and the clinical observations (discussed previously) substantiated.[17] Technetium Tc 99m–nanocolloid was injected into 1 of 6 specified non–tumor-bearing sites of the bladder to minimize the risk of artifacts by blocked lymph vessels or nodes in the case of lymphangiosis. The primary lymphatic landing sites were located by preoperative single-photon emission CT (SPECT) combined with CT. They were verified intraoperatively with a gamma probe and double-checked by a backup extended PLND. If the identified primary landing sites from all 6 injection sites in the bladder were added, a median of 28 nodes per patient was found. Ninety-two percent of all LNs were found distal and caudal to where the ureter crosses the common iliac arteries and 8% proximal thereof. No proximal nodes were detected without simultaneous detection of additional radioactive LNs within the endopelvic region. In a similar study on 40 patients with unilateral bladder cancer, technetium Tc 99m–nanocolloid was injected into the non–tumor-bearing lateral bladder wall.[18] All patients had at least one radioactive LN on the ipsilateral side and 40% of patients had at least one additional radioactive LN on the contralateral side. This study, as others, relies on the operative procedure (PLND) for verification and a few LNs may have been missed despite preoperative SPECT/CT, intraoperative gamma probe verification, and extended backup PLND. The risk of error, however, is much lower than in conventional mapping studies, making this the most accurate description of the bladder's lymphatic drainage pattern to date.

What Can Be Learned From This Technetium-Based Mapping Study?

First the idea of sentinel node, as observed in cancers of other organs, may not be valid for the bladder. Because a median of 4 primary lymphatic landing sites was found in 1 of 6 bladder sites, the median number of primary lymphatic landing sites per bladder is approximately 28. This implies a more complex lymphatic drainage pattern in the bladder than in other organs, such as the breast, a finding also described by other investigators.[10,19,20] The removal of one sentinel node to determine if pelvic lymphadenectomy is necessary or not does not seem applicable for the bladder. Instead, removal of multiple nodes, potentially on both sides of the pelvis, is required. In this setting, removal of nodes/lymphatic tissue from a well-defined template may be more reliable and cost effective. This was supported by Liedberg and colleagues'[19] observations that, when applying intraoperative sentinel node detection in invasive bladder cancer, 19% of LN-positive patients proved false negative and would have been missed. Technetium seems reliable for the detection of normal but not metastatic nodes.

Second, a basis to discuss the template, which can be considered appropriate, was given. In 1962, Whitmore and Marshall[14] described a standard template for bilateral PLND, which included all tissue from the pelvis up to the proximal third of the common iliac artery, at the level of the ureteric crossing. This standard template corresponds to what was defined as an extended PLND. Based on the mapping study (discussed previously), the percentage of primary landing sites left in situ, between where the ureter crosses the common iliac artery and the IMA, would be 8%. Is it worthwhile to resect the remaining 8% to 10% of potential primary lymphatic landing sites between the uretero-iliac junction and the IMA?

Cure is achieved only in patients with a limited number of metastases in normal-sized nodes, a situation not commonly found limited to locations outside of the pelvis.[3] The potential benefit of extending PLND up to the IMA can be calculated. The prevalence of histologically positive LNs in patients with clinically negative LNs is approximately 25%.[1–6] Of patients with positive LNs, 35%[3] will survive, which corresponds to approximately 8 of 100 cystectomy patients. Because at most 8% to 10% of patients can be expected to have positive LNs above the uretero-iliac junction, at most 1 to 2 of 100 cystectomy patients would benefit from a superextended PLND up to the IMA. It is questionable whether overtreatment in 99% of cystectomy patients is justifiable. In patients receiving an ileal orthotopic bladder substitute, there is also a potential risk of impaired continence through damage to the hypogastric nerves after higher resection as well as a potentially increased complication rate.[21,22]

Before resecting the para-aortic/paracaval LNs, the LNs of the fossa of Marcille should be removed. Four percent of all technetium Tc 99m–positive LNs or 12% of all technetium Tc 99m–positive LNs along the external iliac vessels were found in the fossa of Marcille (ie, the presciatic nodes), which are dorsal to the external iliac vein and dorsolateral to the bifurcation of the common iliac vessels.[17] This approach is easier and faster and may be of greater benefit to patients. Meticulous dissection of the internal iliac vessels is also important; 10% of all technetium Tc 99m–positive LNs are found medial to the internal iliac artery (some term these presacral), an area often neglected.

In summary, an adequate or extended PLND is what Whitmore and Marshall already defined as a standard PLND in 1962.

Importance of the Number of Nodes Removed

The number of nodes resected has been proposed as a surrogate for the quality of PLND. This is a difficult proposition because the number of nodes detected not only depends on the extent and meticulousness of dissection but also on the pathologist's dedication to finding and carefully examining the LNs. Subdividing the tissue from a defined template into more separate packages results in a larger number of LNs detected[23] as does requiring a certain number to be submitted by institutional policy.[24] There also is a wide variability in the number of nodes per individual patient.[25] These limitations are underlined by the observations made by Fleischmann and colleagues,[26] who showed that in a single-center series of patients with LN metastases, the number of nodes removed ranged from 10 to 43 after removal of lymphatic tissue from a standardized template. Independent of the number of nodes removed (few or many), recurrence-free survival and overall survival remained unchanged.

These observations all make using the number of nodes as a surrogate for the quality of PLND and consequently for the chance of survival questionable. On the contrary, a standardized template based on a universally accepted nomenclature where the tissue between the defined boundaries is meticulously removed should set the standard for PLND.

Impact of PLND on Prognosis and Outcome

PLND at the time of cystectomy increases the probability of completely removing all cancerous cells. The more complete the PLND, the better the chance of cure. Prognosis further depends on the stage of the primary tumor, the number of positive nodes, LN density, and, most importantly, according to a multivariate analysis, extranodal growth.[26]

In 1950, Kerr and Colby[27] first suggested a benefit for PLND. They reported a 2-year survival in 2 patients after cystectomy and PLND despite nodal disease. Whitmore and Marshall in 1962[14] stated that for patients with only a few pelvic nodal metastases radical cystectomy with PLND has provided some successful 5-year results. Smith and Whitmore[28] and Pagano and colleagues[29] several years later questioned the benefit of PLND for survival. Smith and Whitmore postulated that distant metastases occur at or approximately the same time as does regional nodal spread in the majority of patients, the conclusion being that extrapelvic disease is a significant determinant of survival and interval to recurrence, regardless of the extent of nodal metastases. In contrast, Skinner in 1982[3] stated that a meticulous PLND could provide cure and control of pelvic disease in some patients with regional LN metastases without increasing the morbidity (**Table 1**). Since then, more contemporary data originating from centers, including the University of Southern California in Los Angeles, the Memorial Sloan-Kettering Cancer Center in New York, and the University of Bern, Bern, Switzerland have confirmed that with extended PLND, approximately a third (31%–35%) of bladder cancer patients with LN metastases were alive at 5 years.[2,30–33] In the largest single-center cystectomy series to date, published

Table 1
Survival of bladder cancer patients treated with cystectomy and PLND

Series	No of Patients	Type of PLND	Median No. of Nodes Removed	% of Patients with LN[a]	Median 5-Year RFS (%) of Node-Positive Patients
Pagano et al,[29] 1991	261	En bloc?	—	—	4
Ghoneim et al,[32] 1997	1026[b]	Limited	—	19	23
Poulsen et al,[9] 1998	68	Limited	14	22	56
	126	Extended	25	28	62
Vieweg et al,[30] 1999[d]	686	Extended	—	20	7
Stein et al,[2] 2001	1054	Superextended	—	24	35
Madersbacher et al,[4] 2003	507	Extended	—	24	33
Vazina et al,[1] 2004	176	Extended	25	24	—
Abdel-Latif et al,[11] 2004	417	Limited	—	26	38[c]
Leissner et al,[10] 2004	290[b]	Superextended	43	28	—
Fleischmann et al,[26] 2005	507	Extended	22	24	32
Hautmann et al,[50] 2006	788	Extended	2	18	21
Dhar et al,[33] 2008 (only pT2 and pT3)	336	Limited	12	13	7
	322	extended	22	26	35
Zehnder et al,[34] 2011 (only pT2 and pT3)	405	Extended	22	28	55
	554	Superextended	38	35	57
Park et al,[45] 2011	450	Superextended	18	29	25

Abbreviation: RFS, recurrence-free survival.
[a] Only pT2 and pT3.
[b] Mixed urothelial, squamous, and adenocarcinoma.
[c] 3-Year RFS.
[d] Preoperative radiotherapy.

by Stein and colleagues,[2] using superextended PLND, 31 of the 246 (23%) patients who were node positive were alive at 5 years.

Survival benefit is dependent on the extent of the template applied for lymphadenectomy. This was illustrated in 2 recent interinstitutional comparative studies assessing the survival benefit associated with the extent of the PLND performed. Dhar and colleagues[33] compared the outcome of well-defined patient groups (pT2/3, clinically N0M0, no neoadjuvant chemotherapy) at 2 high volume centers performing either a limited or an extended PLND. LN-positive patients in the limited LND group demonstrated significantly decreased 5-year recurrence-free survival when compared with the extended LND group (7% vs 35%). There was also a 2-fold increase in the rate of LN-positive disease in the extended LND group, suggesting significant understaging in patients undergoing limited LND. Zehnder and colleagues[34] compared 2 well-defined patient groups (pT2/3, clinically N0M0, no neoadjuvant therapy). One group was from the same institution as the study (discussed previously) of extended PLND. The other group was comprised of patients from another high-volume institution routinely performing a superextended PLND. Despite more nodes being removed and more positive nodes detected in the patients who underwent superextended PLND, no significant differences in survival outcome were seen. Five-year recurrence-free survival and overall survival rates in LN-positive patients after superextended versus extended PLND were 40% versus 42% and 34% and 38%, respectively. The lack of difference was consistent irrespective of nodal status or receipt of adjuvant chemotherapy. A partial explanation may be that solitary or few metastases directly to these extrapelvic nodes is rare and prognosis in general is poor for patients with nodal disease outside the pelvis. Therefore, the removal of these nodes hardly affects outcome.[35]

So, at a first glance it seems that approximately 35% of patients with positive LNs could benefit from an extended PLND. But which patients will ultimately benefit?

It seems that patients with LN metastases as well as patients without any identifiable sign of LN metastases may profit from PLND. Herr[36] reported that survival after cystectomy for both patients with LN-negative and node-positive disease was improved (reduced local recurrence rate) when a higher number of nodes was removed. Similarly, a study by Leissner and colleagues[5] demonstrated that of patients without or with 5 or fewer positive nodes who had more than 16 LNs removed, 65% were disease-free and alive at 5 years. In contrast,

51% of the patients who had fewer than 16 LNs resected were alive and disease-free at 5 years. A large collaborative study of the Southwestern Oncology Group evaluating patients treated at 4 high-volume centers found that removal of more than 10 nodes increased 5-year overall survival from 44% to 61% in comparison with removal of fewer than 10 nodes.[37] Recently, Vazina and colleagues[1] reported that enforcing an institutional policy requiring removal of at least 16 nodes improved survival from 40% to 52% in patients with a greater than 2-year follow-up. These data suggest that a greater number of nodes removed (implicating a more extended template) at the time of cystectomy is beneficial for some patients. Using an extended field for PLND increases the number of nodes removed and the probability of removing positive nodes. The removal of nodes found pathologically negative seems equally important, however. Data based on reverse transcription–polymerase chain reaction studies have shown that 20% to 30% of pathologically negative nodes may harbor micrometastatic disease. In this sense, removal of histologically negative nodes harbouring occult metastatic disease may have a significant impact on outcome.[38–40]

Lerner and colleagues[41] was one of the first to report an increased risk of cancer-related progression and death associated with 6 or more LN metastases identified at the time of cystectomy. Similarly, Mills and colleagues[21] from Bern, Switzerland demonstrated that patients with fewer than 5 involved nodes had a statistically significant survival advantage compared with those with greater than or equal to 5 involved nodes. Herr[42] and Stein and colleagues[43] almost simultaneously proposed the number of positive–to–total number of LNs (LN density) removed ratio as a significant prognostic variable. The hypothesis was based on LN density incorporating both the extent of disease based on the number of positive LNs as well as the extent of LN dissection based on the number of nodes removed. Stein and colleagues[43] from the University of Southern California found that patients with less than or equal to 20% LN metastases density had a 43% 10-year recurrence-free survival compared with a 17% 10-year survival for those with greater than 20% density. Furthermore, recent studies support the observation that LN density may be an independent predictor of survival in patients with muscle invasive bladder cancer.[44,45] Density reflects the extent of nodal dissection, however. If 1 of 5 nodes is positive, the ratio is 20%. If 1 of 50 nodes is positive, then the ratio is 2%. This patient may well have a better chance to survive because it is likely that there really are no further positive nodes. Patients with 1 positive node of 5 nodes removed have a high probability of having additional occult positive nodes left behind. Another factor having an impact on outcome is the tumor volume in affected nodes. Of patients with grossly node-positive bladder cancer treated with surgery alone, 24% survived and 76% died of disease. The median survival time for all patients was 19 months and 10 years for surviving patients.[46] Skinner[3] reported a 36% improvement in 5-year survival in bladder cancer patients with limited nodal burden. The conclusion was, "patients who probably benefit most from a meticulous dissection are those with undetectable micrometastases to a few nodes." The authors' group found that patients with maximal nodal metastasis up to 0.5 cm had a median survival of 84 months compared with only 16 months in those with metastases greater than 0.5 cm.[21]

More recently, the authors demonstrated that although the number of positive nodes and volume of metastatic disease are important prognosticators for survival, the strongest predictive factor in multivariate analysis is extracapsular growth.[26] These more aggressive tumors, which present with extracapsular growth in the LNs, are also the ones that involve multiple nodes and develop metastases more rapidly.

One remaining point of discussion is the role of chemotherapy. In a study from the University of Southern California and the University of Bern comparing superextended and extended PLND, no difference in outcome was observed despite removal of more nodes and more patients undergoing chemotherapy in the superextended PLND group.[47] In multivariate analysis, adjuvant chemotherapy did not affect recurrence-free survival. In an initial report from a randomized prospective multicenter trial to determine the effect of neoadjuvant chemotherapy in patients with stage T2-T4 urothelial bladder cancer, neoadjuvant chemotherapy was associated with a significant survival benefit.[48] On a repeated evaluation, however, the extent of surgery was found a more highly significant predictor of survival.[49]

SUMMARY

The conclusions that can be made based on the available literature are that if a cystectomy is indicated, then an extended PLND should be performed and corresponds by in large to Whitmore and Marshall's definition of a standard PLND in 1962. The boundaries should be lateral, the genitofemoral nerve; medial, bladder wall; distal, inguinal ligament; inferior, caudal pelvic floor; dorsal, hypogastric vessels on both the medial (considered presacral by some) and the lateral side; and proximal, common iliac artery up to where the ureter crosses the common iliac vessels, including the tissue in the fossa Marcille (considered presciatic by some). There is no place for a limited PLND and evidence supporting a superextended PLND in bladder cancer is scarce. The patients most likely to profit from the extended PLND are the ones with limited metastases to normal-sized nodes. Skinner's statement from 1982, that not removing the palpable nodes or gross nodal metastatic disease but meticulously removing normal-sized nodes is beneficial, still holds true.

REFERENCES

1. Vazina A, Dugi D, Shariat SF, et al. Stage specific lymph node metastasis mapping in radical cystectomy specimens. J Urol 2004;171:1830–4.
2. Stein JP, Lieskovsky G, Cote R, et al. Radical cystectomy in the treatment of invasive bladder cancer: long-term results in 1,054 patients. J Clin Oncol 2001;19:666–75.
3. Skinner DG. Management of invasive bladder cancer: a meticulous pelvic node dissection can make a difference. J Urol 1982;128:34–6.
4. Madersbacher S, Hochreiter W, Burkhard F, et al. Radical cystectomy for bladder cancer today—a homogeneous series without neoadjuvant therapy. J Clin Oncol 2003;21:690–6.
5. Leissner J, Hohenfellner R, Thuroff JW, et al. Lymphadenectomy in patients with transitional cell carcinoma of the urinary bladder; significance for staging and prognosis. BJU Int 2000;85:817–23.
6. Herr HW, Bochner BH, Dalbagni G, et al. Impact of the number of lymph nodes retrieved on outcome in patients with muscle invasive bladder cancer. J Urol 2002;167:1295–8.
7. Ficarra V, Dalpiaz O, Alrabi N, et al. Correlation between clinical and pathological staging in a series of radical cystectomies for bladder carcinoma. BJU Int 2005;95:786–90.
8. Kibel AS, Dehdashti F, Katz MD, et al. Prospective study of [18F]fluorodeoxyglucose positron emission tomography/computed tomography for staging of muscle-invasive bladder carcinoma. J Clin Oncol 2009;27:4314–20.
9. Poulsen AL, Horn T, Steven K. Radical cystectomy: extending the limits of pelvic lymph node dissection improves survival for patients with bladder cancer confined to the bladder wall. J Urol 1998;160: 2015–9 [discussion: 2020].
10. Leissner J, Ghoneim MA, Abol-Enein H, et al. Extended radical lymphadenectomy in patients with urothelial bladder cancer: results of a prospective multicenter study. J Urol 2004;171:139–44.

11. Abdel-Latif M, Abol-Enein H, El-Baz M, et al. Nodal involvement in bladder cancer cases treated with radical cystectomy: incidence and prognosis. J Urol 2004;172:85–9.

12. Shariat SF, Palapattu GS, Amiel GE, et al. Characteristics and outcomes of patients with carcinoma in situ only at radical cystectomy. Urology 2006;68:538–42.

13. Palapattu GS, Shariat SF, Karakiewicz PI, et al. Cancer specific outcomes in patients with pT0 disease following radical cystectomy. J Urol 2006;175:1645–9 [discussion: 1649].

14. Whitmore WF Jr, Marshall VF. Radical total cystectomy for cancer of the bladder: 230 consecutive cases five years later. J Urol 1962;87:853–68.

15. Abol-Enein H, El-Baz M, Abd El-Hameed MA, et al. Lymph node involvement in patients with bladder cancer treated with radical cystectomy: a pathoanatomical study—a single center experience. J Urol 2004;172:1818–21.

16. Dangle PP, Gong MC, Bahnson RR, et al. How do commonly performed lymphadenectomy templates influence bladder cancer nodal stage? J Urol 2010;183:499–503.

17. Roth B, Wissmeyer MP, Zehnder P, et al. A new multimodality technique accurately maps the primary lymphatic landing sites of the bladder. Eur Urol 2010;57:205–11.

18. Roth B, Zehnder P, Birkhauser FD, et al. Does the lymphatic drainage pattern of the lateral bladder wall make a bilateral pelvic lymph node dissection (PLND) unnecessary in strictly laterally localized invasive bladder cancer? Results of a multimodality mappping study. J Urol 2011;185:e562.

19. Liedberg F, Chebil G, Davidsson T, et al. Intraoperative sentinel node detection improves nodal staging in invasive bladder cancer. J Urol 2006;175:84–8 [discussion: 8–9].

20. Knapp DW, Adams LG, Degrand AM, et al. Sentinel lymph node mapping of invasive urinary bladder cancer in animal models using invisible light. Eur Urol 2007;52:1700–8.

21. Mills RD, Turner WH, Fleischmann A, et al. Pelvic lymph node metastases from bladder cancer: outcome in 83 patients after radical cystectomy and pelvic lymphadenectomy. J Urol 2001;166:19–23.

22. Kessler TM, Burkhard FC, Studer UE. Clinical indications and outcomes with nerve-sparing cystectomy in patients with bladder cancer. Urol Clin North Am 2005;32:165–75.

23. Stein JP, Penson DF, Cai J, et al. Radical cystectomy with extended lymphadenectomy: evaluating separate package versus en bloc submission for node positive bladder cancer. J Urol 2007;177:876–81 [discussion: 881–2].

24. Fang AC, Ahmad AE, Whitson JM, et al. Effect of a minimum lymph node policy in radical cystectomy and pelvic lymphadenectomy on lymph node yields, lymph node positivity rates, lymph node density, and survivorship in patients with bladder cancer. Cancer 2010;116:1901–8.

25. Weingartner K, Ramaswamy A, Bittinger A, et al. Anatomical basis for pelvic lymphadenectomy in prostate cancer: results of an autopsy study and implications for the clinic. J Urol 1996;156:1969–71.

26. Fleischmann A, Thalmann GN, Markwalder R, et al. Extracapsular extension of pelvic lymph node metastases from urothelial carcinoma of the bladder is an independent prognostic factor. J Clin Oncol 2005;23:2358–65.

27. Kerr WS, Colby FH. Pelvic lymphadenectomy and total cystectomy in the treatment of carcinoma of the bladder. J Urol 1950;63:842–51.

28. Smith JA Jr, Whitmore WF Jr. Regional lymph node metastasis from bladder cancer. J Urol 1981;126:591–3.

29. Pagano F, Bassi P, Galetti TP, et al. Results of contemporary radical cystectomy for invasive bladder cancer: a clinicopathological study with an emphasis on the inadequacy of the tumor, nodes and metastases classification. J Urol 1991;145:45–50.

30. Vieweg J, Gschwend JE, Herr HW, et al. Pelvic lymph node dissection can be curative in patients with node positive bladder cancer. J Urol 1999;161:449–54.

31. Kassouf W, Agarwal PK, Herr HW, et al. Lymph node density is superior to TNM nodal status in predicting disease-specific survival after radical cystectomy for bladder cancer: analysis of pooled data from MDACC and MSKCC. J Clin Oncol 2008;26:121–6.

32. Ghoneim MA, el-Mekresh MM, el-Baz MA, et al. Radical cystectomy for carcinoma of the bladder: critical evaluation of the results in 1,026 cases. J Urol 1997;158:393–9.

33. Dhar NB, Klein EA, Reuther AM, et al. Outcome after radical cystectomy with limited or extended pelvic lymph node dissection. J Urol 2008;179:873–8 [discussion: 878].

34. Zehnder P, Studer U, Skinner E, et al. Extended lymph node dissecton for patients undergoing radical cystectomy for cancer: how high? J Urol 2011;185:e563.

35. Dorin RP, Eisenberg ME, Cai J. Proximal extent of lymph node (LN) metastasis and other independent prognositc indicators in 162 LN positive patients undergoing radical cystectomy with extended LN dissection for bladder cancer. In: 2010 ASCo Genitourinary Cancers Symposium. San Francisco (CA); March 5–7, 2010. p. 139 [abstract nr.: 299].

36. Herr HW. Extent of surgery and pathology evaluation has an impact on bladder cancer outcomes after radical cystectomy. Urology 2003;61:105–8.

37. Herr H, Lee C, Chang S, et al. Standardization of radical cystectomy and pelvic lymph node

dissection for bladder cancer: a collaborative group report. J Urol 2004;171:1823–8 [discussion: 1827–8].

38. Retz M, Lehmann J, Szysnik C, et al. Detection of occult tumor cells in lymph nodes from bladder cancer patients by MUC7 nested RT-PCR. Eur Urol 2004;45:314–9.

39. Marin-Aguilera M, Mengual L, Burset M, et al. Molecular lymph node staging in bladder urothelial carcinoma: impact on survival. Eur Urol 2008;54:1363–72.

40. Autenrieth M, Nawroth R, Semmlack S, et al. Muscle-invasive urothelial carcinoma of the bladder. Detection and topography of micrometastases in lymph nodes. Urologe A 2008;47:1157–61 [in German].

41. Lerner SP, Skinner DG, Lieskovsky G, et al. The rationale for en bloc pelvic lymph node dissection for bladder cancer patients with nodal metastases: long-term results. J Urol 1993;149:758–64 [discussion: 764–5].

42. Herr HW. Superiority of ratio based lymph node staging for bladder cancer. J Urol 2003;169:943–5.

43. Stein JP, Cai J, Groshen S, et al. Risk factors for patients with pelvic lymph node metastases following radical cystectomy with en bloc pelvic lymphadenectomy: concept of lymph node density. J Urol 2003;170:35–41.

44. Wiesner C, Salzer A, Thomas C, et al. Cancer-specific survival after radical cystectomy and standardized extended lymphadenectomy for node-positive bladder cancer: prediction by lymph node positivity and density. BJU Int 2009;104:331–5.

45. Park J, Kim S, Jeong IG, et al. Does the greater number of lymph nodes removed during standard lymph node dissection predict better patient survival following radical cystectomy? World J Urol 2011; 29(4):443–9.

46. Herr HW, Donat SM. Outcome of patients with grossly node positive bladder cancer after pelvic lymph node dissection and radical cystectomy. J Urol 2001;165:62–4 [discussion: 64].

47. Zehnder P, Studer UE, Skinner EC, et al. Super extended versus extended pelvic lymph node dissection in patients undergoing radical cystectomy for bladder cancer: a comparative study. J Urol 2011;186(4):1261–8.

48. Grossman HB, Natale RB, Tangen CM, et al. Neoadjuvant chemotherapy plus cystectomy compared with cystectomy alone for locally advanced bladder cancer. N Engl J Med 2003;349:859–66.

49. Herr HW, Faulkner JR, Grossman HB, et al. Surgical factors influence bladder cancer outcomes: a cooperative group report. J Clin Oncol 2004;22:2781–9.

50. Hautmann RE, Gschwend JE, de Petriconi RC, et al. Cystectomy for transitional cell carcinoma of the bladder: results of a surgery only series in the neobladder era. J Urol 2006;176:486–92 [discussion: 491–2].

Feasibility of Minimally Invasive Lymphadenectomy in Bladder and Prostate Cancer Surgery

A. Ari Hakimi, MD, Reza Ghavamian, MD*

KEYWORDS

- Lymphadenectomy • Robotic prostatectomy
- Robotic cystectomy • Bladder cancer • Prostate cancer

This article is not certified for *AMA PRA Category 1 Credit*™ because product brand names are included in the educational content. The Accreditation Council for Continuing Medical Education requires the use of generic names and or drug/product classes as the required nomenclature for therapeutic options in continuing medical education.
For more information, please go to www.accme.org and review the Standards of Commercial Support.

There has been a dramatic increase in the number of minimally invasive procedures (laparoscopic and robotic) for the treatment of prostate and bladder cancers in the last decade. In the United States, robotic-assisted radical prostatectomy (RALP) is the most commonly performed surgical treatment for prostate cancer. The pure laparoscopic technique was never adopted as it was in Europe, due to its technical challenges and because of the rapid increase in use of the Da Vinci surgical system in the United States. As more prostate procedures are being performed, interest in bladder cancer surgery using the robot has also increased recently. For the surgeon adept at performing RALP, robotic cystectomy presented itself as the next pelvic operation to be tackled robotically. Both radical prostatectomy and radical cystectomy have been shown to be volume dependent, with better surgical and oncologic outcomes expected for experienced and high-volume surgeons. In both procedures, but more so in cystectomy, the quality of the oncologic operation is often judged by the extent and adequacy of the lymph node dissection. It has been recently shown that for both cancers, the number and extent of the lymph node dissection leads to better oncologic outcomes. This improvement is achieved by surgical cure with the procedure alone, as in the case of micrometastases detected, while in those in whom surgical cure is not achieved, detection of occult positive nodes can lead to better selection of patients for adjuvant treatment modalities.

The author have nothing to disclose.
Statement of originality: This article is the original work of the authors.
Department of Urology, Montefiore Medical Center, Albert Einstein College of Medicine, Bronx, NY, USA
* Corresponding author. Montefiore Medical Center, 3400 Bainbridge Avenue, Bronx, NY 10467.
E-mail address: rghavami@montefiore.org

Urol Clin N Am 38 (2011) 407–418
doi:10.1016/j.ucl.2011.07.003
0094-0143/11/$ – see front matter © 2011 Elsevier Inc. All rights reserved.

With the rapid and widespread adoption of mini- mally invasive procedure (specifically robotic assistance in the United States) for these two cancers, concerns have been raised regarding whether the technique can emulate the time- tested gold standard open procedures. These concerns are not only directed to the surgical margins and resection of the primary tumor, but also question whether an adequate node dissec- tion along the same defined "extended" templates and hence nodal counts can be achieved rob- otically. Rightfully so, concerns have been raised by the urologic oncology community regarding whether lymph node dissection is even performed in every case for which it is indicated, especially in prostate cancer.

In this article the authors briefly review the indi- cations for lymph node dissection for bladder and prostate cancer, and review the role of extended lymphadenectomy (LND) in each procedure. Other articles elsewhere in this issue are dedicated to the role of LND for both prostate and bladder cancer. Therefore, much of the focus of this review is on minimally invasive approaches and the technical aspects of the procedures, the feasibility of the robotic technique, and early oncologic outcomes.

ROLE OF LYMPHADENECTOMY IN PROSTATE CANCER

The role of LND in prostate cancer remains a contro- versial one, both in terms of the indications as well as the extent. Most investigators agree that LND offers significant pathologic and prognostic infor- mation, which affects the use of adjuvant therapy.[1] Prostate-specific antigen (PSA) screening has re- sulted in a downward stage migration in prostate cancer within the past several years. By detecting disease at an earlier stage, the likelihood of lymph node metastases has decreased and most contemporary series place the lymph node detec- tion rate at 5%[2,3] for the conventional standard lymph node dissection (obturator/external iliac). Many surgeons currently omit LND in patients with low-grade (Gleason score $\leq$6), low-stage (cT2a or less) prostate cancer, or when the likeli- hood of lymph node metastases is less than 2% based on the Partin tables or Kattan nomograms.[4,5]

OVERALL DECLINE IN LYMPHADENECTOMY FOR PROSTATE CANCER

This stage migration likely explains the overall decline in the performance of LND in the United States over the past few decades. For example, the Prostate Strategic Urologic Research Endeavor database previously demonstrated a trend toward

omitting pelvic LND (PLND) for low-risk and intermediate-risk prostate cancer from 94% in 1992 to 80% in 2004,[6,7] with a mean lymph node yield of 5.7 (median 5). The use of LND in the minimally invasive prostate literature has declined even more rapidly, as is evidenced by two recent population-based studies. Prasad and colleagues[8] reviewed the Surveillance, Epidemiology, and End Results (SEER) from 2003 to 2005 to assess factors correlating with the performance of LND. The inves- tigators looked at both laparoscopic radical prosta- tectomy (LRP) and robotic-assisted laparoscopic prostatectomy (RALP), although the time frame correlated with the early adoption of RALP. A multivariate analysis assessing surgical approach, volume, patient demographics, comorbidity, and geographic region was conducted. Overall, 68% of men underwent PLND, with the rates varying signif- icantly by surgical approach (17% vs 83% for mini- mally invasive vs open prostatectomy, respectively, P<.001). High-volume surgeons were more likely to perform PLND in both groups. Of note, minimally invasive surgeons performed PLND in only 28% of cases. The investigators offered several reasons for this discrepancy in performing PLND during the early RALP era, including the new approach and the desire to shorten the operating times, reduce complications, and lessen costs. Another overriding factor suggested was that most patients undergoing surgery in the present era have low-risk cancer pre- dicted to have a low rate of nodal metastases, persuading many surgeons to adopt the attitude that PLND is simply unnecessary.

Feifer and colleagues[9] recently reviewed the SEER database for PLND trends for both open and minimally invasive prostatectomy from 2003 to 2007. The investigators found that the use of PLND declined over time both overall and within subgroups (including those with high-risk features). PLND was 5 times more likely in men undergoing radical retropubic prostatectomy (RRP) compared with the minimally invasive cohort (both laparo- scopic and robotic approaches). While elevated PSA and Gleason sum were significant predictors of LND in both groups, the magnitude was signifi- cantly greater for RRP. Only 60% of patients in the minimally invasive cohort with PSA greater than 10 underwent LND, compared with 86% of those in the open group. The investigators were not able to assess the number of lymph nodes removed or the anatomic extent of LND.

EXTENDED LYMPHADENECTOMY FOR HIGH- RISK DISEASE

Despite this trend against LND for men with lower risk of disease, there has been a movement in performing more extended LNDs for those patients deemed worthy based on risk stratification,[2,10] with significantly higher lymph node/positive lymph node yields. The rationale is that higher-risk patients are more likely to harbor disease that has spread to regional lymph nodes. Further, many of these nomograms and tables are based on a PLND, consisting of the obturator fossa and external iliac regions. Briganti and colleagues[11] have published nomograms predicting the probability of lymph node metastasis among patients undergoing extended PLND (ePLND), which await external validation.

Schumacher and colleagues[12] analyzed their technique regarding long-term outcomes of 122 patients undergoing ePLND ($\geq$10 nodes removed) followed by RRP for high-risk disease (median PSA 16 ng/mL). The lymphatic tissue is taken from 3 distinct locations: the external iliac vein, obturator fossa, and internal iliac artery. Seventy-six percent had Stage pT3 disease or greater and 50% had seminal vesicle invasion. Positive lymph nodes were located exclusively along the external iliac vein in 9% of patients, in the obturator fossa in 16.4%, and along the internal iliac artery (presacral lymph nodes) in 21.3%. In approximately half of the patients, positive lymph nodes were found along the internal iliac vessels, along with positive lymph nodes in the area of the obturator fossa and/or the external iliac vein. Overall, positive internal iliac lymph nodes alone or combined with positive lymph nodes in other locations were found in 70.5% of patients. The median cancer-specific survival rate at 5 and 10 years was 84.5% and 60.1%, respectively. For patients with 2 or less or 3 or more positive lymph nodes removed, the median cancer-specific survival rate at 10 years was 78.6% and 33.4%, respectively ($P<.001$).

LYMPHADENECTOMY IN LAPAROSCOPIC PROSTATECTOMY

Despite a lower incidence of PLND in the minimally invasive literature, there are several studies assessing the outcomes for both standard PLND (sPLND) and ePLND. LRP was introduced in the late 1990s, with several larger series and reviews showing comparable oncologic outcomes to the RRP.[13–15] Most LRP series report sPLNDs performed in similar fashion to the RRP, with comparable results and complications.

Eden and colleagues[16] evaluated 374 patients who underwent LRP with an LND. Two hundred and fifty-three men had an sPLND and 121 had an ePLND for intermediate-risk or high-risk prostate cancer. An extraperitoneal approach was used in all patients having sPLND and a transperitoneal approach in patients having ePLND. The investigators found that the ePLND group had a greater percentage of patients with cT3 disease (9.9% vs 4.2%, $P = .046$), and was associated with a longer operating time of 206.5 versus 180.0 minutes ($P<.001$) and a higher node count of 17.5 versus 6.1 ($P = .002$). Blood loss, hospital stay, transfusion, and complication rates were similar in the two groups.

Wyler and colleagues[17] reported on their experience with ePLND in 123 patients undergoing LRP for high-risk prostate cancer. The boundaries of the pelvic lymph node dissection were the bifurcation of the common iliac artery superiorly, the node of Cloquet inferiorly, the external iliac vein laterally, and the bladder wall medially. The mean number of lymph nodes removed was 21 (range 9–55) in a mean PLND time of 47 minutes. A total of 21 patients (17%) had lymph node metastases. The overall complication rate was 4%. Associated complications occurred in 1 patient (0.8%) with an iliac hematoma and postoperative paresis of the leg that resolved spontaneously, and 1 patient (0.8%) with a lymphocele (after extraperitoneal laparoscopic operation with no primary drainage) that was drained. Two patients (1.6%) had lymphedema of the right leg that resolved spontaneously within 2 and 4 months. Similarly, Lattouf and colleagues[18] showed that ePLND was feasible in 35 patients undergoing LRP for high-risk prostate cancer (median PSA 16.5). The template included the genitofemoral nerve up to the bifurcation of the common iliac artery and down to the epigastric artery. The investigators retrieved a median of 13 lymph nodes. In 5 of the 11 patients with positive lymph nodes, the nodes were detected exclusively outside the obturator fossa. The complications were 2 temporary and reversible neurapraxias (ischiatic nerve and obturator nerve), 1 deep vein thrombosis, and 2 lymphoceles. One lymphocele healed conservatively; the second was marsupialized laparoscopically.

In the United States there has been a significant increase in the number of RALPs performed in the past decade. As surgeons have become more familiar with RALP, a larger volume of patients with greater PSA values, Gleason scores, and clinical stages are being offered robotic surgery. In these patients with more aggressive disease characteristics, concomitant PLND is traditionally performed for the aforementioned reasons.

LYMPHADENECTOMY IN ROBOTIC PROSTATECTOMY

The feasibility of LND within RALP is well established, with several large series demonstrating comparable yield and perioperative outcomes to the RRP. Zorn and colleagues[19] compared 296 RALP patients undergoing standard PLND (external iliac and obturator fossa) with 859 patients undergoing RALP alone. The investigators removed a mean number of 12.5 lymph nodes. The mean operative time (224 vs 216 minutes; $P = .09$), estimated blood loss (206 vs 229 mL; $P = .14$), and hospital stay (1.32 vs 1.24 days; $P = .46$) were comparable between the two groups. The rate of intraoperative complications (1% vs 1.5%; $P = .2$), overall postoperative complications (9% vs 7%; $P = .8$), and lymphocele formation (2% vs 0%; $P = .9$) were not significantly different. The rates compared well with the historical RRP experience. These investigators and many others hypothesize that the low rate of lymphoceles in the RALP literature may be due to increasing technical experience as well as the transperitoneal nature of RALP, which allows for easier egress of the lymphatic fluid, thus preventing collection formation. It has to be noted, however, that because routine imaging is not performed after prostatectomy, the incidence of subclinical lymphoceles might be higher than expected. Even in transperitoneal procedures, there is a "resealing" of the peritoneum expected after 48 to 72 hours in an uncomplicated procedure, which can still potentially mediate lymphocele formation by preventing transperitoneal absorption of lymphatic fluid.

In a feasibility study using graded complications, Yee and colleagues[20] assessed the complications and nodal yield of ePLND for 32 patients undergoing RALP for localized disease (all risk categories). The investigators included the obturator, hypogastric, external iliac, and common iliac lymph nodes up to the bifurcation of the aorta in their dissection. The median number of lymph nodes retrieved was 18, with 4 patients having lymph node metastases. Median operative time for the ePLND was 72 minutes (interquartile range 66–86). Graded complications included 13 grade 1 events and 1 grade 2 event, with 1 grade 1 event being considered related to ePLND. No clinically presenting lymphoceles or thrombotic events were encountered.

Feicke and colleagues[21] also reported the feasibility of ePLND in 99 patients undergoing RALP for PSA of 10 or more or Gleason score greater than 7. The surgeons operated for an average of 51 minutes with a median number of 19 lymph nodes removed. Lymphedema was observed in 2 patients: in one patient, a bilateral lymphedema of the lower leg resolved after physical therapy with supportive lymphatic drainage; the other patient showed persistent unilateral lymphedema at a 3-month follow-up visit. In 2 patients, a symptomatic lymphocele was treated conservatively, and 2 patients required percutaneous drainage (Table 1).

The extent of the lymph node dissection for prostate cancer with robotic prostatectomy can easily emulate the open operation (discussed in an article by La Rochelle and Amling elsewhere in this issue). The robotic camera allows for excellent visualization and identification of individual lymphatic channels for ligation or bipolar cauterization (Fig. 1). The cephalad extent of the dissection is often the iliac bifurcation. The distal extent is the node of Cloquet. The posterior extent is below the obturator vein. Laterally the dissection extends to the external iliac artery. In this fashion the obturator nodes, internal and external iliac nodes, and the common iliac nodes up to the iliac bifurcation can be removed (Fig. 2).

MINIMALLY INVASIVE LYMPHADENECTOMY IN RADICAL CYSTECTOMY

The ubiquity and presumed short-term benefits of robotic prostatectomy have translated to the increase use of robotic-assisted radical cystectomy (RARC) for the surgical treatment of bladder cancer in the United States. The operation has now been shown to be technically feasible, and to offer potential advantages limited not only to less pain and blood loss but also to the actual convalescence of the patient.

Open radical cystectomy can be a morbid catabolic operation with long hospital stays, and medical and surgical complications are in excess of 25%. The prolonged recovery poses a problem for patients in whom adjuvant chemotherapy will prove to be indicated. Performance of the operation through minimally invasive techniques can potentially lead to faster recovery through less bowel manipulation, decreased fluid shifts, and third spacing by limiting the patients' insensible losses, which lead to decreased gastrointestinal, nutritional, and cardiovascular morbidity. In a recent study comparing the robotic versus open approach in 187 patients, robotic cystectomy was associated with a statistically significant decrease in overall (41 vs 51%; $P = .04$) and major (10 vs 30%; $P<.007$) complications at 30 days.[22] The difference in major complications persisted at 90 days, with high American Society of Anesthesiologists (ASA) scores (3–4) and longer surgical times being independent predictors of major complications.

EARLY EXPERIENCE WITH MINIMALLY INVASIVE RADICAL CYSTECTOMY

Laparoscopic radical cystectomy (LRC) for bladder cancer was performed in 1993 with the main intent

Table 1
Extended pelvic lymph node dissection in the minimally invasive prostatectomy literature

Authors,[Ref.] Year	Approach	No. of Patients	Median No. of LNs Removed (Range)	Proximal Extent of Dissection	Minutes for ePLND (Range)	Lymphadenectomy-Specific Complications
Feicke et al,[21] 2009	RALP	99	19 (8–53)	Iliac bifurcation	51 (29–81)	Lymphocele (4) Lymphedema (2)
Yee et al,[20] 2010	RALP	32	18 (IQR 12–28)	Aortic bifurcation	72 (IQR 66–86)	Grade 1 (1)
Eden et al,[16] 2010	LRP	121	17.5 (2–23)	Iliac bifurcation	Additional 26 min (compared with sPLND)	Obturator nerve injury (2)
Wyler et al,[17] 2006	LRP	123	21 (9–55)	Iliac bifurcation	47 min	Iliac hematoma (1) Lymphocele requiring intervention (1) Temporary lymphedema (2)

Abbreviations: ePLND, extended pelvic lymphadenectomy; IQR, interquartile range; LN, lymph node; LRP, laparoscopic radical prostatectomy; RALP, robotic-assisted laparoscopic prostatectomy; sPLND, standard pelvic lymphadenectomy.

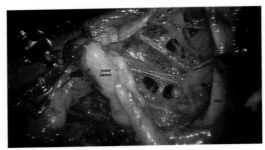

Fig. 1. Obturator and internal iliac nodal packet. Note individual lymphatic channels visualized for ligation. REIV, right external iliac vein.

of lowering overall morbidity.[23] Most of the early literature on LRC focuses on technique and short-term perioperative outcomes, such as decreased morbidity and blood loss. Hrouda and colleagues[24] reviewed the early literature on oncologic outcomes of LRC and RARC. More than 100 patients were reviewed from 9 studies, with no positive margins reported. Regarding LND, all series performed limited lymph node dissection, and only one article reported on the actual lymph node yield, which was only between 2 and 4 nodes.[25]

The first report of ePLND in LRC was in 2004 by Finelli and colleagues[26] The investigators looked at 11 patients with invasive bladder cancer, and the LND included bilaterally skeletonizing the genitofemoral nerve, external iliac artery, external iliac vein, obturator nerve, hypogastric artery, common iliac artery, and pubic bone. The investigators found that ePLND added 1.5 hours of operative time. The median number of nodes removed was 21 in the extended LND group compared with 3 for their initial experience with limited dissection. Three patients were found to have positive nodal disease. At a mean follow-up of 11 months (range: 2–43), there were no port-site recurrences.

Haber and Gill[27] reported their 5-year follow-up with LRC, including their results with LND. A limited LND was used in the initial 11 patients (29%), with a median yield of 6 (range: 2–15) nodes, whereas an ePLND (up to the aortic bifurcation) was used in the next 26 patients (70%), which increased their yield to 21 (range: 11–24) nodes. Overall, the median number of lymph nodes excised was 14 (range: 2–24). Seven patients (17%) had positive nodes.

Several studies have compared the results of lymph node yield in open radical cystectomy versus LRC. In a prospective, nonrandomized Italian study of LRC, Porpiglia and colleagues[28] demonstrated equal lymph node yield between open and laparoscopic approaches (18.4 vs 19.6), with no significant differences in operative time (260 vs 284 min) or surgical morbidity. Hemal and Kolla[29] reported on a single-surgeon series with a total of 55 open and laparoscopic cystectomies. All patients underwent lymph node dissection using their "modified" extended template (proximal extent of dissection was 2.5 cm proximal to the bifurcation of the common iliac artery). Total operative time was significantly higher in the LRC group; however, total blood loss, transfusion, and analgesic requirement were significantly less in the LRC cohort. The positive surgical margin rates were 1% in each cohort, with similar complication rates. The total lymph node yield was 14 in the open group versus 12 in the LRC group. Three-year survival outcomes were similar.

ROBOTIC APPROACHES

Due to the steep and extensive learning of curve of LRC, robotic assistance has fueled an increased interest in minimally invasive approaches. In 2003, the first series of robotic cystectomies was published by Menon and colleagues.[30] In this

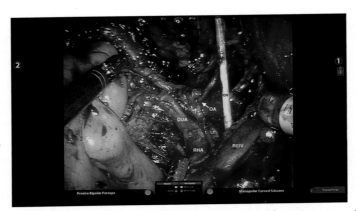

Fig. 2. Completed obturator node and internal iliac node dissection. OA, obturator artery; ON, obturator nerve; OUA, obliterated umbilical artery; REIV, right external iliac vein; RHA, right hypogastric artery.

feasibility study of 17 patients, "standard lympha-denectomy" was successfully performed in all patients with an average lymph node yield of between 4 and 27 nodes. One patient was N1 and all margins were negative.

The first series comparing open cystectomy versus RARC in a single-surgeon experience was published from Cornell University in 2007.[31] Fifty-four consecutive single-surgeon cystectomies were performed, 21 open versus 33 robotic. The open cohort had more patients with extravesical disease (57% vs 28%) and nodal metastasis (34% vs 19%). There were 3 patients in the open group and 2 in the robotic with positive margins. Lymphadenectomy was performed by including all tissue between the external iliac vessels anteriorly and the pelvic side wall, including the node of Cloquet distally, the upper common iliac artery proximally, the obturator nerve posteriorly, and the genitofemoral nerve laterally. The median number of lymph nodes removed was similar in the open and robotic cohorts (20 vs 17).

Pruthi and Wallen[32] reported their initial experience with 20 patients receiving RARC plus ileal conduit versus 24 open cystectomies. The investigators had higher lymph node yields with the robotic approach than with the open approach (mean number of 19 vs 16). There were no cases of positive margins in either group. Guru and colleagues[33] reported their experience of 67 cases of RARC with PLND and extracorporeal urinary diversion, observing that robotic PLND yielded a mean number of 18 lymph nodes with a margin-positive rate of 9%.

Pruthi and colleagues[34] updated the data from their first 100 patients. The investigators initially performed LND using standard dissection for patients with noninvasive disease or extended LND (up to and including common iliac dissection) for patients with muscle invasive disease and lymphovascular invasion. Recently all patients have undergone extended dissection. The investigators reported a mean lymph node yield of 19 (range: 8–40), with no difference between yields in the first 50 cases and the last 50 (18.9 vs 19.3, $P = .733$). There were no positive margins.

Nix and colleagues[35] conducted a prospective, randomized, nonblinded study comparing 21 RARC with 20 open cystectomy patients in single center. There were no statistical differences between the two cohorts in terms of age, sex, body mass index, ASA classification, anticoagulation regimen of aspirin, clinical stage, or diversion type. There was no significant difference in regard of overall complication rate or hospital stay. On surgical pathology, in the robotic group 14 patients had pT2 disease or higher; 3 patients had pT3/T4 disease; and 4 patients had node-positive

disease. In the open group, 8 patients had pT2 disease or higher; 5 patients had pT3/T4 disease; and 7 patients had node-positive disease. The mean number of lymph nodes removed was 19 in the robotic group versus 18 in the open group.

The International Robotic Cystectomy Consortium (IRCC) recently addressed the issue of LND.[36] The IRCC is a pooled cohort of multiple surgeons (>20) from several institutions. In a retrospective review of 527 patients from 15 centers, 437 (82.9%) underwent LND. A mean of 17.8 (range: 0–68) lymph nodes were obtained. High-volume surgeons (>20 cases) were almost 3 times more likely to perform LND than lower-volume surgeons, all other variables being constant (odds ratio = 2.37; 95% confidence interval = 1.39–4.05; $P = .002$]. There was no standardization of LNDs, nor were the specimens reviewed by a central pathology team.

EXTENDED NODAL DISSECTION IN RARC

Extending both the boundaries and degree of dissection in bladder carcinoma has been linked to improved nodal yield, staging, and cancer-specific survival.[37–39] Pruthi and Wallen[40] described their experience with limited and extended lymph node dissection in RARC. In total, 28 patients underwent a standard dissection with a mean of 19 lymph nodes removed (range: 8–33). Extended lymph node dissection was performed in 22 patients with a mean of 30 lymph nodes removed (range: 12–39). No surgical complications occurred related to the LND. There were no positive margins and the rate of positive lymph nodes was 20%. **Table 2** summarizes some of the lymph node dissection details of some of the larger studies with RARC.

Lavery and colleagues[41] assessed the nodal yield in a small series of patients using extended nodal dissection as described by Skinner[42] on 15 patients. Nodal packets were dissected en bloc on each side and both packets extracted together in one laparoscopic pouch. All nodal tissue was submitted to pathology and evaluated as one specimen. Nodes were counted grossly in pathology by finger separation from fat before fixation. No clearing techniques or solvents were used to identify lymph nodes. The mean nodal yield was 41.8 (range: 18–67) and the mean LND time was 107 minutes (range: 66–160). There were no lymph node–related complications at 30 days.

ISSUES OF LEARNING CURVE

Within RARC data, a few studies have examined the influence of experience and lymph node yield

Table 2
Summary of the lymph node dissection details of some of the larger studies with RARC

Authors,[Ref.] Year	No. of Patients	Median No. of LNs Removed (Range)	Proximal Extent of Dissection	Other Data
Pruthi et al,[34] 2010	100	19 (8–40)	Standard, then extended (aortic bifurcation)	No positive margin, no difference in LN yield between first 50 and last 50 cases (18.9 vs 19.3, $P = .733$)
Guru et al,[33] 2008	67	18 (6–43)	Aortic bifurcation	Submitted in packets, 9 patients excluded with advanced disease; 10% positive margin; 29% positive lymph nodes
Lavery et al,[41] 2011	15	41.8 (18–67)	2 cm above aortic bifurcation	No LND related complications, OR for LND was 107 min, included presacral nodes
Hellenthal et al,[36] 2011	437	17.8 (0–68)	Mix of approaches	Consortium of multiple institutions. Surgeon volume and experience correlated with LN yield

Abbreviations: LND, lymphadenectomy; OR, odds ratio; RARC, robotic-assisted radical cystectomy.

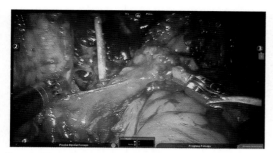

Fig. 3. The obturator nodal packet is mobilized to start the dissection.

in RARC. Pruthi and colleagues[43] examined their initial 50 RARC patients by quintiles for clinically localized (Stage cT2 or less) bladder cancer and evaluated the estimated blood loss, operative time, pathologic outcomes, and complication rate. The operative time declined between each quintile for the first 30 patients and then stabilized. No differences were noted in the complication rate, lymph node yield, or positive margin rate. The investigators reported an average of 19 lymph nodes in all quintiles with "extended dissection" (range: 17–21).

Guru and colleagues[44] divided their first 100 consecutive RARC patients into quartiles, and reported a decrease in operative time and an increase in lymph node yield between the first and fourth quartiles. The investigators performed an extended lymph node dissection to the aortic bifurcation and found that the mean lymph node yield went from 14 in the first cohort to 23 in the fourth quartile. The amount of time spent on the LND increased as well across the cohorts from a mean of 44 to 77 minutes in the first and fourth quartiles, respectively. The lymph node yield seemed to peak by the 30th case.

The impact of prior experience with RALP and outcomes of RARC was recently reported by the IRCC.[45] In a study of 496 patients the surgeons were divided into 4 groups according to their previous robotic-assisted radical prostatectomy (RARP) experience (≤50, 51–100, 101–150, and >150 cases). The mean lymph node yield was 18 nodes (range: 0–68). When divided by RARP volume, the mean lymph node yield was 13.7, 19.8, 19.6, and 11.8 for a surgeon volume of 50 or less, 51 to 100, 101 to 150, and more than 150 cases ($P<.001$). The mean lymph node yield increased by 31% between those surgeons who had performed 50 or less RARPs and those who had done between 51 and 100 RARPs. The margin status was available for 482 patients, and the positive margin rate for the entire cohort was 7% (34 of the 482 patients). A trend was seen toward increased positive margins with increasing surgeon volumes, but this did not reach statistical significance ($P = .089$).

There is no question that the oncologic efficacy of robotic cystectomy is yet to be established in comparison with open cystectomy. Especially early in the surgeon's experience, patients should be carefully selected for the robotic technique. Patients with bulky tumors adherent to the pelvic side wall and the iliac vessels or with grossly positive nodes are probably better suited to the open approach. Tactile sensation is quite helpful in dissecting the difficult cleavage planes around the major vessels, the pelvic side wall, and the prerectal space. Large pelvic masses are difficult to maneuver robotically in the tight confines of the bony pelvis.

TECHNIQUE OF ROBOTIC LYMPH NODE DISSECTION

Concerns have been raised regarding the Da Vinci surgical system's ability in accessing the cephalad borders of the dissection as well as nodes inferior and below the level of the obturator nerve. However, experience with robotic cystectomy has revealed that there are no limitations

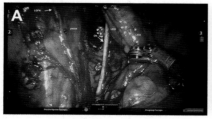
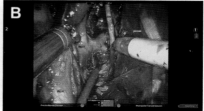

Fig. 4. (A) The triangle of Marcille. The external iliac vessels are medially retracted. All lymph-bearing tissues at the origin of the obturator nerve are accessed easily. (B) The origin of the obturator nerve is visualized. Often large tributaries of the vein are seen, warranting careful dissection. LEIA, left external iliac artery; LEIV, left external iliac vein; LGFN, left genitofemoral nerve; ON, obturator nerve; REIA, right external iliac artery; REIV, right external iliac vein.

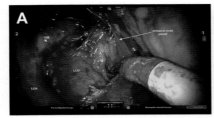
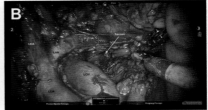

Fig. 5. (*A*) Presacral nodal packet is easily accessed. (*B*) Surface of the sacrum exposed after dissection. LCIA, left common iliac artery; LCIV, left common iliac vein; LEIA, left external iliac artery; LHA, left hypogastric artery.

pertaining to these locations. Cephalad access to the aortic bifurcation can be limited with the first-generation, standard non-S robot. This cephalad limitation can be easily overcome with a slightly higher positioning of the trocars than a robotic prostatectomy. However, the S series and especially the newer SI series of the Da Vinci surgical system provide far more flexibility and hence improved cephalad range of motion of the robotic arms. Therefore, the SI system provides for excellent meticulous dissection of the lymph-bearing tissue, to the accepted cephalad boundaries of extended node dissection and the aortic bifurcation. The downward 30° lens could further aid in the lymph node dissection, allowing excellent visualization of the proximal boundary. In addition, the longer arms that equip the newer system allow for easy access to the deep pelvis, thereby not compromising the deep pelvic dissection if the trocars are placed higher for a radical cystectomy. A complete LND can be achieved, fully abiding by the boundaries and extents discussed in this article. Meticulous bipolar electrocautery of the lymphatic vessels in addition to careful application of Hem-o-lok clips allows for excellent lymphostasis. Some of the paravesical nodes are removed with the cystectomy specimen en bloc. The remaining lateral paravesical nodes that merge with the medial batch of the obturator nodes are separately dissected during the LND portion of the operation, removing all lymph-bearing tissue in the lateral pararectal sulcus adjacent to the pelvic side wall. The lateral border of the nodal dissection is the ipsilateral genitofemoral nerve. Initially, the obturator nodal packet is mobilized (**Fig. 3**). The obturator nodal packet along with the internal iliac packet is meticulously dissected. Recently, attempts have been made to remove all nodes in the triangle of Marcille while the external iliac vessels are skeletonized, removing all lymph-bearing tissue around them. The external iliac vessels are mobilized and reflected medially, exposing the origin of the obturator nerve, the medial aspect of the psoas muscle allowing for

meticulous removal of internal iliac nodal chain posterior to the vessels, which would be difficult to dissect from the front, as in open LND, without medial mobilization of the iliac vessels (**Fig. 4**). Internal iliac, common iliac, and presacral nodes[46,47] are easily accessed with the standard and SI robot (**Fig. 5**). A 30° downward lens is crucial for use with a standard system. The fourth arm aids in retraction of the base of the sigmoid mesentery to the contralateral side, exposing the field of dissection (**Fig. 6**). The nodes are separated in each side and sent to pathology in separate endobags. Port-site metastasis is always a concern with urothelial carcinoma and, therefore, the authors recommend use of meticulous technique and removal through endobags.[35]

One issue is whether the lymph node dissection should be performed before or after the cystectomy. In the authors' experience, the node dissection is easier to perform after the cystectomy portion, as the true pelvis is well exposed without

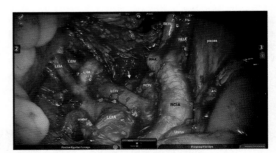

Fig. 6. Completed extended lymph node dissection for bladder cancer. Note the extent of the dissection to the aortic bifurcation. The sigmoid colon is retracted to the left, exposing the completed dissection. All vessels are skeletonized. Arrow points to the sacral promontory. Note the left ureter delivered to the right side. LCIA, left common iliac artery; LCIV, left common iliac vein; LEIA, left external iliac artery; LHA, left hypogastric artery; RCIA, right common iliac artery; RCIV, right common iliac vein; REIA, right external iliac artery; REIV, right external iliac vein; RHA, right hypogastric artery.

the bladder. In this era of neoadjuvant chemotherapy for bladder cancer, a patient who comes to cystectomy usually needs the cystectomy. The historical situation whereby large bulky nodes are detected intraoperatively is rarely encountered in this era of cross-sectional imaging.

As with any surgical procedure, the experience of the operating surgeon is of paramount importance. There is great variability in the extent of lymph node dissection and the definition of "standard" or "extended" lymph node dissections in various open and robotic series. Using the number of lymph nodes as a surrogate for adequacy of the lymph node dissection is fraught with difficulty. Removal of all lymph-bearing tissue in the boundaries outlined previously is the best means to ensure oncologic efficacy. Perhaps one possibility would be to perform the lymph node dissection robotically and then to assess the adequacy in an open fashion when an incision is made to perform the urinary diversion.[46]

SUMMARY

In this era of increasing use of the robotic platform for the surgical management of bladder and certainly prostate cancer, there is a clear role for robotic extended and standard lymph node dissection for both malignancies. The procedures can emulate their open counterparts in terms of both feasibility and efficacy. There is a significant learning curve for the performance of a thorough extended node dissection. Meticulous dissection around the iliac vessels allows for a complete dissection while minimizing complications. However, the indications to perform the LND are the same for the open and robotic operation. It is paramount that the actual attempt and minimally invasive surgery should not jeopardize the oncologic principles of bladder cancer and prostate cancer surgery.

REFERENCES

1. Cheng L, Zincke H, Blute ML, et al. Risk of prostate carcinoma death in patients with lymph node metastasis. Cancer 2001;91:66–73.
2. Allaf ME, Palapattu GS, Trock BJ, et al. Anatomical extent of lymph node dissection: impact on men with clinically localized prostate cancer. J Urol 2004;172:1840–4.
3. Masterson TA, Bianco FJ Jr, Vickers AJ, et al. The association between total and positive lymph node counts, and disease progression in clinically localized prostate cancer. J Urol 2006;175:1320–4.
4. Partin AW, Kattan MW, Subong EN, et al. Combination of prostate-specific antigen, clinical stage, and Gleason score to predict pathological stage of localized prostate cancer. A multi-institutional update. JAMA 1997;277(18):1445–51.
5. Kattan MW, Eastham JA, Stapleton AM, et al. A preoperative nomogram for disease recurrence following radical prostatectomy for prostate cancer. J Natl Cancer Inst 1998;90(10):766–71.
6. Wagner M, Sokoloff M, Daneshmand S. The role of pelvic lymphadenectomy for prostate cancer–therapeutic? J Urol 2008;179(2):408–13.
7. Kawakami J, Meng MV, Sadetsky N, et al, CaPSURE Investigators. Changing patterns of pelvic lymphadenectomy for prostate cancer: results from CaPSURE. J Urol 2006;176(4 Pt 1):1382–6.
8. Prasad SM, Keating NL, Wang Q, et al. Variations in surgeon volume and use of pelvic lymph node dissection with open and minimally invasive radical prostatectomy. Urology 2008;72(3):647–52.
9. Feifer AH, Elkin EB, Lowrance WT, et al. Temporal trends and predictors of pelvic lymph node dissection in open or minimally invasive radical prostatectomy. Cancer 2011. [Epub ahead of print].
10. Heidenreich A, Varga Z, Von Knobloch R. Extended pelvic lymphadenectomy in patients undergoing radical prostatectomy: high incidence of lymph node metastasis. J Urol 2002;167:1681–6.
11. Briganti A, Chun FK, Salonia A, et al. Validation of a nomogram predicting the probability of lymph node invasion among patients undergoing radical prostatectomy and an extended pelvic lymphadenectomy. Eur Urol 2006;49:1019–26.
12. Schumacher MC, Burkhard FC, Thalmann GN, et al. Good outcome for patients with few lymph node metastases after radical retropubic prostatectomy. Eur Urol 2008;54(2):344–52.
13. Rassweiler J, Seemann O, Schulze M, et al. Laparoscopic versus open radical prostatectomy: a comparative study at a single institution. J Urol 2003;169(5):1689–93.
14. Tooher R, Swindle P, Woo H, et al. Laparoscopic radical prostatectomy for localized prostate cancer: a systematic review of comparative studies. J Urol 2006;175(6):2011–7.
15. Ficarra V, Novara G, Artibani W, et al. Retropubic, laparoscopic, and robot-assisted radical prostatectomy: a systematic review and cumulative analysis of comparative studies. Eur Urol 2009;55(5):1037–63.
16. Eden CG, Arora A, Rouse P. Extended vs standard pelvic lymphadenectomy during laparoscopic radical prostatectomy for intermediate- and high-risk prostate cancer. BJU Int 2010;106(4):537–42.
17. Wyler SF, Sulser T, Seifert HH, et al. Laparoscopic extended pelvic lymph node dissection for high-risk prostate cancer. Urology 2006;68(4):883–7.
18. Lattouf JB, Beri A, Jeschke S, et al. Laparoscopic extended pelvic lymph node dissection for prostate cancer: description of the surgical technique and initial results. Eur Urol 2007;52(5):1347–55.

19. Zorn KC, Katz MH, Bernstein A, et al. Pelvic lympha-denectomy during robot-assisted radical pro-statectomy: assessing nodal yield, perioperative outcomes, and complications. Urology 2009;74(2): 296–302.

20. Yee DS, Katz DJ, Godoy G, et al. Extended pelvic lymph node dissection in robotic-assisted radical prostatectomy: surgical technique and initial experience. Urology 2010;75(5):1199–204.

21. Feicke A, Baumgartner M, Talimi S, et al. Robotic-assisted laparoscopic extended pelvic lymph node dissection for prostate cancer: surgical technique and experience with the first 99 cases. Eur Urol 2009;55(4):876–83.

22. Ng CK, Kauffman EC, Lee MM, et al. A comparison of postoperative complications in open versus robotic cystectomy. Eur Urol 2010;57(2):274–81.

23. Sánchez de Badajoz E, Gallego Perales JL, Reche Rosado A, et al. Radical cystectomy and laparo-scopic ileal conduit. Arch Esp Urol 1993;46:621–4.

24. Hrouda D, Adeyoju AA, Gill IS. Laparoscopic radical cystectomy and urinary diversion: fad or future? BJU Int 2004;94:501–5.

25. Gupta NP, Gill IS, Fergany A, et al. Laparoscopic radical cystectomy with intracorporeal ileal conduit diversion: 5 cases with a 2-year follow-up. BJU Int 2002;90:391–6.

26. Finelli A, Gill IS, Desai MM, et al. Laparoscopic extended pelvic lymphadenectomy for bladder cancer: technique and initial outcomes. J Urol 2004;172:1809–12.

27. Haber GP, Gill IS. Laparoscopic radical cystectomy for cancer: oncological outcomes at up to 5 years. BJU Int 2007;100:137–42.

28. Porpiglia F, Renard J, Billia M, et al. Open versus laparoscopy-assisted radical cystectomy: results of a prospective study. J Endourol 2007;21:325–9.

29. Hemal AK, Kolla SB. Comparison of laparoscopic and open radical cystoprostatectomy for localized bladder cancer with 3-year oncological followup: a single surgeon experience. J Urol 2007;178:2340–3.

30. Menon M, Hemal AK, Tewari A, et al. Nerve-sparing robot-assisted radical cystoprostatectomy and urinary diversion. BJU Int 2003;92:232–6.

31. Wang GJ, Barocas DA, Raman JD, et al. Robotic vs. open radical cystectomy: prospective comparison of perioperative outcomes and pathological measures of early oncological efficacy. BJU Int 2008;101:89–93.

32. Pruthi RS, Wallen EM. Robotic assisted laparoscopic radical cystoprostatectomy: operative and pathological outcomes. J Urol 2007;178(3):814–8.

33. Guru KA, Sternberg K, Wilding GE, et al. The lymph node yield during robot-assisted radical cystectomy. BJU Int 2008;102:231–4.

34. Pruthi RS, Nielsen ME, Nix J, et al. Robotic radical cystectomy for bladder cancer: surgical and pathological outcomes in 100 consecutive cases. J Urol 2010;183(2):510–4.

35. Nix J, Smith A, Kurpad R, et al. Prospective random-ized controlled trial of robotic versus open radical cystectomy for bladder cancer: perioperative and pathologic results. Eur Urol 2010;57(2):196–201.

36. Hellenthal NJ, Hussain A, Andrews PE, et al. Lym-phadenectomy at the time of robot-assisted radical cystectomy: results from the International Robotic Cystectomy Consortium. BJU Int 2011;107(4): 642–6.

37. Leissner J, Ghoneim MA, Abol-Enein H, et al. Extended radical lymphadenectomy in patients with urothelial bladder cancer: results of a prospec-tive multicenter study. J Urol 2004;171:139–44.

38. Stein JP, Cai J, Groshen S, et al. Risk factors for patients with pelvic lymph node metastases following radical cystectomy with en bloc pelvic lym-phadenectomy: concept of lymph node density. J Urol 2003;170:35–41.

39. Herr HW, Bochner BH, Dalbagni G, et al. Impact of the number of lymph nodes retrieved on outcome in patients with muscle invasive bladder cancer. J Urol 2002;167:1295–8.

40. Pruthi RS, Wallen EM. Robotic-assisted laparo-scopic pelvic lymphadenectomy for bladder cancer: a surgical atlas. J Laparoendosc Adv Surg Tech A 2009;19(1):71–4.

41. Lavery HJ, Martinez-Suarez HJ, Abaza R. Robotic extended pelvic lymphadenectomy for bladder cancer with increased nodal yield. BJU Int 2011; 107(11):1802–5.

42. Skinner DG. Management of invasive bladder cancer: a meticulous pelvic node dissection can make a difference. J Urol 1982;128:34–6.

43. Pruthi RS, Smith A, Wallen EM. Evaluating the learning curve for robot-assisted laparoscopic radical cystectomy. J Endourol 2008;22:2469–74.

44. Guru KA, Perlmutter AE, Butt ZM, et al. The learning curve for robot-assisted radical cystectomy. JSLS 2009;13:509–14.

45. Hayn MH, Hellenthal NJ, Hussain A, et al. Does previous robot-assisted radical prostatectomy expe-rience affect outcomes at robot-assisted radical cystectomy? Results from the International Robotic Cystectomy Consortium. Urology 2010;76(5): 1111–6.

46. Wiesner C, Salzer A, Thomas C, et al. Cancer-specific survival after radical cystectomy and standardized extended lymphadenectomy for node-positive bladder cancer: prediction by lymph node positivity and density. BJU Int 2009;104(3):331–5.

47. Davis JW, Gaston K, Anderson R, et al. Robot assis-ted extended pelvic lymphadenectomy at radical cystectomy: lymph node yield compared with second look open dissection. J Urol 2011;185(1): 79–83.

The Role of Lymph Node Dissection in Renal Cell Carcinoma

Scott E. Delacroix Jr, MD, Brian F. Chapin, MD,
Christopher G. Wood, MD*

KEYWORDS

- Lymph node dissection • Lymphadenectomy
- Renal cell carcinoma • Staging • Therapeutic

The role of lymph node dissection (LND) in the staging and treatment of renal cell carcinoma (RCC) has been a topic of debate since Robson and colleagues[1] first reported a survival advantage in patients undergoing concomitant radical nephrectomy and complete retroperitoneal LND (RPLND) from the crus of the diaphragm to the bifurcation of the great vessels. The debate has focused on whether LND is purely an adjunctive staging procedure or has a therapeutic role in the management of this disease. The potential benefits of LND include enhanced staging, better selection for adjuvant therapies/clinical trials, a decrease in recurrence rates, and improved disease specific and overall survival.

Approximately 30% to 40% of patients with RCC will either present with distant metastatic disease or develop distant disease after nephrectomy. The presence of lymph node metastasis in patients with locally advanced RCC is one of the strongest prognostic factors influencing survival. The 5-year survival rate of patients with lymph node–only metastasis ranges from 5% to 38%.[2–6] Depending on the extent of local disease and presence or absence of distant metastatic disease, lymphadenopathy (short-axis size ≥ 1 cm) detected in the retroperitoneum on cross-sectional imaging harbors metastatic disease in 30% to 70% of patients.[7–9] In the absence of distant metastatic disease, the incidence of isolated regional lymphatic metastases (pN+M0) in patients staged as clinically node-negative (cN0) with modern cross-sectional imaging is rare and estimated to occur in only 1% to 5% of patients.[9,10] However, these pathologic rates (pN+) vary considerably based on multiple clinical and pathologic features, whether the patient actually undergoes an LND, and the extent of LND performed.[11,12] In the absence of distant metastatic disease, nodal metastasis can be detected at higher rates in patients with high stage and grade primary tumors and those with clinical lymphadenopathy.[4,11]

Because of the infrequent occurrence of isolated lymph node metastasis along with the significant stage migration that has occurred in RCC, using an "all or none" practice will either expose a majority of patients to an unnecessary and potentially morbid procedure or may preclude a portion of patients from undergoing a potentially therapeutic procedure. Although level one evidence does show LND is unnecessary in patients with low-risk primary tumors with clinically negative regional lymph nodes, multiple investigators have attempted to quantify an individual's risk for nodal metastases based on adverse features.[4,11–13] The authors believe that a risk/benefit approach should be applied when deciding on the applicability of a LND in a given patient. This article reviews the available literature on LND and discusses specific subsets of patients for whom aggressive surgical resection involving a lymphadenectomy may be beneficial.

PROSPECTIVE EVIDENCE

The European Organisation for Research and Treatment of Cancer (EORTC) trial 30881 is the

Department of Urology, University of Texas MD Anderson Cancer Center, 1515 Holcombe Boulevard, Unit 1373, Houston, TX 77030, USA
* Corresponding author.
E-mail address: cgwood@mdanderson.org

Urol Clin N Am 38 (2011) 419–428
doi:10.1016/j.ucl.2011.07.008
0094-0143/11/$ – see front matter © 2011 Published by Elsevier Inc.

only large prospective randomized trial assessing the role of LND in RCC.[10] The investigators randomized 772 patients with $cT_{any}N0M0$ RCC to radical nephrectomy with or without LND. Patients were excluded if clinically node-positive disease was detected on preoperative CT. The right-sided template included the paracaval, retrocaval, precaval, and interaortocaval nodes, whereas the left side dissection included the preaortic, para-aortic, and left diaphragmatic nodes. With respect to morbidity, recurrence, and survival end points, no differences were found with the addition of LND to a standard radical nephrectomy. Several important characteristics of the study population must be highlighted. This trial did not use a risk-based protocol to guide performance of an LND, and most patients enrolled had low-risk primary tumors (approximately 70% pT2 and 70%–80% grade 1–2). The median tumor size in the LND group was 5.5 cm. Not surprisingly, only 4% of patients were found to harbor clinically occult lymph node disease (only 1% if cN0 by imaging and nonpalpable at surgery).

The EORTC 30881 study provides level one evidence that LND does not have a role in patients presenting with low-risk primary tumors. Because of the stage migration that has occurred in RCC, these results will apply to most contemporary patients. However, it may not be prudent to liberally apply these findings to all patients, and particularly those with high-risk primary tumors, clinically node-positive disease, or those being considered for adjuvant clinical trials.

STAGING

If the potential therapeutic role of a properly performed LND is discounted, its use still provides more accurate staging and consequently a more accurate assessment of prognosis. Although multiple trials of contemporary adjuvant therapies are underway, omitting the staging LND in high-risk locally advanced disease may impede the selection of patients for adjuvant therapy and represents a confounding factor when assessing the results of these trials.[14,15]

In the current American Joint Committee on Cancer staging system (AJCC version 7), lymph nodes are categorized as either pNx, pN0, or pN1.[16] Any positive lymph node, regardless of the number positive, is assigned the pN1 designation, whereas the former pN2 ($\geq$2 + nodes) designation has been removed. The change in version 7 occurred as a result of several series showing a lack of prognostic significance between the pN1 and pN2 designations.[17,18] In contrast, a recent analysis of patients with isolated retroperitoneal lymph node metastases showed a significant difference in overall (median time not reached vs 21.8 months) and recurrence-free survival (54.7 vs 4.4 months) between the former N1 and N2 designations.[5] Additional prognostic factors of lymph node disease have been implicated, including extranodal extension, size of lymph node, lymph node density, and total number of nodes removed, but are not incorporated into the current staging system.[17–19]

The number of lymph nodes necessary or the minimal template required to be categorized as pN0 is not defined by the AJCC. As expected, the total number of lymph nodes removed (and examined) correlates with the identification of node-positive disease. Terrone and colleagues[20] examined this relationship in 725 patients undergoing radical nephrectomy for RCC; 84% of the patients also received a variable template lymphadenectomy, with a median number of 9 nodes removed. The rate of pN+ disease was significantly increased when the pathologist examined 13 or more nodes (20.8% N+ vs 10.2% N+ for $\leq$12 nodes; $P = .001$). The only independent factor related to the number of nodes removed was the surgeon, with the surgeon performing the highest median number of nephrectomies also having the highest lymph node count. The authors advocated that a minimum of 13 nodes should be excised to adequately stage a patient. Although node count has been advocated as a surrogate marker to define the extent of dissection, multiple technical factors related to pathologic processing can lead to significant variability in total node counts independent of the template of dissection.[21]

Ward and colleagues[22] at the Mayo clinic evaluated whether including pNx with patients staged as pN0 was appropriate when creating prediction models for outcomes after radical nephrectomy in clear cell RCC. On univariate analysis, patients staged as pN0 were more likely to die of RCC than those staged as pNx. However, when accounting for tumor stage and grade in a multivariate model, no difference was seen in cancer-specific survival between patients staged as pNx and those as pN0. The practice at this center has been to use the presence of multiple adverse features in the primary tumor to determine individual risk and whether to perform an LND. Therefore, patients undergoing LND were probably more likely to have adverse features, which prompted the surgeon to stage the retroperitoneum. With the use of this clearly defined approach, the grouping of patients with pNx and those with pN0 seems appropriate. However, this may not be valid in an understaged population when LND is underused. These findings have been further replicated and highlight the role of the primary tumor in defining subsequent disease biology.[18]

ANATOMY AND TEMPLATES

The lymphatic drainage of the kidneys was first described in a cadaveric series by Parker[23] in 1935. These pathways can be highly variable, with occasional primary drainage sites located in the pelvis or intrathoracic regions.[24,25] Most importantly, the renal hilar lymph nodes are not the initial landing sites in most patients with regional lymphatic metastasis, and therefore isolated sampling of the hilar lymph nodes is inadequate when an LND is being performed.[26] As a general rule, both kidneys will drain to interaortocaval lymph nodes.[11] In addition, the right kidney has primary drainage to the precaval, retrocaval, and paracaval regions, whereas the left kidney drains to the preaortic, retroaortic, and paraaortic regions.

Crispen and colleagues[11] examined the location of positive lymph nodes in a series of 169 patients with high-risk clear cell RCC. Patients were defined as high-risk if they had two adverse primary tumor features. This high-risk protocol uses intraoperative pathologic assessment of the primary tumor for nuclear grade 3 or 4, presence of sarcomatoid dedifferentiation, size of 10 cm or greater, stage T3 or higher, and the presence of histologic tumor necrosis.[4] Of these high-risk patients, 64 (38%) were found to have pathologic

positive nodes (pN+) within the retroperitoneum. Disease was never present in a contralateral landing zone without first involving one of the ipsilateral sites or the interaortocaval lymph nodes (**Fig. 1**). Again, simply performing a hilar LND would have missed most of a significant proportion of pN+ disease.

Based on these data, the authors proposed a standardized template for lymph node dissection in RCC encompassing the nodes from the ipsilateral great vessel and interaortocaval regions down to the bifurcation of the great vessels while using intraoperative frozen section of the lymph nodes to guide the expansion of the template to a full bilateral RPLND. An important caveat to this study was that 66% of these patients had clinically enlarged lymph nodes in addition to high-risk primary tumors. Although intraoperative frozen section does seem to be efficacious in providing reliable pathologic diagnoses in patients with clinically positive lymph nodes (≥ 1 cm), the negative predictive value when assessing for occult lymphatic disease in nonpalpable nonenlarged lymph nodes is unknown.[8]

In an older study by Herlinger and colleagues,[27] the authors examined the outcomes of 511 patients with localized and regionally advanced RCC to determine whether an extended rather than a facultative LND provided any therapeutic benefit. A total of 320 patients received a systematic extended dissection (≥ 17 lymph nodes removed per patient), whereas 191 had only a facultative dissection (0 nodes in 50%; 1–5

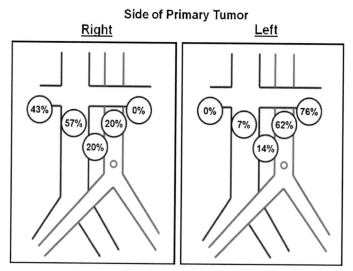

Fig. 1. Percentage frequency of involved locations of pathologic lymph node–positive disease based on the side of the primary tumor. (*From* Crispen PL, Breau RH, Allmer C, et al. Lymph node dissection at the time of radical nephrectomy for high-risk clear cell renal cell carcinoma: indications and recommendations for surgical templates. Eur Urol 2011;59(1):18–23; with permission.)

nodes in 30%; >5 nodes in 10%). The incidence of pathologic positive nodes in the extended and facultative groups was 17.5% and 10%, respectively. The 5- and 10-year overall survival rates were significantly different, with a large benefit shown in the extended LND group (5-year, 66% vs 58%; 10-year, 56.1% vs 40.9%). The authors reported that the survival advantage was most pronounced in patients with lower-stage disease (Robson stage 1 and 2). In addition, morbidity was not increased in patients undergoing extended versus facultative LND.

Bex and colleagues[25] recently reported on the feasibility of sentinel node detection in RCC. The investigators used preoperative single-photon emission CT (SPECT) to identify the sentinel lymph node (SN) followed by intraoperative identification with a gamma probe and camera. Although this was a feasibility study of only 20 patients, the SN was identified in 70% of cases. Excision of the SN was performed through either an open (80%) or laparoscopic (20%) approach. Whether this approach can be replicated and would be feasible in patients with regionally advanced RCC to detect clinically occult lymphatic disease will require further investigation.

MORBIDITY/TECHNIQUE

Although the EORTC 30881 trial did not show any significant differences in operative or postoperative complications,[10] we believe that the addition of an LND to a standard radical nephrectomy conveys a higher risk of lymphadenectomy-specific complications over nephrectomy alone. Multiple factors may contribute to the development of a complication, including the extent of dissection, the presence of bulky clinically positive lymph nodes, medical comorbidities, and individual surgeon experience. Complications associated with LND include injury to major vessels or adjacent organs, bleeding, lymphocele, chylous ascites, and postoperative small bowel obstruction. A standardized system for assessing complications has not been used in comparable cohorts to provide a valid estimation of risk for these procedural-specific complications.

Minimally invasive techniques for treating RCC have increased tremendously over the past 15 years. When compared with its open counterpart, minimally invasive radical nephrectomy may be associated with a decrease in morbidity, particularly postoperative pain and convalescence.[28] As shown by Chapman and colleagues,[29] laparoscopic RPLND is technically feasible in patients with clinically negative regional nodes. Although the template of LND was variable and gradually increased in scope with increasing experience, no differences in complications were noted in patients undergoing laparoscopic nephrectomy versus laparoscopic nephrectomy with LND. Although this seems feasible, considerable experience with minimally invasive techniques is necessary to laparoscopically replicate the LND templates, as recently described by Crispen and colleagues.[11]

Surgical approach does seem to influence the use of LND in patients undergoing radical nephrectomy for RCC. In an analysis of the U.S. Kidney Cancer Study, Filson and colleagues[30] evaluated 730 patients with RCC undergoing open (n = 427, 58%) or laparoscopic (n = 303, 42%) radical nephrectomy for RCC. Lymphadenectomy was performed in only 11% of cases and seemed to be a limited dissection in most of these cases. LND was performed more frequently in patients undergoing open radical nephrectomy versus laparoscopic radical nephrectomy (14.1% vs 5.9%; $P<.01$) and those with higher-stage, higher-grade, and larger-sized tumors. The potential staging or therapeutic benefit of LND in highly selected cases may be further obfuscated if clinical decisions are based on technique alone. Like in the not-so-uncommon case of patients undergoing laparoscopic nephrectomy in lieu of open partial nephrectomy for T1a masses, surgeons must be wary of supplanting potential oncologic benefits (staging or therapeutic) with the desire to use minimally invasive techniques.

PROTOCOLS AND NOMOGRAMS FOR PREDICTING LN+ DISEASE

Determining an individual patient's risk of occult lymph node metastasis would help surgeons in planning for LND and, at the very least, improve the staging in high-risk patients. As shown in the recent EORTC trial, most patients presenting with RCC are at low risk for lymph node metastasis. The question is whether a template LND would benefit the subset of patients at the highest risk for metastasis. This issue has yet to be properly addressed with an adequate prospective study designed specifically for high-risk patients.

Blute and colleagues[4] retrospectively reviewed a cohort of 1584 patients with M0 RCC from Mayo Clinic with an average follow-up of 9.6 years. Most patients underwent a staging LND (variable template), and included 43.5% (n = 882) who were staged as pNx and thus had no lymph nodes removed with surgical specimen; 52.1% (n = 1057) staged as pN0; 3.6% (n = 51) who had a single positive lymph node (pN1); and 0.8% (n = 17) who were pN2 with metastasis in more than one regional lymph node. In those staged as pN0/pNx, 24.6% (n = 390) died of their disease compared with 88.2% (n = 68) of the patients with pN1/pN2 RCC. Estimated disease-specific survival is shown in **Fig. 2**. The authors examined multiple pathologic features obtained on frozen section at nephrectomy and developed an intraoperative protocol using five adverse features. On multivariate analysis, each of the following were shown to be independent risk factors for lymph node involvement: Fuhrman grade 3 or 4 ($P<.001$); sarcomatoid component ($P<.001$); tumor 10 cm or greater ($P = .005$); pathologic T3 or greater ($P = .017$); and histologic evidence of tumor coagulative necrosis ($P = .051$). A patient was defined as high risk when at least two adverse features were identified. Among the 621 patients with at least two adverse features, 10% (n = 62) had regional lymph node involvement detected through LND. These data have yet to be validated in an external series, and this intraoperative protocol requires a frozen section analysis at nephrectomy to determine risk.

In a recent publication, Crispen and colleagues[11] identified 415 patients with clear cell RCC undergoing radical nephrectomy between 2002 and 2006 at Mayo Clinic. Using the previously described protocol by Blute and colleagues,[4] 169 (41%) high-risk patients (two or more adverse features) were identified and targeted for LND. The incidence of lymph node–positive disease (overall, 38% of high-risk; 64/169) correlated with the number of high-risk features. Unfortunately, this protocol has been developed solely based on intraoperative collection of data from the primary tumor, and completely discounts the clinical node

status of the patient. Clinically positive lymph node disease was apparent preoperatively based on CT findings in 66% (42/64) of patients later found to have pN+ disease. At many centers, these patients with cN+ disease with regionally advanced primary tumors would undergo a LND without the need for intraoperative frozen section analysis. In addition, this analysis included 59 patients with metastases (M1) in the high-risk category, which is likely the reason for the higher incidence of pathologic nodal disease compared with the prior publication from Blute and colleagues.[4] This high incidence of pN+ disease is surely influenced by the clinical node status and the presence of distant metastases.

In an effort to provide a preoperative assessment of the risk of lymph node disease, several investigators have developed nomograms based on clinical factors. Hutterer and colleagues[12] developed a preoperative nomogram using patient age, symptom classification, and tumor size to predict probability of lymph node metastases in 4658 patients without metastatic disease ($cT_{any}N_{any}cM0$). The nomogram was produced using the data from seven European centers (n = 2522), and externally validating against patients from five other centers (n = 2136) (**Fig. 3**). Symptoms were classified as asymptomatic, local (flank pain, palpable mass, or hematuria), or systemic (anorexia, asthenia, weight loss). Unfortunately, the clinical node status assessed with preoperative CT was not used or analyzed for inclusion in this nomogram. On multivariate analysis, only tumor size and symptom classification were independent predictors of lymph node disease. External validation

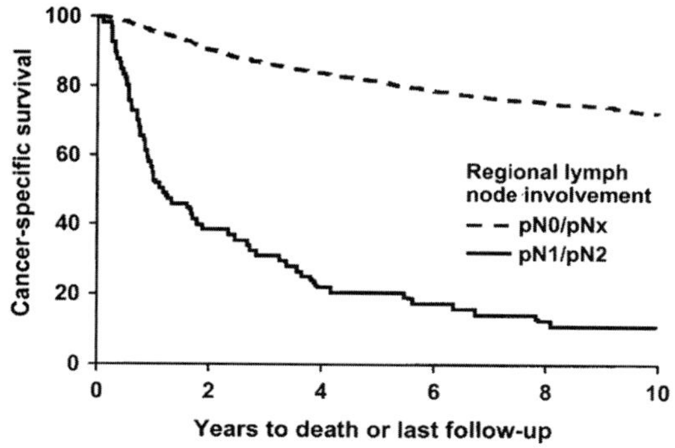

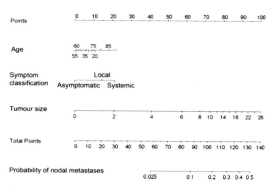

Fig. 2. Estimated disease-specific survival according to regional lymph node involvement. (*From* Blute ML, Leibovich BC, Cheville JC, et al. A protocol for performing extended lymph node dissection using primary tumor pathologic features for patients treated with radical nephrectomy for clear cell renal cell carcinoma. J Urol 2004;172(2):465–9; with permission.)

Fig. 3. Preoperative nomogram to predict for pathologic positive lymph nodes. Clinical nodal status not included. (*From* Hutterer GC, Patard JJ, Perrotte P, et al. Patients with renal cell carcinoma nodal metastases can be accurately identified: external validation of a new nomogram. Int J Cancer 2007;121(11):2556–61; with permission.)

showed an area under the curve of 0.78. The incidence of positive lymph nodes was only 4.2%, which is lower than the incidence reported by Blute and colleagues[4] (10%) and could be from the limited hilar dissection performed in most of these patients, which, as previously shown, does not represent the primary landing zone for RCC.

Thompson and colleagues[13] pooled patients from Mayo Clinic and Memorial Sloan-Kettering Cancer Center in an attempt to define a completely preoperative clinical nomogram. The authors identified 4844 patients with M0 RCC, of whom 139 (2.9%) were found to have lymph node–positive disease. Predictive variables for lymph node metastases included lymphadenopathy, tumor size, and the presence of hematuria or other symptoms. Internal validation showed a concordance index of 0.76. This nomogram has not yet been published in manuscript form but could provide a basis for the prospective preoperative evaluation of a high-risk cohort.

THE THERAPEUTIC ROLE OF LND

Although the available literature on LND leaves many questions unanswered, particularly regarding the optimal patient selection for LND, multiple retrospective series suggest a therapeutic benefit of LND in select patients.

Low-Risk Localized RCC

As shown in the EORTC 30881 trial and numerous retrospective studies, patients with clinically localized low-risk RCC ($cT_{1-2}cN0M0$) have a very low risk of harboring micrometastatic disease.[10] Therefore, in patients with low-risk primary tumors and clinically node-negative regional lymph nodes, the understaging rate of omitting an LND seems to be approximately 1% and does not justify its inclusion. In clinically localized, low-risk, clinically node-negative RCC, LND does not seem to have a therapeutic or suitable staging benefit.

High-Risk Localized RCC

Although only based on retrospective data, patients with high-risk clinical and pathologic features are a select group who may benefit therapeutically from resection of isolated nodal metastasis (**Box 1**). RCC-specific survival in patients with exclusive nodal metastases shows important variability. In addition to the potential therapeutic effects of LND, these patients may warrant further therapeutic intervention and are prime candidates for novel adjuvant clinical trials.

Box 1
Adverse/high-risk clinical and pathologic features

Clinical lymphadenopathy[13]

Tumor size of 10 cm or greater[4,12,13]

Primary tumor stage of pT3 or greater[4]

Presence of sarcomatoid features[4]

Nuclear grade of 3 or more[4]

Presence of histologic tumor necrosis[4]

Systemic symptoms[12]

Gross hematuria[13]

In a series of 200 consecutive radical nephrectomies performed at the University of Genoa with extensive LND, Giuliani and colleagues[31] showed survival in patients with pN+ disease was intermediate between those in whom the tumor was confined to the kidney and those with distant metastatic disease. Of the patients in this series, 10% had positive lymph nodes without distant metastases, and the 5-year survival rate in this group was 52% compared with 7% in those with distant metastases. Similar to Herrlinger and colleagues,[27] the authors rationalized that this very high survival rate was from the extensive LNDs (mean lymph node count, 30–40) that were performed. A later analysis of 328 patients confirmed the intermediate prognosis of patients with nodal-only metastasis and further suggested a benefit to surgical resection.

At the University of California, Los Angeles, Pantuck and colleagues[32] reviewed a large series of nephrectomies with suspected nodal involvement. This series included 535 patients with N0M0 disease, 129 patients with pN+ disease, and 236 patients with distant metastasis only (N0M+). Of the 129 pN+ patients, 43 had isolated nodal metastases without distant metastatic disease ($T_{any}N1-2M0$). Patients with isolated clinical node involvement ($T_{any}N+M0$) who received the benefits of an LND had significantly longer survival despite having a worse predicted prognosis after adjusting for Fuhrman grade and T stage.

In a recent publication, investigators from the University of California, San Francisco (UCSF) identified 9586 patients with $pT_{any}N_{any}M0$ RCC through the SEER database.[33] Patients were divided into two cohorts: node-negative (n = 8321) and node-positive (n = 1265). At a median follow-up of 3.5 years, 58% (n = 736) of the node-positive patients and 20% (n = 1646) of the node-negative patients had died of RCC. An increase in disease-specific survival was seen with the extent of lymphadenectomy in patients with lymph node–positive disease. An increase of 10 lymph nodes in a patient with one positive lymph node was significantly associated with a 10% absolute increase in disease-specific survival at 5 years. Clinical risk factors (including lymphadenopathy) were not assessed. In addition, only 25% of the patients with pN+ disease had more than five nodes removed. Whether a more extensive dissection would result in a more significant survival advantage is unknown. The authors concluded patients at high risk for nodal disease should be considered for LND with this potential therapeutic benefit.[33]

Delacroix and colleagues[5] reported on the outcomes of patients with isolated nodal metastases (pT$_{any}$N1–2M0) treated at the University of Texas MD Anderson Cancer Center. Of the 68 patients with nodal metastasis (T$_{any}$N+M0), 22.1% were disease-free at a median follow-up of 43.5 months. The Kaplan Meier estimated 5-year overall and disease-specific survival rates were 37% and 39%, respectively. Characteristics of the cohort included a median tumor size of 11 cm, 88% with stage pT3 or higher, 80% clinically node-positive, and the median number of nodes removed was six. In patients who experienced recurrence (n = 49), disease was detected between 0 and 4 months in 51%, from 4 to 12 months in 16%, and more than 12 months postoperatively in 33%. The median time to recurrence was 10.8 months. Almost all recurrences were multifocal and not amenable to solitary metastasectomy. Patients with papillary RCC lymph node metastases had a delayed time to recurrence (median, 37.21 months), and the median overall survival was not reached, suggesting a significant variability in the biology of disease based on histologic findings. Differences in outcomes between clear cell and papillary RCC may be explained by a more indolent biology in the latter, or these differences may be from a lower incidence of clinically undetectable hematogenous metastases at nephrectomy and LND.[34] Predictors of a favorable and durable outcome included an ECOG performance status of 0, single-node involvement (N1 vs N2 AJCC, version 6), absence of sarcomatoid features, and papillary histology. Despite the lack of a standardized template in these patients, the investigators concluded that a therapeutic benefit exists for LND with nephrectomy in patients with regionally advanced RCC with limited lymph node metastases.

The authors believe that clinical node-positive disease without distant metastases (T$_{any}$N+M0) mandates aggressive surgical resection and, when possible, template lymphadenectomy as described by Crispen and colleagues.[11] A therapeutic benefit is implied based on numerous retrospective series. Because of the high recurrence rates within short intervals, patients with node-positive (pN+M0) disease are a unique cohort for which adjuvant therapies can be tested in an expeditious fashion.

Salvage RPLND

Some patients with isolated regional recurrences after radical nephrectomy may benefit from salvage RPLND. In an analysis of 1503 patients who underwent nephrectomy, Kwon and colleagues[18] reported a 2.4% (36/1503) incidence of regional recurrence in the absence of distant metastatic disease. Most of these recurrences (30/36) were in the regional lymph nodes. In a study by Boorjian and colleagues,[35] the 4-year progression-free and cancer-specific survival rates after salvage RPLND for regional lymph node recurrence were 15% and 35%, respectively. Significant complications occurred in 27% of patients, indicating the technically challenging nature of salvage resection. Patients who underwent full resection with isolated regional lymph node recurrences had worse outcomes than patients with presumable isolated hematogenous recurrences. Although salvage RPLND is associated with worse cancer-specific outcomes than resection of metachronous distant recurrence, it seems to benefit a small proportion of patients and should be considered in this rare situation.

M1 Disease

The presence of concomitant nodal and distant metastatic disease has been shown to be a significant predictor of overall survival in patients undergoing cytoreductive nephrectomy.[36–38] In a series of 1153 metastatic patients undergoing cytoreductive nephrectomy, the cancer-specific mortality rates of those with pNxM1, pN0M1, and pN+M1 were significantly different (66%, 65%, and 86%, respectively).[37] Lughezzani and colleagues[37] showed lymph node status to be an informative predictor of outcomes after cytoreductive nephrectomy and suggested including this variable in future prognostic models. These significant findings are in contrast with prior investigators and have yet to be externally validated.

The therapeutic role of LND in the setting of cytoreductive nephrectomy has been evaluated in several retrospective series from the cytokine era. The National Cancer Institute evaluated a cohort of 154 patients who underwent cytoreductive nephrectomy in preparation for interleukin 2 (IL-2)–based regimens.[38] Among 82 patients with clinically negative lymph nodes (cN0M1) and 72 patients with clinically positive lymph nodes (cN+M1). Median survivals for patients with clinically node-negative and node-positive RCC were 14.7 and 8.5 months ($P = .0004$). No statistically significant difference in survival was noted between patients with clinical N0 disease and those with retroperitoneal lymphadenopathy completely resected (cN+ made NED by resection) (14.7 vs 8.6; $P = .07$). Although this data suggested a therapeutic effect of LND, the study was underpowered to make any conclusive statements. Patients whose nodes were incompletely resected still maintained an overall survival of 8.5 months (comparable with those with cN+ disease), whereas those with unresectable lymph node disease had a dismal 3.3-month survival. Response rates to IL-2 therapy were not significantly different between those with resected lymphadenopathy and those with residual unresected lymph node disease. Because resection did not change the response to systemic therapy, whether a more complete cytoreduction with resection of lymphadenopathy changes the natural history of disease is unknown.

Pantuck and colleagues[2] assessed the impact of lymph node–positive disease on a large cohort of metastatic patients (n = 322 M1) treated with cytoreductive nephrectomy at UCLA. In this study, 236 patients with clinical N0M1 RCC were compared with 86 patients with clinical N+M1 disease. Both groups received postoperative immunotherapy at the same rate (65%). The median survival was 20.4 months for patients with N0M1 disease versus 10.5 months in those with N+M1 disease. In a separate analysis including patients with N+M0 disease, the authors found no perceived survival benefit to IL-2 in patients with unresected clinically positive lymph nodes.[32] Patients undergoing nephrectomy with synchronous LND (n = 129) had a significant survival advantage (5-month improvement) over patients with clinically positive nodes left in situ. The analysis included patients with N+M0 disease (n = 43), and whether this perceived survival advantage is from the heterogeneous population studied is unclear. Although no strong conclusions can be made in patients with M1 disease, these retrospective series suggest that the natural history of disease in patients with metastatic RCC treated with immunotherapy may be altered with LND.

SUMMARY

Regional LND as a standard practice for low-grade, low-stage RCC is neither supported nor recommended. Level one data supporting LND for patients with locally advanced or clinical lymphadenopathy do not exist. The prognostic/staging benefit of LND is supported and its role as a therapeutic intervention is apparent in high-risk patients with clinically enlarged lymph nodes. Level one evidence for the high-risk M0 patient population will never be available for patients with clinically node-positive RCC, because this would inappropriately (in the authors' opinion) require these patients to be randomized to nephrectomy alone. After critical review of the limited data on clinical node-negative patients, being dogmatic with respect to the use of lymph node dissection risks depriving a high-risk patient of a potential therapeutic benefit or risks exposing a lower-risk patient to unnecessary morbidity. Despite this, no significant evidence-based recommendations can be made for the high-risk clinically node-negative presentation. As technology advances, physicians may be able to better predict which patients would most benefit from LND through using a combination of preoperative nomograms, more advanced imaging, and potentially with the use of biomarkers. For the foreseeable future, however, the controversies over when to perform an LND in RCC will persist.

REFERENCES

1. Robson CJ, Churchill BM, Anderson W. The results of radical nephrectomy for renal cell carcinoma. J Urol 1969;101(3):297–301.
2. Pantuck AJ, Zisman A, Dorey F, et al. Renal cell carcinoma with retroperitoneal lymph nodes. Impact on survival and benefits of immunotherapy. Cancer 2003;97(12):2995–3002.
3. Karakiewicz PI, Trinh QD, Bhojani N, et al. Renal cell carcinoma with nodal metastases in the absence of distant metastatic disease: prognostic indicators of disease-specific survival. Eur Urol 2007;51(6):1616–24.
4. Blute ML, Leibovich BC, Cheville JC, et al. A protocol for performing extended lymph node dissection using primary tumor pathological features for patients treated with radical nephrectomy for clear cell renal cell carcinoma. J Urol 2004;172(2):465–9.
5. Delacroix SE, Chapin BF, Chen JJ, et al. Can a durable disease free survival be achieved with surgical resection in patients with pathologic node positive renal cell carcinoma? J Urol, in Press.
6. Capitanio U, Jeldres C, Patard JJ, et al. Stage-specific effect of nodal metastases on survival in patients with non-metastatic renal cell carcinoma. BJU Int 2009;103(1):33–7.

7. Studer UE, Scherz S, Scheidegger J, et al. Enlargement of regional lymph nodes in renal cell carcinoma is often not due to metastases. J Urol 1990; 144(2 Pt 1):243–5.

8. Ming X, Ningshu L, Hanzhong L, et al. Value of frozen section analysis of enlarged lymph nodes during radical nephrectomy for renal cell carcinoma. Urology 2009;74(2):364–8.

9. Johnsen JA, Hellsten S. Lymphatogenous spread of renal cell carcinoma: an autopsy study. J Urol 1997; 157(2):450–3.

10. Blom JH, van Poppel H, Marechal JM, et al. Radical nephrectomy with and without lymph-node dissection: final results of European Organization for Research and Treatment of Cancer (EORTC) randomized phase 3 trial 30881. Eur Urol 2009; 55(1):28–34.

11. Crispen PL, Breau RH, Allmer C, et al. Lymph node dissection at the time of radical nephrectomy for high-risk clear cell renal cell carcinoma: indications and recommendations for surgical templates. Eur Urol 2011;59(1):18–23.

12. Hutterer GC, Patard JJ, Perrotte P, et al. Patients with renal cell carcinoma nodal metastases can be accurately identified: external validation of a new nomogram. Int J Cancer 2007;121(11):2556–61.

13. Thompson R, Raj G, Leibovich B, et al. Preoperative nomogram to predict positive lymph nodes during nephrectomy for renal cell carcinoma. Presented at the American Urological Association Annual Meeting. Orlando, May 17–22, 2008 [abstract: 603].

14. Bex A, Jonasch E, Kirkali Z, et al. Integrating surgery with targeted therapies for renal cell carcinoma: current evidence and ongoing trials. Eur Urol 2010; 58(6):819–28.

15. Jonasch E, Tannir NM. Adjuvant and neoadjuvant therapy in renal cell carcinoma. Cancer J 2008; 14(5):315–9.

16. Kidney cancer. In: Edge SB, Byrd DR, Compton CC, et al, editors. AJCC Cancer staging manual. 7th edition. New York: Springer-Verlag; 2010. p. 479–89.

17. Terrone C, Cracco C, Porpiglia F, et al. Reassessing the current TNM lymph node staging for renal cell carcinoma. Eur Urol 2006;49(2):324–31.

18. Kwon T, Song C, Hong JH, et al. Reassessment of renal cell carcinoma lymph node staging: analysis of patterns of progression. Urology 2011;77(2): 373–8.

19. Dimashkieh HH, Lohse CM, Blute ML, et al. Extranodal extension in regional lymph nodes is associated with outcome in patients with renal cell carcinoma. J Urol 2006;176(5):1978–82 [discussion: 1982–3].

20. Terrone C, Guercio S, De Luca S, et al. The number of lymph nodes examined and staging accuracy in renal cell carcinoma. BJU International 2003;91(1): 37–40.

21. Parkash V, Bifulco C, Feinn R, et al. To count and how to count, that is the question: interobserver and intraobserver variability among pathologists in lymph node counting. Am J Clin Pathol 2010; 134(1):42–9.

22. Ward JF, Blute ML, Cheville JC, et al. The influence of pNx/pN0 grouping in a multivariate setting for outcome modeling in patients with clear cell renal cell carcinoma. J Urol 2002;168(1):56–60.

23. Parker A. Studies in the main posterior lymph channels of the abdomen and their connections with the lymphatics of the genitourinary system. Am J Anat 1935;56:409–43.

24. Assouad J, Riquet M, Foucault C, et al. Renal lymphatic drainage and thoracic duct connections: implications for cancer spread. Lymphology 2006; 39(1):26–32.

25. Bex A, Vermeeren L, Meinhardt W, et al. Intraoperative sentinel node identification and sampling in clinically node-negative renal cell carcinoma: initial experience in 20 patients. World J Urol. DOI: 10.1007/s00345-010-0615-6.

26. Saitoh H, Nakayama M, Nakamura K, et al. Distant metastasis of renal adenocarcinoma in nephrectomized cases. J Urol 1982;127(6):1092–5.

27. Herrlinger A, Schrott KM, Schott G, et al. What are the benefits of extended dissection of the regional renal lymph nodes in the therapy of renal cell carcinoma. J Urol 1991;146(5):1224–7.

28. Tan HJ, Wolf JS Jr, Ye Z, et al. Population-level comparative effectiveness of laparoscopic versus open radical nephrectomy for patients with kidney cancer. Cancer 2011;117(18):4184–93.

29. Chapman TN, Sharma S, Zhang S, et al. Laparoscopic lymph node dissection in clinically node-negative patients undergoing laparoscopic nephrectomy for renal carcinoma. Urology 2008;71(2):287–91.

30. Filson CP, Miller DC, Colt JS, et-al. Surgical approach and the use of lymphadenectomy and adrenalectomy among patients undergoing radical nephrectomy for renal cell carcinoma. Urol Oncol 2011. [Epub ahead of print].

31. Giuliani L, Giberti C, Martorana G, et al. Radical extensive surgery for renal cell carcinoma: long-term results and prognostic factors. J Urol 1990; 143(3):468–73.

32. Pantuck AJ, Zisman A, Dorey F, et al. Renal cell carcinoma with retroperitoneal lymph nodes: role of lymph node dissection. J Urol 2003;169(6): 2076–83.

33. Whitson JM, Harris CR, Reese AC, et al. Lymphadenectomy improves survival of patients with renal cell carcinoma and nodal metastases. J Urol 2011; 185(5):1615–20.

34. Delacroix SE Jr, Wood CG. The role of lymphadenectomy in renal cell carcinoma. Curr Opin Urol 2009;19(5):465–72.

35. Boorjian SA, Crispen PL, Lohse CM, et al. Surgical resection of isolated retroperitoneal lymph node recurrence of renal cell carcinoma following nephrectomy. J Urol 2008;180(1):99–103 [discussion: 103].

36. Culp SH, Tannir NM, Abel EJ, et al. Can we better select patients with metastatic renal cell carcinoma for cytoreductive nephrectomy? Cancer 2010;116(14):3378–88.

37. Lughezzani G, Capitanio U, Jeldres C, et al. Prognostic significance of lymph node invasion in patients with metastatic renal cell carcinoma: a population-based perspective. Cancer 2009;115(24):5680–7.

38. Vasselli JR, Yang JC, Linehan WM, et al. Lack of retroperitoneal lymphadenopathy predicts survival of patients with metastatic renal cell carcinoma. J Urol 2001;166(1):68–72.

The Emerging Role of Lymphadenectomy in Upper Tract Urothelial Carcinoma

Christopher J. Weight, MD, Mathew T. Gettman, MD*

KEYWORDS

- Lymphadenectomy • Urothelial carcinoma
- Lymph node dissection

Within the last decade, there has been an increased focus on the utility of lymphadenectomy or lymph node dissection (LND) in patients with upper tract urothelial carcinoma (UTUC). UTUC is generally defined as urothelial carcinoma originating from the renal collecting system, renal pelvis, or ureter. Part of this excitement surrounding the issue stems from the abundant and growing literature about the importance of LND in other genitourinary (GU) malignancies, such as bladder cancer, testicular cancer, and penile cancer. However, although the data with regards to LND in UTUC are sparse, investigators are beginning to evaluate the role and define the anatomy to understand how LND may ultimately affect outcomes in patients with UTUC. This article will review the history of LND for UTUC, outline the relative anatomy, and evaluate the arguments and the evidence for, and against, LND in patients with UTUC.

UTUC is a relatively rare site of urothelial cancer, with an incidence of approximately 3500 cases per year, compared with 70,000 cases of urothelial bladder cancer in the United States.[1] This relative rarity has made it difficult to study, and although it may share a histologic origin with bladder cancer, it has some unique features with regards to anatomy, lymph drainage patterns, and etiologic causes that have demanded study in its own right. These differences also prevent blind extrapolation from what is known in urothelial carcinoma of the bladder to UTUC. Nevertheless, LND in patients with UTUC is becoming increasingly important. Large urologic organizations that made no mention

of LND in UTUC just 7 years ago[2] now recommend its consideration for all patients with UTUC, although they acknowledge that the evidence is lacking.[3] The application of LND in patients with UTUC is by no means universal. Among 13 large tertiary, referral, academic medical centers around the world, close to 50% of patients with UTUC will not get an LND.[4] Furthermore, in the United States, 73.6% of patients with UTUC undergo some level of LND,[5] demonstrating the lack of consensus.

ANATOMY

Unfortunately, the anatomy of the lymph drainage of UTUC has not been well studied or described, and templates used from institution to institution have varied widely. This lack of uniformity, coupled with the differing drainage patterns observed depending on where the tumor originates, only muddies the debate.

The lymph drainage of the kidneys/renal pelvises appears to predominantly collect in a predictable pattern, following the blood supply. Kondo and colleagues[6] mapped the location of regional lymph node metastasis and found that right renal pelvis tumors most often metastasize to the hilar nodes, followed by equal proclivity for the paracaval and retrocaval nodes. Tumors of the upper- and mid-right ureter most often go to the retrocaval and interaortocaval nodes, and tumors of the lower ureter on either side go to their respective common iliac, obturator, and internal iliac nodes. Left-sided renal pelvic tumors metastasize to the left hilar nodes,

Department of Urology, Mayo Clinic, Rochester, MN 55905, USA
* Corresponding author.
E-mail address: anderson.carol@mayo.edu

Urol Clin N Am 38 (2011) 429–437
doi:10.1016/j.ucl.2011.07.012

followed by the para-aortic nodes, followed by in-teraortocaval nodes. This mapping study was one of the most complete studies to date, but was limited to a total of 42 patients, of which only 23 were actually confirmed pathologically. Although the study was small, it follows the patterns well recognized in lymph drainage, namely the drainage follows the blood supply. These authors should also be commended for accurate communication about their dissection borders. Based on these findings, they proposed that LND for right-sided renal pelvic and mid- and upper-ureteral tumors should include the hilar nodes, the paracaval, inter-aortocaval, and retrocaval lymph nodes, from the level of the renal hilus to the aortic bifurcation. For left-sided renal pelvic tumors and mid- and upper ureters, dissection should include para-aortic and hilar nodes from the renal hilus to the aortic bifurca-tion.[6] This is a similar dissection scheme proposed by others[7]; however, it should be mentioned that there are widely variable templates and practices and no standard dissection. It seems clear that if an LND is to be performed, the hilar nodes must be included. Others have confirmed that the hilar nodes are the primary site of metastasis for renal pelvic tumors, accounting for between 30% and 50% of nodal metastasis.[8,9] The other regional sites (such as para-aortic, retrocaval, paracaval and interaortocaval) are involved less frequently, although some have found higher lymph node (LN) involvement to these regions than even the hilar nodes.[10] Various authors recommend varying degrees of aggressiveness from templates, nearly mirroring RPLND templates for testis cancer on 1 extreme, to less aggressive templates where they only remove hilar nodes. These data, or lack thereof, indicate an opportunity for improvement with more lymph node mapping studies, clear defi-nitions of anatomic boundaries used in LND, and larger series.

The overall incidence of LN involvement in patients with UTUC is between 12% and 25%.[4,5] LN involvement increases with pathologic stage and grade.[11] For example, 1 study showed that as pathologic T stage increased from T1, T2, T3 to T4, the frequency of nodal involvement was 4.5%, 8.9%, 28.7%, and 70.6%, respectively.[12] Although the percentages were not identical, a similar pattern was observed in another large population-based study with + LNs in 1.8%, 5.7%, 19%, and 20% of patients, respectively.[10]

LYMPHADENECTOMY

To build a rational argument for LND, one must be convinced that the extra effort, time, and increased risk of complications associated with LND are rewarded by some measurable benefit to the patient. These benefits may be realized by better staging, better local control, reduced risk of local or regional nodal relapse, or ultimately better cancer-specific or overall survival. The remainder of this article will address each of these points in turn.

IMPROVED STAGING

There appears to be little debate that LND in patients with UTUC will be staged better than those without LND. The knowledge of LN metastases allows more complete patient counseling because it is recognized that patients with positive nodes (pN1/2) have a 2.5- to 3.0-fold worse survival compared with pN0 (pathologically negative lymph node) patients.[2,13] Computed tomography (CT) Imaging of LNs often misses between 40% and 50% of small lymph node metastases in patients with UTUC.[7,9] Even with modern imaging tech-niques such as positron emission tomography (PET), CT, and PET magnetic resonance imaging (MRI), about 20% of patients with nodal metas-tases will still be missed on radiographic imaging.[14]

Routine pathologic staging may not even identify all metastases. Recent data from a multi-institutional study found that the more lymph nodes removed in pN0 patients, the better the cancer-specific survival (CSS).[15] The authors suggested that there may have been micrometastatic disease removed during the LND that contributed to the survival advantage. This phenomenon has also been observed in bladder cancer,[16,17] strength-ening the argument. Further evidence to support this theory comes from Japan, where investigators found that 14% of patients with negative nodes by hematoxylin and eosin (H&E) staining were positive on immunohistochemical staining.[12]

It seems fair to conclude that LND will undoubt-edly allow for the most accurate predictions of survival, remove micrometastatic disease not identified by routine H&E staining, and identify those who may benefit from immediate systemic therapy.[9] However, if LND does not improve patient outcomes, it is not clear that this extra information is worth the increased operative time, effort, and complications associated with LND.

LOCAL CONTROL/NODAL RELAPSE

To answer the question of whether LND prevents locoregional relapse is somewhat challenging, although the answer based on biologic plausibility alone is probably yes. The challenge in answering this question stems from the quality of the studies. In general, the studies are relatively few and often underpowered (and only univariate); the methodology of the existing studies is not rigorous, and the application of LND is not universal (which introduces confounding). The various studies report subset analyses and use differing definitions of survival, and the dissection templates are not uniform. The end result is a mixture of arguments for and against LND preventing local/nodal relapse in all patients with UTUC.

In patients with lower-risk UTUC (ie, those with Ta, Tis and T1 disease), the risk of nodal involvement at initial surgery is quite low, probably between 0% and 5% (**Table 1**) and 82% lower than the risk of nodal involvement in patients with invasive disease.[11] Although the authors were unable to find the risk of local/nodal recurrence in this low-risk cohort, it stands to reason that the rates would be so low that no study would be powered to detect a difference given the rarity of this disease. Furthermore, the 5-year cancer-specific survival in this cohort is 92%.[13]

In higher-risk patients, there seems to be less ambiguity. Abe and colleagues[12] found in a subset analysis of 214 patients with T1 or higher UTUC, the risk of local/regional relapse was nearly fourfold higher for those not undergoing LND compared with those who did and was found to be pN0 (hazard ratio [HR] 3.96, 95% CI:1.6–11.2). However, they did not compare the risk of relapse for those without an LND versus those with an LND in all patients with UTUC. Other groups were unable to demonstrate that any LND prevents local/nodal relapse.[18–20] In one of these studies however, the crude rates were lower in those patients undergoing a compete LND versus no LND (6.7% vs 9.0%), and the authors hypothesized that an incomplete LND may be no better than no LND.[20]

EFFECTS ON SURVIVAL

Increasing pathologic T stage has consistently been associated with decreased CSS.[13,21] Lymph node involvement has also long been a strong negative prognostic factor, increasing the risk of cancer-specific death by 2.5- to 3.0-fold.[2,13] Patients with positive lymph nodes have a dismal 5-year CSS between 0% and 39%.[7] However, some patients with pN1/2 disease appear to be cured by surgery,[9,12] leading to increased evaluation of the role of LND in UTUC.

Unfortunately, the evidence supporting the use of LND in UTUC is level 3 at best. There are only a few retrospective studies comparing LND versus no LND in patients with UTUC.[4,8,20,22] All of these studies are retrospective; none applied uniform preoperative criteria to determine when LND was to be preformed. Therefore, they are therefore prone to confounding. None of the studies used a standardized LND dissection template or identified a CSS advantage for those undergoing LND in patients with UTUC (**Table 2**). All of these studies have been based on a series of post-hoc, subset analyses and have eventually found a subset of patients who appear to benefit from LND. These subsets, however, have always been based on pathologic criteria and therefore not applicable to preoperative planning. For example, Brausi and colleagues[22] found a survival advantage on univariate analysis for CSS, but it was limited to patients pT2 (pathologic stage T2 [organ confined]) or higher. Additionally, they did not report a multivariate model. Miyake and colleagues[8] found an advantage in CSS for patients with lymphatic vessel invasion, but again this was only based on univariate analysis. Kondo and colleagues[20] observed an advantage only when comparing complete LND versus no LND, but when comparing any LND versus no LND the advantage was lost. Finally, the largest study, by Roscingo and colleagues[4] with 1130 patients, reported no difference in actuarial 5-year CSS, and the authors turned their attention to comparing pNx versus pN0 patients. This paucity of data gives the diligent practitioner no solid direction as to whether LND will benefit a patient in terms of survival and calls attention to the need for better studies. Although a randomized trial would be best, even prospective cohort studies with uniformly applied, preoperative selection criteria and defined dissection templates would greatly improve upon the understanding of the role of LND in patients with UTUC.

Another question that has risen from the bladder cancer paradigm[17,23,24] is whether LND offers any survival advantage in patients who are found to have no positive pathologic lymph nodes (pN0) compared with patients who did not undergo a LND (pNx) (**Table 3**). A similar and related question asks if the probability of survival increases as the number of lymph nodes removed increases.

The balance of the data seems to suggest that with the context of selection bias and variable dissection templates, most retrospective reviews have been unable to measure a survival advantage for patients with pN0 compared with pNx disease (see **Table 3**). Most notably, the US Surveillance, Epidemiology and End Results (SEER) population database found no significant difference in CSS in 2582 patients on multivariate analysis (hazard ratio [HR] = 0.99, P = 0.9) when comparing pN0 with pNx disease.[5] These data should be contrasted with the study of Roscingo and colleagues,[4] where there was a significant survival advantage noted with the pN0 cohort on multivariate analysis (HR = 0.7, P = .007). The reasons for

Table 1
Incidence of lymph node metastasis by pT stage in patients with upper tract urothelial carcinoma

Study	Population	Number in Study	Overall LN+/Total	pTa/pTis	pT1	pT2	pT3	pT4
Lughezzani et al[5]	United States	2077	242/2077 (11.7%)	—	12/651 (1.8%)	22/383 (5.7%)	84/432 (19%)	124/611 (20%)
Roscigno et al[4]	Combined	552	140/552 (25%)	—	7/111 (6.3%)	21/125 (17%)	112/316 (35%)[b]	—
Kondo et al[6]	Japan	181	42/181 (23%)[a]	0/11 (0%)	0/31 (0%)	2/36 (5.6%)	19/78 (24%)	17/20 (85%)
Abe et al[12]	Japan	152	22/152 (14.5%)	0/25 (0%)	0/35 (0%)	1/32 (3.0%)	13/36 (27%)	8/10 (80%)
Secin et al[10]	United States	133	28/133 (21.1%)	1/33 (3.0%)	1/19 (5.3%)	0/20 (0%)	18/49 (37%)	4/6 (67%)
Komatsu et al[9]	Japan	36	11/36 (31%)	0/13 (0%)[b]		2/5 (40%)	8/17 (47%)	1/1 (100%)

Abbreviation: pT, pathologic T stage.
[a] Both radiographic and pathologic positive nodes.
[b] Reported together.

Table 2
Comparison of lymphadenectomy versus no lymphadenectomy

| Study | Median Follow-up (mo) | Cohort | Number of Patients | | HR Cancer-Specific Death (95% Confidence Interval)[a] | Crude Rates Reported 5-year Survival LND + vs LND − |
			LND +	LND −		
Kondo et al[20]	37	Any T	81	88	0.55 (0.27–1.11)[a]	Not Reported
Miyake et al[8]	Not Reported	Any T	35	37	Not Reported	58% vs 50%[a]
Brausi et al[22]	65	pT2–pT4	40	42	Not Reported	82% vs 45%[b]
Roscingo et al[4]	NR[c]	pT1–pT4	552	578	Not Reported	66% vs 69%[a]

Abbreviations: HR, hazard ratio; LND, lymph node dissection.
[a] No significant difference.
[b] *P* = .03 on univariate analysis, time of estimate not reported, multivariate analysis not reported.
[c] Median follow-up not reported, median follow-up for those still alive = 49 months.

Table 3
Comparison of cancer specific survival and relapse free survival in patients with upper tract urothelial carcinoma who are pN0 versus pNx

Study	Median Follow-up (mo)	Cohort	Median LNs Removed (IQR)	Number of Patients pN0	Number of Patients pNx	Cancer-Specific Death N0/Nx HR (95% CI)	Actuarial 5-year Survival N0 vs Nx	Relapse-free Survival N0/Nx HR (95% CI)
Abe et al[12]	NR[a]	pT2–pT4	NR	130	141	NR	NR	0.35 (0.17–0.70)
Favaretto et al[18]	23[b]	Any T	8 (4–15)	124	37	NR	NR	0.66 (0.40–1.10)[c]
Secin et al[10]	37[b]	Any T	4 (2–10)	133	119	1.23 (0.74–2.08)[c]	56% vs 73%[c]	NR
Roscingo et al[4]	48[b]	pT1–pT4	5	412	578	0.69[d]	77% vs 69%	0.86[d]
Lughezzani et al[5]	43[b]	pT1–pT4	NR	1835	747	0.99[c]	81% vs 78%[c]	NR

Abbreviations: CI, confidence interval; HR, hazard ratio; IQR, interquartile range; NR, not reported; pN0, pathologically node negative; pNx, no nodes removed at surgery/not assessed.
[a] Mean follow-up reported 60.5.
[b] Median follow-up for survivors, median follow-up for entire cohort not reported.
[c] No significant difference.
[d] CI not reported but both values significant, *P*<.05.

these differences could be due to different patient populations, different dissection templates, or different levels of bias. The populations treated in these 2 analyses appear to be different. The cohort described by Roscingo and colleagues[11] represents patients from 13 tertiary, referral, academic centers at various locations throughout the world. The incidence of stage-specific lymph node metastasis is twofold to fivefold higher stage by stage than that observed in the SEER database. This suggests either the populations are quite different, or possibly that the LND in the Roscingo cohort is more complete and detects lymph node metastases that may have been otherwise missed. The median number of nodes removed in the Roscingo cohort was five but the median number of LNs removed in the SEER paper was not reported.

Addressing the question of whether the number of LNs removed is important in pN0 patients, the Roscingo cohort found that if eight or greater lymph nodes were removed, there was a 49% increased likelihood of finding positive LN metastases even when controlling for pathologic stage and grade (HR = 1.49 95% confidence interval [CI]: 1.28–2.19).[11] They also identified a CSS advantage for patients (pT2–pT4) with eight or greater nodes resected (HR = 0.42, $P<.01$).[4] However, others have not been able to replicate those results, and Kondo and colleagues[25] suggest that it is the dissection template rather than the number of nodes removed that makes a difference in survival. So while some of these analyses find survival advantage for subsets of patients, these subsets are identified after surgery, precluding the authors from making definitive statements about who truly will benefit from an LND in the preoperative setting.

OPEN VERSUS LAPAROSCOPIC NEPHROURETERECTOMY

Some have used the argument that the need for LND necessitates an open approach over a laparoscopic approach. In several reported studies, LND is less likely in those undergoing laparoscopic nephroureterectomy (LNUx) compared with open (ONUx).[12,18,26] However, in centers of excellence, there appears to be no indication that ONUx offers any advantage over LNUx in terms of cancer-specific survival or ability to do an LND. In one recent comparison,[18] the median node counts between the 2 methods were identical (n = 8), and there was no difference in CSS, while those undergoing LNUx lost less blood and had a shorter hospital stay. In addition, a large multi-institutional trial found no significant difference in lymph node counts between those treated by open versus lap surgery,[15] and on multivariate analysis LNUx

did not compromise CSS.[26] Furthermore, in a randomized single-surgeon trial of 80 patients, there was no difference in CSS or metastasis-free survival, although LND was not performed in any of these cases.[15] Taken as a whole, these data seem to conclude that the surgeon should proceed as his or her comfort level dictates with regards to laparoscopic or open surgery, but there is certainly no standard of care that mandates ONUx.

COMPLICATIONS

The complications of LND in patients with UTUC is rarely discussed or reported. The authors were unable to find any reports on complication rates in any of the series in this review. Therefore it makes an already difficult debate nearly impossible. Since the authors do not know the risks of LND in UTUC, they cannot evaluate whether the risks outweigh the benefits. The LND in UTUC is performed in and around the great vessels, and there is potential for high-volume blood loss, retrograde ejaculation, and deep vein thrombosis. Although one should not expect the complications to be as high as a full-template RPLND for testis cancer, it should be noted that perioperative complication rates for primary RPLND are 29%.[27] Furthermore, the increased operative time and cost should be factored into the decision.

SUMMARY AND RECOMMENDATIONS

The evidence to support the role of LND in patients with UTUC is level 3 at best. All the reported studies are flawed with confounding bias. There are no uniform preoperative criteria to determine when LND should be preformed, and there are no standardized LND dissection templates. Given the flaws and limitations in the current literature, one can conclude the following:

1. LND improves staging.
2. There is biologic plausibility that LND improves survival.
3. LND to date does not offer any measurable survival advantage to patients with UTUC.
4. There may be subsets of patients that benefit from LND (pT2–pT4, pN0).
5. Unfortunately, these subsets appear to only be identified pathologically, and current clinical staging precludes definitive identification of the cohorts that may benefit from LND.
6. There are virtually no data regarding the complications, costs, and extra time added by including LND.
7. LND cannot be considered a standard of care in patients with UTUC.

8. There is a huge opportunity for researchers and clinicians to evaluate the role of LND in patients with UTUC.

Although there appears to be excitement in the urologic community surrounding the idea that LND improves survival in several GU cancers, there continues to be very little evidence currently in other solid organ tumors that this is true. In an exhaustive review of solid tumors from the neck to the pelvis, Gervasoni and colleagues[28] failed to find evidence that LND affects survival and conclude that once it reaches the lymph nodes, the disease is systemic. Taken in this larger context and given the limitations for the current evidence in UTUC, there appears to be a great opportunity for the urologic community to evaluate the risks and the benefits of LND in a systematic way among patients with UTUC.

REFERENCES

1. Jemal A, Siegel R, Xu J, et al. Cancer statistics, 2010. CA Cancer J Clin 2010;60:277.
2. Oosterlinck W, Solsona E, Van Der Meijden AP, et al. EAU guidelines on diagnosis and treatment of upper urinary tract transitional cell carcinoma. Eur Urol 2004;46:147.
3. Roupret M, Zigeuner R, Palou J, et al. European guidelines for the diagnosis and management of upper urinary tract urothelial cell carcinomas: 2011 update. Eur Urol 2011;59:584.
4. Roscigno M, Shariat SF, Margulis V, et al. Impact of lymph node dissection on cancer specific survival in patients with upper tract urothelial carcinoma treated with radical nephroureterectomy. J Urol 2009;181:2482.
5. Lughezzan G, Jeldres C, Isbarn H, et al. A critical appraisal of the value of lymph node dissection at nephroureterectomy for upper tract urothelial carcinoma. Urology 2010;75:118.
6. Kondo T, Nakazawa H, Ito F, et al. Primary site and incidence of lymph node metastases in urothelial carcinoma of upper urinary tract. Urology 2007;69: 265.
7. Eggener SE, Kundu SD. Retroperitoneal lymph nodes in transitional cell carcinoma of the kidney and ureter. Adv Urol 2009;181927. Available at: http://www.hindawi.com/journals/au/2009/181927/cta/. Accessed July 7, 2011.
8. Miyake H, Kara I, Gohji K, et al. The significance of lymphadenectomy in transitional cell carcinoma of the upper urinary tract. Br J Urol 1998;82:494.
9. Komatsu H, Tanabe N, Kubodera S, et al. The role of lymphadenectomy in the treatment of transitional cell carcinoma of the upper urinary tract. J Urol 1997;157:1622.
10. Secin FP, Koppie TM, Salamanca JI, et al. Evaluation of regional lymph node dissection in patients with upper urinary tract urothelial cancer. Int J Urol 2007;14:26.
11. Roscigno M, Shariat SF, Freschi M, et al. Assessment of the minimum number of lymph nodes needed to detect lymph node invasion at radical nephroureterectomy in patients with upper tract urothelial cancer. Urology 2009;74:1070.
12. Abe T, Shinohara N, Harabayashi T, et al. The role of lymph node dissection in the treatment of upper urinary tract cancer: a multi-institutional study. BJU Int 2008;102:576.
13. Novara G, De Marco V, Gottardo F, et al. Independent predictors of cancer-specific survival in transitional cell carcinoma of the upper urinary tract: multi-institutional dataset from 3 European centers. Cancer 2007;110:1715.
14. Jensen TK, Holt P, Gerke O, et al. Preoperative lymph-node staging of invasive urothelial bladder cancer with 18F-fluorodeoxyglucose positron emission tomography/computed axial tomography and magnetic resonance imaging: correlation with histopathology. Scand J Urol Nephrol 2011;45:122.
15. Roscigno M, Shariat SF, Margulis V, et al. The extent of lymphadenectomy seems to be associated with better survival in patients with nonmetastatic upper-tract urothelial carcinoma: how many lymph nodes should be removed? Eur Urol 2009;56:512.
16. Herr H, Lee C, Chang S, et al. Standardization of radical cystectomy and pelvic lymph node dissection for bladder cancer: a collaborative group report. J Urol 2004;171:1823.
17. Koppie TM, Vickers AJ, Vora K, et al. Standardization of pelvic lymphadenectomy performed at radical cystectomy: can we establish a minimum number of lymph nodes that should be removed? Cancer 2006;107:2368.
18. Favaretto RL, Shariat SF, Chade DC, et al. Comparison between laparoscopic and open radical nephroureterectomy in a contemporary group of patients: are recurrence and disease-specific survival associated with surgical technique? Eur Urol 2010;58:645.
19. Ozsahin M, Zouhair A, Villà S, et al. Prognostic factors in urothelial renal pelvis and ureter tumours: a multicentre rare cancer network study. Eur J Cancer 1999;35:738.
20. Kondo T, Nakazawa H, Ito F, et al. Impact of the extent of regional lymphadenectomy on the survival of patients with urothelial carcinoma of the upper urinary tract. J Urol 2007;178:1212.
21. Batata MA, Whitmore WF Jr, Hilaris BS. Primary carcinoma of the ureter: a prognostic study. Cancer 1975;35:1626.
22. Brausi MA, Gavioli M, De Luca G, et al. Retroperitoneal lymph node dissection (RPLD) in conjunction with nephroureterectomy in the treatment of infiltrative

transitional cell carcinoma (TCC) of the upper urinary tract: impact on survival. Eur Urol 2007;52:1414.

23. Stein JP, Skinner DG. The role of lymphadenectomy in high-grade invasive bladder cancer. Urol Clin North Am 2005;32:187.

24. Herr HW, Bochner BH, Dalbagni G, et al. Impact of the number of lymph nodes retrieved on outcome in patients with muscle invasive bladder cancer. J Urol 2002;167:1295.

25. Kondo T, Hashimoto Y, Kobayashi H, et al. Template-based lymphadenectomy in urothelial carcinoma of the upper urinary tract: impact on patient survival. Int J Urol 2010;17:848.

26. Capitanio U, Shariat SF, Isbarn H, et al. Comparison of oncologic outcomes for open and laparoscopic nephroureterectomy: a multi-institutional analysis of 1249 cases. Eur Urol 2009;56:1.

27. Subramanian VS, Nguyen CT, Stephenson AJ, et al. Complications of open primary and post-chemotherapy retroperitoneal lymph node dissection for testicular cancer. Urol Oncol 2010; 28:504.

28. Gervasoni JE Jr, Sbayi S, Cady B. Role of lymphadenectomy in surgical treatment of solid tumors: an update on the clinical data. Ann Surg Oncol 2007; 14:2443.

The Role of Lymphadenectomy for Testicular Cancer: Indications, Controversies, and Complications

Tatum Tarin, MD, Brett Carver, MD, Joel Sheinfeld, MD*

KEYWORDS
- Lymphadenectomy • Testicular cancer
- Lymph node dissection • Germ cell tumor

GERM CELL TUMORS OF THE TESTIS

Testicular germ cell tumors (GCTs) are the most common solid malignancy in young men ages 20 to 35. The incidence of testis tumors is rising, with 8480 new diagnoses in 2010, resulting in 350 deaths.[1] With survival rates exceeding 90%, the multidisciplinary management of testicular cancer serves as a model for the treatment of other solid tumors.[2] Surgery, cisplatin-based chemotherapy, and radiotherapy play integral roles in the treatment of this disease and have contributed to these excellent cure rates. This article discusses the surgical management of testicular cancer, focusing on retroperitoneal lymphadenectomy (RPLND) for nonseminomatous GCT treatment (NSGCT), specifically addressing the indications, controversies, and complications of lymphadenectomy for both low-stage and high-stage disease.

DEVELOPMENT OF THE CONTEMPORARY RPLND

Retroperitoneal lymph node dissection was first performed in the 1950s using a surgical template based on the initial lymphatic drainage studies described by Jamieson and Dobson in 1910.[3] Further mapping studies performed by Donohue

and colleagues,[4] Weissbach and colleagues,[5] and Ray and colleagues,[6] established specific anatomic regions within the retroperitoneum described as "primary landing zones" for right-sided and left-sided tumors.[4–6] Right-sided testicular tumors most commonly metastasize to the interaortocaval lymph nodes followed by precaval and paracaval lymph nodes, whereas left-sided testicular tumors most commonly spread to the para-aortic and preaortic lymph nodes. Contralateral involvement occurs more commonly with right-sided primary tumors, especially with higher-stage tumors.[7]

The role of RPLND has been well established in the management of NSGCT; however, surgical templates have become the focus of considerable debate. In an era where clinical staging was limited and effective chemotherapy was not available, emphasis for RPLND was placed on extensive dissection and removal of all lymph nodes in the retroperitoneum.[8] Initial templates, as described by Donohue and colleagues,[9] included bilateral suprahilar dissection as well as removal of all nodal tissue between both ureters down to the bifurcation of the common iliac arteries. Several investigators confirmed therapeutic effectiveness with this extended template RPLND; however, suprahilar dissection was associated with

Memorial Sloan-Kettering Cancer Center, 1275 York Avenue, New York, NY 10065, USA
* Corresponding author.
E-mail address: sheinfej@mskcc.org

Urol Clin N Am 38 (2011) 439–449
doi:10.1016/j.ucl.2011.07.010
0094-0143/11/$ – see front matter © 2011 Elsevier Inc. All rights reserved.

increased pancreatic injury, lymphatic injury, and renovascular complications.[4,10] Given the morbidity of performing suprahilar dissection, Donohue and colleagues[9] investigated relapse rates for patients with low-stage NSGCT and found that relapse was independent of whether or not the patient underwent a suprahilar node dissection. Thus, bilateral infrahilar dissection, with boundaries set superiorly by the renal hilum, laterally by the ureters, and inferiorly by the bifurcation of the common iliac vessels, decreased the morbidity of RPLND while maintaining oncologic efficacy and has been established as the standard of care.

With the modification of the RPLND template to an infrahilar dissection, the most common long-term complication was infertility secondary to retrograde ejaculation from injury to the sympathetic nerve fibers. Normal antegrade ejaculation requires sympathetic innervation to trigger the coordinated processes of closure of the bladder neck, seminal emission, and expulsion of semen. Efferent impulses originate in the preganglionic fibers at the T12 to L3 thoracolumbar spinal cord. After leaving the lumbar sympathetic trunks, these fibers converge near the inferior mesenteric artery just above the aortic bifurcation and form the hypogastric plexus. From the hypogastric plexus, these fibers innervate the seminal vesicles, prostate, vas deferens, and bladder neck through the pelvic plexus.[12] Ejaculation is triggered by nerves originating at the lumbosacral spinal cord levels, primarily S2 to S4. The coordinated event of antegrade ejaculation requires sympathetic innervation to close the bladder neck and sacral somatic innervation to cause external urethral sphincter relaxation and rhythmic contractions of the bulbourethral and perineal muscles.[7,8,13,14]

Preservation of the paravertebral sympathetic ganglia, postganglionic sympathetic fibers from T2 to L4, and the hypogastric plexus during RPLND are critical to prevent ejaculatory dysfunction.[13,15] Through an improved understanding of neuroanatomy, unilateral metastatic distribution patterns, and surgical mapping studies, surgeons began developing strategies to minimize the risk of retrograde ejaculation and subsequent infertility.[4–6] Thus, two strategies were developed to preserve these structures, unilateral modified template RPLND and nerve-sparing RPLND.

Modified template RPLND was initially introduced for carefully selected patients with low-stage disease and eliminated contralateral dissection below the inferior mesenteric artery.[9] Several different modified templates have been used and have reported excellent functional outcomes, ranging from 51% to 88% preserved antegrade

ejaculation.[16–19] Despite varying surgical boundaries, unilateral modified templates share the common goals of (1) dissection of the interaortocaval and ipsilateral lymph nodes between the renal hilum and the bifurcation of the common iliac artery ipsilateral to the primary tumor, and (2) minimizing contralateral dissection, especially below the level of the inferior mesenteric artery, thereby preserving the contralateral sympathetic trunk, postganglionic sympathetic fibers, and hypogastric plexus.[8,15]

Further understanding of the sympathetic innervation and anatomy has led to the development of the modern nerve-sparing bilateral template RPLND. Prospective identification and meticulous preservation of the sympathetic trunks, postganglionic sympathetic fibers, and hypogastric plexus have resulted in antegrade ejaculation in more than 95% of patients undergoing primary RPLND in high-volume centers.[20] Using a similar technique in select patients undergoing a more challenging postchemotherapy (PC)-RPLND, Pettus[21] at Memorial Sloan-Kettering Cancer Center (MSKCC) reported a 79% success rate for antegrade ejaculation in patients with involved lymph nodes. Although bilateral nerve-sparing RPLND is feasible in experienced hands, oncologic outcome should never be compromised to preserve antegrade ejaculation and fertility. The issue of decreasing template size and potential risks of extratemplate disease is discussed later.

With further modifications to RPLND templates, lymph node count, as with other malignancies,[22,23] has been evaluated in an effort to establish benchmarks in surgery. Thompson and colleagues[24] evaluated the lymph node counts of 255 patients who underwent primary RPLND at MSKCC and reported a median node count of 48 lymph nodes. These investigators reported that increasing lymph node count increased the odds of identifying a positive lymph node; and on multivariate analysis, a lymph node count greater than 40 retained a significant association with identifying positive lymph nodes, even after adjusting for year of surgery, clinical stage (CS), and surgeon (odds ratio 2.0; 95% CI, 1.1–3.7; $P = .026$). In the postchemotherapy setting, Carver and colleagues[25] evaluated the number of lymph nodes obtained in 628 patients who underwent PC-RPLND and were found to have fibrosis or teratoma. The investigators reported decreasing lymph node count as a significant predictor of disease recurrence ($P = .04$) and a 2-year relapse-free survival of 97% when greater than 50 lymph nodes were removed. These data suggest that lymph node counts during RPLND may be an independent predictor of disease recurrence and, thus, may have important implications in determining adequacy of surgical quality and pathologic assessment.

INDICATIONS FOR RETROPERITONEAL LYMPH NODE DISSECTION
Clinical Stage I NSGCT

Approximately one-third of patients with testicular cancer present with CS I disease, defined as normal postorchiectomy tumor markers (β-human chorionic gonadotropin, α-fetoprotein, and lactate dehydrogenase) and absence of metastatic disease on imaging studies of the chest, abdomen, and pelvis. Treatment options for patients with stage I NSGCT include surveillance, 2 cycles of cisplatin-based adjuvant chemotherapy, and retroperitoneal lymph node dissection. The management of stage I NSGCT has been risk-adapted based on pathologic features (histology and presence or absence of vascular invasion) of the primary tumor with a trend toward surveillance for compliant patients with low-risk features and chemotherapy for patients with high-risk features.[26] Recent data questioning the long-term morbidities of imaging-related ionizing radiation exposure, however, as well as the long-term morbidities of chemotherapy, have re-emphasized the importance of surgery.[27,28] Some of the advantages provided by RPLND include (1) definitive pathologic nodal staging, (2) removal of chemoresistant teratoma, and (3) therapeutic removal of viable GCT.

Despite advances in modern radiographic imaging techniques, the accurate staging of these patients remains challenging. Approximately 30% of patients who present with CS I disease harbor occult metastasis in the retroperitoneum after orchiectomy, and up to 35% of patients presenting with CS IIa disease have negative nodes at the time of RPLND.[29] This inaccuracy in staging results in both the undertreatment and the overtreatment of these patients and increases their long-term morbidity. RPLND allows for definitive nodal pathologic staging of patients with CS I or CS IIa NSGCT and provides critical information to guide further treatment and minimize treatment-related long-term morbidity.

In addition to improved staging, RPLND removes chemoresistant teratomatous elements. Failure to control the retroperitoneum during the initial treatment phase may compromise overall patient curability.[29] Additionally, retroperitoneal relapse is rare (2%) after a properly performed RPLND, thus eliminating the need for routine postoperative CT scanning, aside from a baseline scan. Although histologically described as benign, teratoma is biologically unpredictable and, when left unresected, possesses the potential to invade into adjacent organs (growing teratoma syndrome), undergo malignant transformation, and increase the risk of late relapse.[30–32] Late relapse is defined as disease recurrence more than 2 years after primary therapy and occurs in 2% to 3% of all patients with testicular cancer. Late relapse is associated with relatively poor survival, with approximately 50% of patients remaining free of disease.[32–34]

The therapeutic benefit of RPLND has been well established, providing a cure rate of 99% for patients with CS I NSGCT.[9,35,36] The retroperitoneum is the first site of metastatic spread in more than 90% of patients and metastatic testicular cancer to the retroperitoneum can be cured with surgery alone.[37] In a review of the literature, Stephenson and Sheinfeld[29] found RPLND, without subsequent chemotherapy, to be curative in 60% to 92% of patients with pathologic N1 disease. In patients with pathologic N2 disease, cure rates with surgery alone decreased to 50%; however, administration of 2 cycles of cisplatin-based adjuvant chemotherapy improved relapse-free survival rates to 98%.[29,35]

Clinical Stage IIa and IIb NSGCT

The management strategy for patients with CS IIa or CS IIb is dependent on many factors, including extent of disease, serum tumor marker levels, and presence or absence of tumor-related back pain.[2,29] Candidates best suited for RPLND include those patients with a single focus of retroperitoneal disease measuring less than or equal to 3 cm at the primary landing zone, patients with normal postorchiectomy markers, and patients without signs of tumor-related back pain.[2,29] Elevated tumor markers or tumor-related back pain may indicate metastatic systemic disease or unresectable disease and these patients should be considered for induction chemotherapy.

Stephenson and colleagues[36] reviewed the experience at MKSCC and identified important selection factors that have an impact on the risk of recurrence for patients undergoing primary RPLND. Elevated postorchiectomy markers ($P<.001$), CS ($P = .0002$), and pre-1999 RPLND ($P = .05$) were identified as independent pretreatment predictors of progression. Excluding patients with elevated tumor markers and patients with CS IIb disease improved 4-year relapse-free survival rates from 83% to 96% (95% CI, 79%–88% and 91%–100%; $P = .005$), increased the percentage of pN1 disease among patients who were pathologic stage II (64% vs 40%, $P = .01$), and did not affect the rate of retroperitoneal teratoma (21 vs

22%, P = .89). Patients with elevated tumor markers or CS IIb should be referred for induction chemotherapy.

After primary RPLND, accurate pathologic assessment is critical to assess prognosis and determine the need for adjuvant therapy. A select group of patients with pathologic stage II disease may benefit from receiving 2 cycles of adjuvant chemotherapy. The Testicular Cancer Intergroup Study randomized 195 patients who underwent RPLND with complete resection and pathologic stage II disease to receive either 2 cycles of adjuvant chemotherapy or observation. Their study showed a significant reduction in the risk of relapse after receiving adjuvant chemotherapy (6% vs 49%) but did not show any survival difference. The investigators were not able to show any difference between pathologic N1 versus N2 disease and attribute this to the small sample size.[38] The majority of other investigators, however, have demonstrated that the risk of relapse is dependent on the size and/or number of lymph node involvement. In general, observation is recommended for compliant patients with completely resected pathologic N1 disease and 2 cycles of adjuvant chemotherapy for patients with pathologic N2 or N3 disease. Chemotherapy cannot compensate for poor quality surgery, however. Two cycles of adjuvant chemotherapy should only be recommended for patients with complete resection of their retroperitoneal disease. Patients with incomplete resection should be referred for induction chemotherapy.[29]

Clinical Stage IIc and III NSGCT

Patients with CS IIc or CS III should receive induction cisplatin-based chemotherapy, based on IGCCG risk criteria.[10] Elevated tumor markers after primary induction chemotherapy often represent viable metastasis and second-line chemotherapy should be administered to these patients. The criteria for use of PC-RPLND have undergone continued refinement; however, most experts agree that PC-RPLND is indicated in the setting of normalized tumor markers with radiographic evidence of a residual retroperitoneal mass. Recent studies have demonstrated a histologic stage migration due to the use of more effective cisplatin-based chemotherapy regimens.[8] The histologic outcomes of patients who underwent induction chemotherapy followed by PC-RPLND have been reported as 45% fibrosis, 40% teratoma, and 15% viable GCT.[8] After second-line chemotherapy, histologic evaluation of PC-RPLND specimens revealed approximately 50% malignant GCT, 40% teratoma, and 10% fibrosis.[8] Several investigators have proposed predictive

models to determine the retroperitoneal pathology and avoid the morbidity of PC-RPLND in patients with necrosis or fibrosis. The accuracy of these models is limited and has ranged from 70% to 90% and, thus, bilateral PC-RPLND (with nerve sparing if feasible) remains the treatment of choice for these patients.[39–41] Similar to RPLND in the primary setting, PC-RPLND provides several advantages, including improved pathologic staging and removal of chemoresistant elements.

Clinicians have had difficulty differentiating between necrosis and teratoma or viable malignant GCT on postchemotherapy imaging. Thus, the radiographic criteria defining the "normal" retroperitoneum have varied widely among institutions. The controversy regarding management of small residual retroperitoneal masses is discussed later. Nonetheless, PC-RPLND provides definitive nodal staging to guide further treatment. Modern imaging cannot accurately stage the postchemotherapy retroperitoneum; thus, surgical resection of any radiographic abnormality is required to evaluate for the presence of malignant GCT or teratoma.

The removal of teratoma in the resected PC-RPLND specimen confers a survival benefit to the patient because of the unpredictable biology of teratoma. As discussed previously, there are several key benefits to removing residual teratoma in the retroperitoneum. First, teratoma may grow, obstruct, or invade into adjacent organs (growing teratoma syndrome) and become unresectable. Secondly, teratoma with malignant transformation is reported in 3% to 6% of men undergoing PC-RPLND. The incidence of malignant transformation increases to 12% to 18% in patients undergoing reoperative PC-RPLND for late relapse. In this scenario, complete surgical resection remains the treatment of choice.[31,42] Lastly, unresected residual teratoma may be associated with late relapse which, as discussed previously, is often chemoresistant, requiring surgical resection, and is often associated with poor outcomes.[42,43]

High-Risk PC-RPLND for NSGCT

Combined modality treatment for advanced GCTs has yielded improved outcomes; however, Donohue and associates have identified surgical scenarios where patients are at higher risk of relapse and experience lower survival rates: (1) PC-RPLND after salvage or second-line chemotherapy, (2) redo RPLND, (3) desperation RPLND, and (4) RPLND with viable cancer in resected specimen.

The first subset of patients includes patients who require salvage or second-line chemotherapy with subsequent normalization of tumor markers. PC-RPLND after salvage chemotherapy is technically difficult, due to desmoplastic reactions, and thus is associated with lower rates of complete resection and higher histologic proportions of viable cancer.[44] Furthermore, additional standard-dose chemotherapy does not seem to benefit the patients in this setting.[45]

The second subset of high-risk patients includes patients who undergo redo RPLND. McKiernan and colleagues[44] reviewed the experience at MSKCC and evaluated 56 patients who underwent redo operations for NSGCT, 22 after primary RPLND and 34 after PC-RPLND. Left-sided recurrence occurred more commonly and the sites of recurrence most commonly identified were at the left renal hilum and para-aortic regions, likely secondary to the technical demands necessary to gain adequate dissection in these regions. The overall 5-year survival rate for patients who underwent redo PC RPLND was 56%, thus underscoring the importance of initial complete resection. Data from MSKCC and Indiana University clearly demonstrate that patients who undergo incomplete initial resection and require redo RPLND are at a severe disadvantage, regardless of other risk factors.[46]

The third subset of high-risk patients includes patients who undergo desperation RPLND in the setting of persistently elevated serum tumor markers after chemotherapy. Elevated tumor markers after cisplatin-based chemotherapy are conventionally considered a contraindication to surgical therapy due to persistent presence of viable GCT. In a select subset of patients, however, RPLND may be curative in the setting of elevated tumor markers. Historic and contemporary series report a 20% to 55% 5-year survival rate after desperation RPLND, thus conferring some therapeutic benefit despite the elevated tumor markers.[47–50] Careful patient selection is critical, however, in determining which patients benefit from desperation RPLND. General indications include (1) stable or declining serum tumor markers, (2) radiographic resectable disease in 1 or 2 sites, and (3) resectable disease after exhausting salvage chemotherapy regimens.[50]

The last subset of high-risk patients includes patients with viable cancer in a resected specimen after RPLND. Patients who undergo first-line chemotherapy followed by complete resection during PC-RPLND with viable GCT currently receive 2 additional cycles of chemotherapy and achieve disease-free survival rates of up to 70%.[45] Fizazi and colleagues[51] recently challenged the role of adjuvant chemotherapy after completely resected GCT during PC-RPLND in a retrospective analysis of 146 patients. They identified 3 independent prognostic variables for

survival: (1) complete resection, (2) good risk IGCCCGT classification, and (3) less than 10% viable malignant cells. They concluded that additional chemotherapy benefited patients with 1 risk factor but not those with 2 or more risk factors. After salvage or second-line therapy, Fox and colleagues[45] reported that 2 additional cycles of chemotherapy, in the setting of viable GCT in the PC-RPLND specimen, did not have any additional therapeutic benefit. For patients with residual teratoma, complete surgical resection remains the treatment of choice.

CONTROVERSIES

Because testis cancer affects a young population with excellent life expectancy, the consideration of long-term toxicity with each treatment modality remains critical in patient management. Success in the multimodality treatment of testis cancer has allowed clinicians to focus their efforts on decreasing treatment-related morbidity. Attempts to minimize morbidity have led to several controversies regarding the surgical treatment of testis cancer: (1) Indications for PC-RPLND for patients with subcentimeter residual mass, (2) utilization of unilateral modified templates, and (3) utilization of laparoscopic (L)-RPLND.

Indications for PC-RPLND for Patients with Subcentimeter Residual Mass

The radiographic criteria defining the normal retroperitoneum vary among institutions and, thus, the radiographic size indication for PC-RPLND has been the subject of debate. Although the upper limit of normal has yet to be defined, several investigators have identified a significant presence of either viable GCT or teratoma in patients with subcentimeter retroperitoneal adenopathy. Steyerberg and colleagues[52] evaluated small retroperitoneal masses and found teratoma or viable GCT in 45% of lesions measuring 11 mm to 20 mm and 28% of lesions measuring 0 mm to 10 mm on CT imaging. In a study from MSKCC, Carver and colleagues[43] identified teratoma in 23% of patients with postchemotherapy masses measuring 1 cm or less.

More recently, Ehrlich and colleagues[53] reviewed their experience with 141 patients who underwent chemotherapy for metastatic NSGCT with radiographic complete response (residual mass <1 cm) and subsequent management with surveillance. Twelve patients experienced relapse with half recurring within the retroperitoneum and 5 patients experiencing late relapse. The investigator reported 15-year recurrence-free survival rates of 95% and 73% for good risk and intermediate-risk or poor-risk patients, respectively.[11] In a separate study, Kollmannsberger retrospectively reviewed 161 patients who achieved a complete response after chemotherapy for metastatic NSGCT and were followed with surveillance. Ten patients experienced relapse and, of these, 8 patients relapsed within the retroperitoneum. These investigators reported 100% disease-specific survival after a median follow-up of 52 months (3–135 months) in this cohort of patients.[54] These investigators conclude that patients who achieve a radiographic complete response after chemotherapy for metastatic NSGCT can be safely managed with surveillance.

Several considerations must be made before omitting PC-RPLND in patients with minimal residual masses after chemotherapy.[55] First, these 2 cohorts of patients include patients who would not routinely be recommended to undergo PC-RPLND, patients with stage III NSGCT without disease in the retroperitoneum before chemotherapy, and patients with CS IS disease. These patients should be excluded from both studies and, thus, the reported relapse rates could actually be higher than reported. Second, RPLND is a therapeutic procedure and, when performed in experienced centers, can be accomplished with minimal morbidity with the added benefit of minimizing the risk of in-field relapse. Unresected GCTs are likely to relapse and when discovered on surveillance after chemotherapy, are likely to be more chemoresistant. PC-RPLND could prevent the need for salvage chemotherapy and its associated morbidities. Third, deferring PC-RPLND until relapse assumes that growing teratoma remains resectable. In these series, 68% of patients who relapsed had teratoma progression, thus demonstrating the capacity of microscopic teratoma to grow. Even though Ehrlich and colleagues[53] reported an impressive median follow-up of 15.5 years, 74% of their cohort did not have teratoma in the primary tumor. Thus, their findings may not be consistent with other reported series. Kollmansberger and colleagues[54] reported the presence of teratoma in 40% of primary tumors; however, limited follow-up suggests that more late relapses are likely to occur. These considerations, as well as the identification of either teratoma or viable GCTs in a significant percentage of residual masses less than 1 cm, have led MSKCC to advocate PC-RPLND in select patients with detectable radiographic mass within the retroperitoneum after chemotherapy.

Unilateral Modified Template RPLND

The main objective of the unilateral modified RPLND template is to preserve the sympathetic innervation required for antegrade ejaculation. Modification of the RPLND template was not based on prospective randomized trials evaluating oncologic efficacy; rather, these modifications were based on retrospective mapping studies that may underestimate the true burden of disease.[56,57] Several studies have reported excellent functional outcomes, ranging from 51% to 88% preserved antegrade ejaculation; however, these studies must be critically evaluated due to limited or absence of follow-up and the administration of adjuvant chemotherapy for patients with viable disease.[9,58]

More recently, 2 studies from MSKCC evaluated the incidence of extratemplate disease in both the primary and the PC-RPLND setting. These studies challenge the oncologic equivalence of modified templates with bilateral RPLND. Eggener and colleagues[57] retrospectively evaluated the incidence of viable GCT or teratoma outside different modified RPLND templates in patients with CS I or CS IIa NSGCT. The distribution of metastases was evaluated in 191 patients with pathologic stage II disease and 3% to 23% of patients were found to have extratemplate disease, depending on the applied template. These results likely underestimate the extent of extratemplate disease because more than half of these patients received adjuvant chemotherapy. Due to the high incidence of extratemplate disease, the investigators concluded that more extensive, nerve-sparing bilateral RPLND templates optimize oncologic outcomes while preserving antegrade ejaculation.

In the postchemotherapy setting, Carver and colleagues[56] analyzed the incidence of extratemplate disease in 269 patients with advanced testis cancer. Viable GCT or teratoma was identified in 7% to 32% of patients depending on the boundaries of the modified template used. Modified template dissection also limits the anatomic regions of dissection. This can result in decreased numbers of lymph nodes removed and evaluated by pathologists, thus potentially increasing the risk for relapse for these patients.[25] The investigators concluded that a full bilateral RPLND should remain the primary surgical treatment after chemotherapy for advanced NSGCT.[43]

Based on these studies, modified template primary and PC-RPLND may leave residual tumor in a subset of patients and may result in an increased risk of disease recurrence and late relapse. The incidence of extratemplate nonteratomatous GCT in patients undergoing modified template RPLND exceeds the incidence of retroperitoneal relapse,[43,57,59] and this finding may be due to several factors. First, residual disease may be partially treated with postoperative adjuvant chemotherapy and thus reduce the incidence of retroperitoneal relapse. Secondly, as discussed previously, cross-sectional imaging of the retroperitoneum using modern CT scan carries a 30% false-negative rate as seen in CS I patients. Lastly, insufficient follow-up may exclude patients who recur as late relapse. In summary, these data indicate an increased risk of unresected retroperitoneal metastasis in patients undergoing unilateral modified template RPLND. Residual disease in the retroperitoneum may increase treatment burden and result in inferior oncologic outcomes. The authors believe that a bilateral template nerve-sparing RPLND increases control while minimizing treatment-related morbidity.

Laparoscopic RPLND

To decrease the morbidity of RPLND, several investigators have advocated the use of minimally invasive techniques in the treatment of testis cancer. L-RPLND is technically feasible in patients with CS I and, more recently, CS II patients; however, it is technically difficult and associated with a steep learning curve. In experienced hands, L-RPLND was associated with less postoperative pain, reduced blood loss, and shorter hospital stays. In its early stages, L-RPLND was performed as a diagnostic procedure without therapeutic intent. The procedure was aborted if positive lymph nodes were identified and virtually all of these patients received adjuvant chemotherapy, including patients with pathologic N1 disease.[60,61] As experience with L-RPLND increased, the procedure evolved from lymph node sampling to the mimicking of described open unilateral modified templates.[62,63] The potential consequences of incomplete RPLND have been discussed previously.[43] Viable GCT or teratoma in the uncontrolled retroperitoneum increases the risk of late relapse and increases the overall treatment burden for these patients.

More recently, L-RPLND has continued to evolve and bilateral nerve-sparing L-RPLND has been described. Steiner and colleagues[64] reported a small series of 42 patients with NSGCT, 23 primary L-RPLND, and 19 PC-L-RPLND, treated with bilateral nerve-sparing RPLND with therapeutic intent. Patients with pathologic N1 disease did not receive adjuvant chemotherapy. The investigators reported preservation of antegrade ejaculation in 85.7% and a relapse rate of 2.3% with no retroperitoneal recurrences. Follow-up was limited, however, to only 17.2 months and, thus, more relapses are likely to occur.

Despite short-term success, L-RPLND, even when using similar anatomic boundaries as open surgery, requires further long-term evaluation. The low lymph node counts in many reports of L-RPLND are concerning. In a recent meta-analysis, Rassweiller and colleagues[65] reported mean lymph node counts for patients undergoing L-RPLND to be 16 (range 5–36 lymph nodes). As discussed previously, the total number of lymph nodes removed is associated with the diagnostic efficacy of RPLND (recommended removal of >40 LNs) and is also an independent predictor of disease recurrence.[24,25] Pizzocaro and colleagues[11] reported the long-term results of L-RPLND and identified 2 unusual cases of liver metastasis a few months after L-RPLND. The effect of pneumoperitoneum on GCTs remains unknown and further investigation is warranted (**Fig. 1**).

The application of L-RPLND is continually evolving and what began as a staging procedure is only now undergoing evaluation for therapeutic efficacy. In its current state, the data supporting L-RPLND are limited by small sample size and short follow-up. The technical equivalence has yet to be established and the unusual sites of metastasis are potentially concerning. In attempting to minimize the morbidity of RPLND, the oncologic outcome of L-RPLND must be compared with the gold standard bilateral nerve-sparing RPLND.

COMPLICATIONS

Contemporary surgical and anesthetic techniques as well as use of standardized postoperative pathways have minimized major complications during primary RPLND, especially when performed at tertiary care centers by experienced surgeons.[52] Historically, overall complication rates for primary RPLND has been reported as 10.6% compared with 20% to 35% for PC-RPLND.[66] The most common major complications encountered with RPLND include chylous ascites, pulmonary complications, renovascular injury, and mechanical small bowel obstruction.

Chylous ascites occurs in 2% to 7% of patients and usually resolves with conservative management, including low-fat diet, diuretics, total parenteral nutrition, or paracentesis.[67,68] In a minority of cases, however, rapid or refractory ascites requires peritoneovenous shunting for definitive treatment.[68]

The majority of pulmonary complications after RPLND are minor in nature and resolve with aggressive pulmonary physiotherapy; however, major pulmonary complications can occur, especially in patients who receive bleomycin. Patients who received bleomycin should undergo preoperative pulmonary function testing and if a diffusion

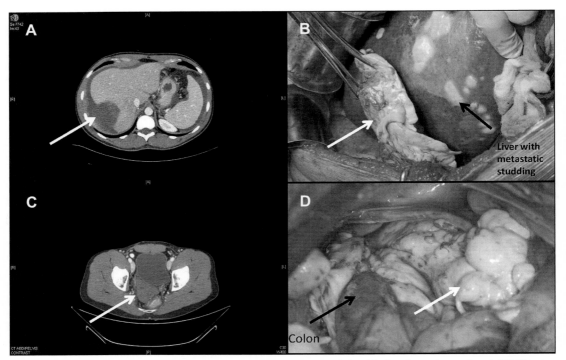

Fig. 1. A 30-year-old man presented with CS IB NSGCT status post. Right-sided unilateral template L-RPLND at an outside facility. At 4 months' postoperatively, patient was found to have diffuse liver metastasis, carcinomatosis, and a frozen pelvis (*white arrows*) (*A, C*). He underwent high-dose chemotherapy and stem cell transplantation followed by desperation surgery (*B, D*), including metastasectomy, partial hepatectomy, right diaphragm resection, splenectomy, ileocecal resection, and intraperitoneal chemotherapy port placement. Pathology revealed multiple nodules of mature teratoma and the patient's current status as no evidence of disease.

defect is identified, should be managed by an experienced anesthesia team using judicious fluid management and the lowest fraction of inspired oxygen possible to maintain oxygenation. Postoperative fluid management should continue to be carefully managed and should preferentially use colloid over crystalloid.[66]

The rates of renovascular injury have decreased after the institution of a bilateral infrahilar surgical template and the rates of small bowel obstruction have remained low over time. Other complications of RPLND include atelectasis, superficial wound infection, retrograde ejaculation, and prolonged ileus. These complications usually resolve with conservative management.

SUMMARY

RPLND is an integral component in the multimodality treatment of testicular cancer. For patients with low-stage or high-stage testicular cancer, RPLND remains a diagnostic as well as a therapeutic procedure. Continued advancements in surgical technique and perioperative care have allowed RPLND to be performed safely with minimal short-term and long-term morbidity, especially in high-volume centers. Future refinements in this technique must evaluate the potential oncologic implications compared with open bilateral nerve-sparing RPLND.

REFERENCES

1. Jemal A, Siegel R, Xu J, et al. Cancer statistics, 2010. CA Cancer J Clin 2010;60(5):277–300.
2. Bosl GJ, Motzer RJ. Testicular germ-cell cancer. N Engl J Med 1997;337(4):242–53.
3. Jamieson JK, Dobson JF. On the injection of lymphatics by prussian blue. J Anat Physiol 1910; 45(Pt 1):7–10.
4. Donohue JP, Zachary JM, Maynard BR. Distribution of nodal metastases in nonseminomatous testis cancer. J Urol 1982;128(2):315–20.
5. Weissbach L, Boedefeld EA. Localization of solitary and multiple metastases in stage II nonseminomatous testis tumor as basis for a modified staging lymph node dissection in stage I. J Urol 1987;138(1):77–82.
6. Ray B, Hajdu SI, Whitmore WF Jr. Proceedings: distribution of retroperitoneal lymph node

metastases in testicular germinal tumors. Cancer 1974;33(2):340–8.

7. Sogani PC. Evolution of the management of stage I nonseminomatous germ-cell tumors of the testis. Urol Clin North Am 1991;18(3):561–73.

8. Sheinfeld JB, Bartsch G, Bosl G. Surgery for testicular tumors. In: Wein AJ, editor. Campbell-Walsh urology. 9th edition. Philadelphia: Saunders Elsevier; 2007. p. 936–64.

9. Donohue JP, Thornhill JA, Foster RS, et al. Retroperitoneal lymphadenectomy for clinical stage A testis cancer (1965 to 1989): modifications of technique and impact on ejaculation. J Urol 1993; 149(2):237–43.

10. International Germ Cell Consensus Classification: a prognostic factor-based staging system for metastatic germ cell cancers. International Germ Cell Cancer Collaborative Group. J Clin Oncol 1997; 15(2):594–603.

11. Pizzocaro G, Schiavo M, Solima S, et al. Long-term results of laparoscopic retroperitoneal lymph node dissection (RPLND) in low-stage nonseminomatous germ-cell testicular tumors (NSGCTT) performed by a senior surgeon: 1999-2003. Urologia 2010; 77(Suppl 17):50–6 [in Italian].

12. Jewett MA, Groll RJ. Nerve-sparing retroperitoneal lymphadenectomy [abstract viii]. Urol Clin North Am 2007;34(2):149–58.

13. Lange PH, Narayan P, Fraley EE. Fertility issues following therapy for testicular cancer. Semin Urol 1984;2(4):264–74.

14. Sheinfeld J. Nonseminomatous germ cell tumors of the testis: current concepts and controversies. Urology 1994;44(1):2–14.

15. Sheinfeld J, Herr HW. Role of surgery in management of germ cell tumor. Semin Oncol 1998;25(2):203–9.

16. Fossa SD, Klepp O, Ous S, et al. Unilateral retroperitoneal lymph node dissection in patients with non-seminomatous testicular tumor in clinical stage I. Eur Urol 1984;10(1):17–23.

17. Pizzocaro G, Salvioni R, Zanoni F. Unilateral lymphadenectomy in intraoperative stage I nonseminomatous germinal testis cancer. J Urol 1985;134(3):485–9.

18. Donohue JP, Foster RS, Rowland RG, et al. Nerve-sparing retroperitoneal lymphadenectomy with preservation of ejaculation. J Urol 1990;144(2 Pt 1):287–91 [discussion: 291–2].

19. Richie JP. Clinical stage 1 testicular cancer: the role of modified retroperitoneal lymphadenectomy. J Urol 1990;144(5):1160–3.

20. Jewett MA, Kong YS, Goldberg SD, et al. Retroperitoneal lymphadenectomy for testis tumor with nerve sparing for ejaculation. J Urol 1988;139(6):1220–4.

21. Pettus J. Preservation of ejaculation in patients undergoing nerve-sparing postchemotherapy retroperitoneal lymph node dissection for metastatic testicular cancer. Urology 2009;73(2):328–31.

22. Koppie TM, Vickers AJ, Vora K, et al. Standardization of pelvic lymphadenectomy performed at radical cystectomy: can we establish a minimum number of lymph nodes that should be removed? Cancer 2006;107(10):2368–74.

23. Ludwig MS, Goodman M, Miller DL, et al. Postoperative survival and the number of lymph nodes sampled during resection of node-negative non-small cell lung cancer. Chest 2005;128(3):1545–50.

24. Thompson RH, Carver B, Bosl G, et al. Evaluation of lymph node counts in primary retroperitoneal lymph node dissection. Cancer 2010;116(22):5243–50.

25. Carver B, Cronin A, Eggener S, et al. The total number of retroperitoneal lymph nodes resected impacts clinical outcome after chemotherapy for metastatic testicular cancer. Urology 2010;75(6):1431–5.

26. Choueiri TK, Stephenson AJ, Gilligan T, et al. Management of clinical stage I nonseminomatous germ cell testicular cancer. Urol Clin North Am 2007;34(2):137–48 [abstract: viii].

27. Tarin TV, Sonn G, Shinghal R. Estimating the risk of cancer associated with imaging related radiation during surveillance for stage I testicular cancer using computerized tomography. J Urol 2009; 181(2):627–32 [discussion: 632–3].

28. Chamie K, Kurzrock EA, Evans CP, et al. Secondary malignancies among nonseminomatous germ cell tumor cancer survivors. Cancer 2011;117(18): 4219–30.

29. Stephenson AJ, Sheinfeld J. The role of retroperitoneal lymph node dissection in the management of testicular cancer. Urol Oncol 2004;22(3):225–33.

30. Logothetis CJ, Samuels ML, Trindade A, et al. The growing teratoma syndrome. Cancer 1982;50(8): 1629–35.

31. Motzer RJ, Amsterdam A, Prieto V, et al. Teratoma with malignant transformation: diverse malignant histologies arising in men with germ cell tumors. J Urol 1998;159(1):133–8.

32. Baniel J, Foster RS, Einhorn LH, et al. Late relapse of clinical stage I testicular cancer. J Urol 1995;154(4): 1370–2.

33. Dieckmann KP, Albers P, Classen J, et al. Late relapse of testicular germ cell neoplasms: a descriptive analysis of 122 cases. J Urol 2005;173(3): 824–9.

34. George DW, Foster RS, Hromas RA, et al. Update on late relapse of germ cell tumor: a clinical and molecular analysis. J Clin Oncol 2003;21(1):113–22.

35. Kondagunta GV, Sheinfeld J, Mazumdar M, et al. Relapse-free and overall survival in patients with pathologic stage II nonseminomatous germ cell cancer treated with etoposide and cisplatin adjuvant chemotherapy. J Clin Oncol 2004;22(3):464–7.

36. Stephenson AJ, Bosl GJ, Motzer RJ, et al. Retroperitoneal lymph node dissection for nonseminomatous germ cell testicular cancer: impact of patient

selection factors on outcome. J Clin Oncol 2005; 23(12):2781–8.

37. Whitmore WF Jr. Surgical treatment of adult germinal testis tumors. Semin Oncol 1979;6(1):55–68.

38. Williams SD, Stablein DM, Einhorn LH, et al. Immediate adjuvant chemotherapy versus observation with treatment at relapse in pathological stage II testicular cancer. N Engl J Med 1987;317(23):1433–8.

39. Debono DJ, Heilman DK, Einhorn LH, et al. Decision analysis for avoiding postchemotherapy surgery in patients with disseminated nonseminomatous germ cell tumors. J Clin Oncol 1997;15(4):1455–64.

40. Donohue JP, Rowland RG, Kopecky K, et al. Correlation of computerized tomographic changes and histological findings in 80 patients having radical retroperitoneal lymph node dissection after chemotherapy for testis cancer. J Urol 1987;137(6):1176–9.

41. Vergouwe Y, Steyerberg EW, Foster RS, et al. Validation of a prediction model and its predictors for the histology of residual masses in nonseminomatous testicular cancer. J Urol 2001;165(1):84–8 [discussion: 88].

42. Baniel J, Foster RS, Gonin R, et al. Late relapse of testicular cancer. J Clin Oncol 1995;13(5):1170–6.

43. Carver BS, Bianco FJ Jr, Shayegan B, et al. Predicting teratoma in the retroperitoneum in men undergoing post-chemotherapy retroperitoneal lymph node dissection. J Urol 2006;176(1):100–3 [discussion: 103–4].

44. McKiernan JM, Motzer RJ, Bajorin DF, et al. Reoperative retroperitoneal surgery for nonseminomatous germ cell tumor: clinical presentation, patterns of recurrence, and outcome. Urology 2003;62(4):732–6.

45. Fox EP, Weathers TD, Williams SD, et al. Outcome analysis for patients with persistent nonteratomatous germ cell tumor in postchemotherapy retroperitoneal lymph node dissections. J Clin Oncol 1993; 11(7):1294–9.

46. Donohue JP, Leviovitch I, Foster RS, et al. Integration of surgery and systemic therapy: results and principles of integration. Semin Urol Oncol 1998; 16(2):65–71.

47. Wood DP Jr, Herr HW, Motzer RJ, et al. Surgical resection of solitary metastases after chemotherapy in patients with nonseminomatous germ cell tumors and elevated serum tumor markers. Cancer 1992; 70(9):2354–7.

48. Eastham JA, Wilson TG, Russell C, et al. Surgical resection in patients with nonseminomatous germ cell tumor who fail to normalize serum tumor markers after chemotherapy. Urology 1994;43(1):74–80.

49. Murphy BR, Breeden ES, Donohue JP, et al. Surgical salvage of chemorefractory germ cell tumors. J Clin Oncol 1993;11(2):324–9.

50. Beck SD, Foster RS, Bihrle R, et al. Pathologic findings and therapeutic outcome of desperation post-chemotherapy retroperitoneal lymph node dissection in advanced germ cell cancer. Urol Oncol 2005;23(6):423–30.

51. Fizazi K, Tjulandin S, Salvioni R, et al. Viable malignant cells after primary chemotherapy for disseminated nonseminomatous germ cell tumors: prognostic factors and role of postsurgery chemotherapy–results from an international study group. J Clin Oncol 2001; 19(10):2647–57.

52. Steyerberg EW, Keizer HJ, Fossa SD, et al. Prediction of residual retroperitoneal mass histology after chemotherapy for metastatic nonseminomatous germ cell tumor: multivariate analysis of individual patient data from six study groups. J Clin Oncol 1995;13(5):1177–87.

53. Ehrlich Y, Brames M, Beck S, et al. Long-term follow-up of cisplatin combination chemotherapy in patients with disseminated nonseminomatous germ cell tumors: is a post-chemotherapy retroperitoneal lymph node dissection needed after complete remission? J Clin Oncol 2010;28(4):531–6.

54. Kollmannsberger C, Daneshmand S, So A, et al. Management of disseminated nonseminomatous germ cell tumors with risk-based chemotherapy followed by response-guided postchemotherapy surgery. J Clin Oncol 2010;28(4):537–42.

55. Bosl GJ, Motzer RJ. Weighing risks and benefits of postchemotherapy retroperitoneal lymph node dissection: not so easy. J Clin Oncol 2010;28(4):519–21.

56. Carver BS, Shayegan B, Eggener S, et al. Incidence of metastatic nonseminomatous germ cell tumor outside the boundaries of a modified postchemotherapy retroperitoneal lymph node dissection. J Clin Oncol 2007;25(28):4365–9.

57. Eggener SE, Carver BS, Sharp DS, et al. Incidence of disease outside modified retroperitoneal lymph node dissection templates in clinical stage I or IIA nonseminomatous germ cell testicular cancer. J Urol 2007;177(3):937–42 [discussion: 942–3].

58. Weissbach L, Boedefeld EA, Horstmann-Dubral B. Surgical treatment of stage-I non-seminomatous germ cell testis tumor. Final results of a prospective multicenter trial 1982–1987. Testicular Tumor Study Group. Eur Urol 1990;17(2):97–106.

59. Beck SD, Foster RS, Bihrle R, et al. Is full bilateral retroperitoneal lymph node dissection always necessary for postchemotherapy residual tumor? Cancer 2007;110(6):1235–40.

60. Janetschek G, Reissigl A, Peschel R, et al. Diagnostic laparoscopic retroperitoneal lymph node dissection for non seminomatous testicular tumor. Ann Urol (Paris) 1995;29(2):81–90.

61. Bhayani SB, Ong A, Oh WK, et al. Laparoscopic retroperitoneal lymph node dissection for clinical stage I nonseminomatous germ cell testicular cancer: a long-term update. Urology 2003;62(2):324–7.

62. Allaf ME, Bhayani SB, Link RE, et al. Laparoscopic retroperitoneal lymph node dissection: duplication of open technique. Urology 2005;65(3):575–7.

63. Nelson JB, Chen RN, Bishoff JT, et al. Laparoscopic retroperitoneal lymph node dissection for clinical stage I nonseminomatous germ cell testicular tumors. Urology 1999;54(6):1064–7.

64. Steiner H, Zangerl F, Sthr B, et al. Results of bilateral nerve sparing laparoscopic retroperitoneal lymph node dissection for testicular cancer. J Urol 2008; 180(4):1348–52.

65. Rassweiller J, Scheitlin W, Heidenreich A, et al. Laparoscopic retroperitoneal lymph node dissection: does it still have a role in the management of clinical stage I nonseminomatous testis cancer?

A European Perspective. Eur Urol 2008;54(5): 1004–15.

66. Baniel J, Foster RS, Rowland RG, et al. Complications of post-chemotherapy retroperitoneal lymph node dissection. J Urol 1995;153(3):976–80.

67. Baniel J, Sella A. Complications of retroperitoneal lymph node dissection in testicular cancer: primary and post-chemotherapy. Semin Surg Oncol 1999;17(4):263–7.

68. Evans JG, Spiess PE, Kamat AM, et al. Chylous ascites after post-chemotherapy retroperitoneal lymph node dissection: review of the M. D. Anderson experience. J Urol 2006;176(4 Pt 1):1463–7.

Minimally Invasive Retroperitoneal Lymph Node Dissection for Testicular Cancer

Ornob P. Roy, MD, MBA, Brian D. Duty, MD*,
Louis R. Kavoussi, MD, MBA

KEYWORDS

- Testicular cancer • Lymph node dissection • Laparoscopy
- Retroperitoneal • Germ cell tumor

This article is not certified for *AMA PRA Category 1 Credit*™ because product brand names are included in the educational content. The Accreditation Council for Continuing Medical Education requires the use of generic names and or drug/product classes as the required nomenclature for therapeutic options in continuing medical education.
For more information, please go to www.accme.org and review the Standards of Commercial Support.

Testicular cancer is the most common solid organ malignancy in young men between the ages of 15 and 35. With proper multimodal therapy, cure rates have increased dramatically over the last 40 years to greater than 90% overall survival.[1] Although much of this increase in survival can be attributed to improvements in systemic chemotherapy, surgery retains a critical role in the diagnostic and therapeutic management of testicular cancer.

Histologically, all testicular cancer can be classified into germ cell and nongerm cell. Nongerm cell tumors do not exhibit typical, predictable retroperitoneal metastasis and are not the focus of this article. Germ cell tumors (GCT) are further divided into 2 groups, seminomatous and nonseminomatous.

The spread of GCTs is well described and highly predictable. Beginning within the parenchyma of the testis, the tumor cells can rapidly metastasize into the retroperitoneal lymph nodes. Laterality does predict which lymph nodes in the retroperitoneum are likely to be affected. This pattern of lymphatic spread allows for the creation of lateralized templates for localized therapy (**Figs. 1–3**).

In seminomatous GCTs, radiotherapy plays a prominent role in treatment of retroperitoneal disease. These tumor cells are highly radiosensitive; therefore, they are often treated with radiation to the retroperitoneum for low-stage disease. Other options for low-stage (American Joint Committee on Cancer Stage 1, 2a, and 2b), seminomatous GCT include close observation protocols and

The authors have nothing to disclose.
Department of Urology, North Shore Long Island Jewish Health System, The Smith Institute for Urology, 450 Lakeville Road, Suite M41, New Hyde Park, NY 11040, USA
* Corresponding author.
E-mail address: dutybd@me.com

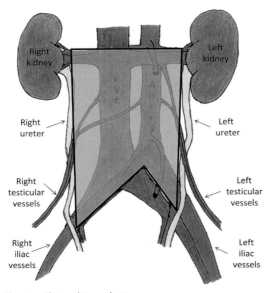

Fig. 1. Bilateral template.

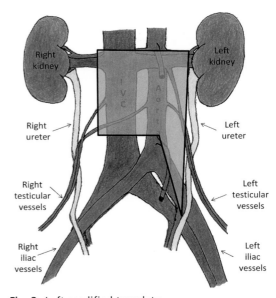

Fig. 3. Left modified template.

single-agent chemotherapy. For higher-stage disease, multiagent chemotherapy is routinely used.

For nonseminomatous GCT's (NSGCT), radiotherapy is not an option. After orchiectomy, therapeutic options are limited to close surveillance,[2] chemotherapy, or retroperitoneal lymph node dissection.[3] In choosing between these options, many factors, such as morbidity, cost, reliability, patient preference, and ability to tolerate surgery or nephrotoxic agents are increasingly important.[4]

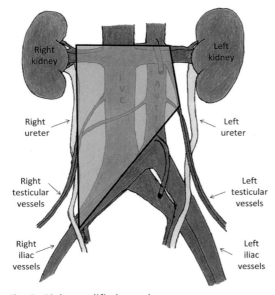

Fig. 2. Right modified template.

Retroperitoneal lymph node dissection (RPLND) provides essential staging information, which will in turn determine further therapeutic options. In certain patients, RPLND can also be therapeutic.[5] For example, it eliminates the primary landing zone in clinical stage 1 patients and ensures complete removal of all residual retroperitoneal tissue after chemotherapy.

However, only 30% of patients who are clinical stage 1 for NSGCT show any positive nodes after RPLND.[5] This could represent considerable overtreatment with a procedure that could cause considerable morbidities. Traditional open RPLND is associated with a large abdominal incision (xyphoid process to pubic symphysis) and several days of postoperative hospital stay. In addition, patients can potentially experience ejaculatory dysfunction due to dissection around the sympathetic nerves, although these rates have significantly decreased with the advent of nerve-sparing RPLND.

With the advent and widespread adoption of laparoscopic surgery, laparoscopic RPLND (L-RPLND) is increasingly being used as a treatment option for NSGCT. Aside from the obvious advantage of improved cosmesis from smaller incisions and shorter postoperative hospital stay,[6] laparoscopy offers a highly magnified view of delicate retroperitoneal structures such as the sympathetic nerve plexuses. A recent meta-analysis suggests equivalent rates of staging accuracy and long-term disease-specific survival to open RPLND.[7] Despite increased operating room time often required for this approach (204 vs 186 minutes in the recent meta-analysis), L-RPLND demonstrates benefits in length of stay, postoperative pain, and overall complication rates.[7] With experience, therapeutic dissections equivalent to open surgery are achievable.

INDICATIONS

All patients with testicular cancer diagnosed after orchiectomy should have a complete metastatic evaluation. This includes comprehensive serum chemistries, liver function tests, bone scan, and computerized tomography of the chest, abdomen, and pelvis. Serum tumor markers specific to testicular cancer, namely α-fetoprotein, β-human chorionic gonadotropin, and lactate dehydrogenase, should be obtained after sufficient time for normalization following orchiectomy.

Current indications for RPLND are for patients with stage 1, stage 2a, and a subset of patients with low-volume stage 2b NSGCT. The procedure serves as a diagnostic procedure to stage the disease. In addition, given that most metastatic disease is confined to the retroperitoneum, excision of all retroperitoneal nodal tissue can be therapeutic. In a diagnostic capacity, RPNLD can identify patients with no evidence of lymphatic disease within the template of nodes removed. This can be very beneficial in patients who wish to avoid the toxicities associated with chemotherapy. However, in these patients, up to 10% will develop extraretroperitoneal recurrences, and they still require long-term imaging follow-up, especially in the chest and mediastinum.[8]

RPLND not only has a role in primary treatment after diagnostic orchiectomy, but also as a salvage treatment option after chemotherapy.[9] A common problem for the clinician is the residual retroperitoneal mass after chemotherapy for testicular cancer. Upon excision of residual masses after chemotherapy, approximately 40% will contain teratoma, and 20% will contain viable tumor, both requiring excision for cure. The remaining 40% will have necrotic tissue. Unfortunately, current imaging techniques are unable to reliably differentiate necrotic tissue from teratoma or viable tumor.

Patients not suitable for RPLND include those who have clinical stage 2 NSGCT with elevated tumor markers, because this usually reflects systemic disease.[1] Also indicative of systemic disease is the presence of enlarged lymph nodes in the suprahilar, retrocrural, pelvic, inguinal, or contralateral areas. In addition, when considering L-RPLND, patients with a bleeding diathesis, bulky lymphadenopathy, or active peritoneal or abdominal wall infection should be avoided. Also, in postchemotherapy patients undergoing L-RPLND, the dense scar tissue can make laparoscopic dissection challenging. Subsequently, higher rates of conversion to open RPLND are seen in this population.[9]

PREPARATION

Patients should be extensively counseled about the various treatment options available, including initial chemotherapy, surgery, and when appropriate, surveillance. A thorough discussion of known complications should include damage to the gastrointestinal tract, kidneys, liver, and pancreas. In addition, manipulation of the sympathetic chain may cause postoperative neurologic complications and ejaculatory disturbance. Consequently, patients should be encouraged to pursue preoperative sperm banking if interested in having biologic children.

Some have advocated starting patients on a low-fat diet 2 weeks before surgery to reduce the chance of chylous ascites. The day before surgery, a mechanical bowel prep is very helpful, and if anticipating multiple adhesions, a full bowel preparation should be considered. Type and screen are essential for all patients.

Postchemotherapy patients present special challenges due to the widespread use of bleomycin, which can put patients at risk for pulmonary fibrosis. This bleomycin-induced pulmonary fibrosis can cause multiple postoperative difficulties with respiration and ventilation, most notably for acute respiratory distress syndrome (ARDS). Thorough screening with pulmonary function testing and possible consultation with a pulmonologist preoperatively should be considered. In these patients, intraoperative intravenous fluid administration should be closely monitored due to the increased postoperative pulmonary difficulties.

It is also important to remember the effects of myelosuppression when planning the timing of surgery after chemotherapy. A period of at least 5 weeks should pass for proper cellular regeneration before surgery. In addition, the use of nephrotoxic agents should be limited in patients who have undergone cisplatin-based chemotherapeutic regimens.

OPERATING ROOM SETUP

The surgeon stands on the contralateral side of dissection and is encouraged to use a self-retaining laparoscopic camera-holding device (robotic or mechanical) to prevent crowding from the assistant. Monitors are placed on each side, so both surgeon and assistant have unobstructed, ergonomic viewing angles of the images. A full laparoscopic tray, including vascular instruments, should be available. In addition, a full open vascular tray should be in the operating room and immediately available for timely conversion to the open procedure if necessary.

PATIENT POSITIONING

As is routine for all transperitoneal laparoscopic surgery, a urethral catheter and oral or nasogastric tube are placed in the intubated patient. Although some advocate for a slight elevation (modified flank) of the ipsilateral side for a unilateral template approach, the authors use supine positioning. An operating table with adequate airplaning or bilateral rotational ability provides sufficient lateral angle to use gravity for bowel retraction. This expedites transition to a full bilateral template without having to reposition the patient if gross lymphatic disease is encountered during exploration. Sequential compression devices are placed on the lower extremities, and both arms are tucked to the sides. The patient is padded appropriately over pressure points and secured to the table with multiple layers of wide adhesive tape over the chest, hips, and lower extremities.

Draping and preparing involve the area from the xyphoid process superiorly to the upper thighs inferiorly and the full girth of the abdomen laterally exposed in the surgical field.

LAPAROSCOPIC ACCESS

Transperitoneal access allows greater working space, a more familiar anatomic view for most urologists, and greater flexibility in placement of additional ports. Either Veress needle or Hasson technique is sufficient for initial peritoneal access. For Veress needle access, the umbilicus is the ideal access point. If there is previous surgery at that site (laparoscopic or otherwise), left upper quadrant and right lower quadrant are excellent alternative access points. The body wall is elevated away from intraperitoneal structures using the surgeon's nondominant hand (or towel clips if this is difficult). The needle is passed through the abdominal wall and after 2 or 3 clicks should slide easily up and down with minimal resistance. To confirm placement before insufflations, a saline water-drop test may be performed. Once insufflation is initiated, the surgeon must carefully follow the intra-abdominal pressure on the insufflation equipment. If initially the pressure is high (>10 mm Hg), consider replacing the needle. Insufflate to a pressure of 15 to 20 mm Hg for placement of additional trocars, and reduce to 15 mm Hg to begin the dissection.

A 1 cm incision is made adjacent to the umbilicus, and subcutaneous fat is bluntly separated. A 10 mm trocar is then placed using the Visiport technique, where a zero-degree laparoscope placed into the clear-tipped trocar is guided into the peritoneum under vision. Once intraperitoneal, this lens is replaced with a 30° angled lens.

For the Hasson technique, a 10 to 12 mm incision is made adjacent to the umbilicus and the subcutaneous tissues bluntly separated. Two 2-0 sutures are placed on opposite sides of the ensuing fascial incision, and these are used to elevated the body wall away from abdominal viscera. The fascia is incised using a scalpel for 1 cm. Careful dissection through the underlying tissue is performed, and metzenbaum scissors are used to incise the underlying fascial layers and peritoneum. Once into the peritoneum, air should rush into this potential space, dropping the viscera below. The Hasson port is then placed through this access site and secured in place using the 2 stay sutures mentioned previously.

Three additional 10 mm laparoscopic ports are then placed in the midline under laparoscopic guidance (**Fig. 4**). They should be spaced approximately equidistant from each other, with the most superior port 2 cm inferior to the xyphoid process and the most inferior port 3 cm above the pubic symphysis. A lateral 5 mm port may be used to assist in dissection of the distal remnant of the spermatic cord.

The ipsilateral side is then elevated to the maximal safe angle by turning the operating table, and slight Trendelenburg is applied to assist with gravitational bowel retraction. In most cases, additional bowel retraction is necessary and can be provided using a paddle placed through the most inferior port.

TECHNIQUE FOR RIGHT TEMPLATE DISSECTION

For unilateral dissections, a modified template is employed (see **Fig. 2**). Borders of the template

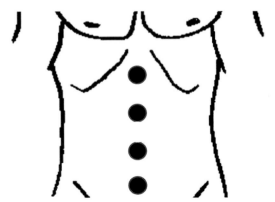

Fig. 4. Trocar placement for L-RPLND. Four 10 mm trocars are placed in the midline evenly spaced from the xyphoid process to the pubic symphysis.

include the right renal vein superiorly, the right ureter laterally, and the bifurcation of the right iliac artery inferiorly. Medially, all paracaval, interaorto-caval, and anterior aortic tissues are removed. First, the ascending colon is mobilized medially by incising the white line of Toldt from the medial umbilical ligament inferiorly to the hepatic flexure. It is important to minimize spread of electrical energy during mobilization. Judicious use of endo-scopic monopolar scissors or a bipolar cutting device minimizes bleeding. Superomedially, the posterior peritoneum is opened subhepatically to the inferior vena cava (IVC). The duodenum is mobilized medially by using a cold scissors to divide the colorenal ligaments, thereby performing the Kocher maneuver.

Next, the spermatic cord (SC) is dissected free. It is easy to identify at the level of the internal inguinal ring, and the peritoneum around it is divided here. The vas deferens is identified, clip-ped, and divided. The SC is then separated from attachments within the inguinal ring and canal until identifying the marking suture left after radical or-chiectomy. It is important to avoid damage to the inferior epigastric vessels during this dissection. Once identified and separated from the inguinal canal, the SC is completely freed distally. Dissect-ing proximally, the SC is traced to and separated from the ureter, then dissected along its lateral border to its insertion into the IVC. At its origin, the testicular vein is clipped and divided. The testicular artery is then followed medially toward the aorta, where it is clipped and divided. The entire SC is then placed in an entrapment sac and extracted.

While at the origin of the right testicular vein, the adventitia of the IVC is elevated and incised. Supe-riorly, this incision of the adventitia is carried toward the renal vein, and inferiorly to the bifurca-tion of the iliac vessels. Beginning at the level of the ureter crossing over the iliacs, lymphatic tissue is then lifted laterally toward the ureter, and its underlying attachments are clipped and divided. While dividing any lymphatic attachments, liberal use of clips is advised. Traveling up the iliacs toward the IVC, the lymphatic tissue is kept intact and lifted off its medial attachments and divided. Next, the packet is retracted cephalad and sepa-rated without the use of any cautery off of the underlying posterior wall and sympathetic trunk and branches. This carries the dissection posterior to the lateral portion of the IVC.

Next, at the bifurcation of the aorta, the left border of the aorta is identified, and the anterior lymphatic tissue is retracted toward the IVC. This dissection is then carried superiorly up the lateral surface of the aorta, taking care to identify and preserve the left renal artery. The tissue is then swept medially off the anterior surface of the aorta and separated from the medial and posterior surface of the aorta. At the superior margin, it is important to identify and preserve the right renal artery. During this dissection, multiple lumber arteries may be encountered; these should be clip-ped and divided. If an accessory right renal artery is identified during the lateral dissection, this should be preserved. Posteriorly, the border of dissection is the anterior spinous ligament.

Next, as the lymphatic packet is swept toward the IVC, the entire IVC is gently elevated anteriorly, and lymphatic channels and lumbar veins are clip-ped and divided. As the dissection moves laterally behind the IVC, the packet's only remaining attachment should be to the previously dissected lateral lymphatic tissue. Finally, the right ureter is lifted laterally; the lymphatic tissue underneath is swept off the ureter medially up to the level of the renal hilum. The packet(s) are placed in an entrapment sac and extracted.

If grossly positive nodes were encountered, the operation should transition and proceed with a left-sided template dissection (see **Fig. 3**). If no grossly positive nodes were encountered, the lymph node dissection ends here. Careful inspec-tion for lymphatic leak should focus on areas of pooling of chylous liquid. Any open lymphatic vessel should be clipped. Suture passers with size 0 absorbable sutures are used with laparo-scopic guidance to close all ports 10 mm or greater. All ports are then removed, port sites closed using the preplaced sutures, and sites vigorously irri-gated. Skin is closed using absorbable 4-0 sutures.

TECHNIQUE FOR LEFT TEMPLATE DISSECTION

The borders of the left modified template dissec-tion are the left ureter laterally, left renal hilum superiorly, vena cava medially, and bifurcation of the iliac arteries inferiorly (see **Fig. 3**). The white line of Toldt is incised from the spleen superiorly to the bifurcation of the iliacs inferiorly. As the colon is mobilized medially, the splenophrenic and splenorenal attachments are divided. In addi-tion, the tail of the pancreas is identified and bluntly moved medially.

Next, the left internal inguinal ring is identified, and the SC remnant with tagging suture is dissected free in a manner similar to the technique in the right-sided dissection, while identifying and separating the SC from the ureter. One difference is as the left testicular vein is dissected superiorly, it is followed to the left renal vein, and clipped and divided here. The SC is then placed in an entrap-ment sac and extracted.

The paraortic node dissection is then initiated by dividing the adventitia overlying the aorta at the level of the renal hilum. This tissue is divided along the anterior surface of the aorta moving inferiorly toward the inferior mesenteric artery (IMA), which is identified and preserved. The dissection continues inferiorly along the left iliac artery until encountering the ureter, which is preserved and is the inferolateral limit of the packet. The dissection then resumes at the renal hilum, where the tissue medial to the anterior surface is split and rolled medially and separated from the medial surface of the aorta and the anterior spinal ligament. Care is taken to preserve sympathetic nerves seen in this location. The right renal artery and any accessory right renal arteries are preserved, while lumbar arteries can be clipped and divided as the dissection moves to the inferior limit of the IMA. Of note, the aorta and IVC can be gently elevated anteriorly to facilitate gathering all the posterior interaortocaval tissue. The tissue is then mobilized medially up to the left margin of the IVC and disconnected here. Next, beginning at the renal hilum, the paraaortic lymphatic tissue is lifted laterally and separated from the lateral surface of the aorta and posterior body wall similar to the dissection of the paracaval lymph nodes described previously, taking care to preserve the sympathetic chain and its branches. Once the packet is freed from all medial, inferior, and superior attachments, it is bluntly swept off the left ureter and placed in an entrapment sac and extracted. After ruling out significant lymphatic leak, the ports and incisions are closed in the same manner as described for the right-side dissection.

POSTOPERATIVE CARE

Peritoneal drains are usually not necessary, but may be placed at the discretion of the surgeon. Unless preoperative issues that could slow return of bowel function are expected or bowel injury is detected and repaired, the orogastric or nasogastric tube can be removed before emergence from anesthesia. Foley catheter removal, advancement of diet, and pain control regimens can proceed in routine fashion. Patients may be discharged when tolerating regular diet, and pain is adequately controlled using oral medications.

RESULTS

Several articles have been published in the scientific literature regarding L-RPLND. Outcomes reflect the evolution and improvement in L-RPLND technique and overall comfort with laparoscopy for urologists by comparing recent (after 2001) to earlier (before 2001) series. A recent meta-analysis has analyzed over 800 patients spanning 34 articles. Operative data in this meta-analysis showed a mean operative time of 204 minutes, with a range of 138 to 261 minutes. This represents a significant improvement from earlier series (before 2001), where the mean published operating room times ranged from 258 to 480 minutes. Accordingly, the mean rate of conversion to open technique is currently only 3.8% (range 1.1% to 5.4%), as compared with a range of 5.8% to 13.3% in earlier series. Currently, the mean hospital length of stay is only 3.3 days (as compared with 6.6 days for recent open series).[7]

In addition, relative to open RPLND, L-RPLND showed reduced postoperative analgesic requirements and less time off from work.[10] In fact, in 1 recent series, LRPLND patients required less than one-half the total amount of postoperative analgesic (31 mg vs 69 mg daily dose of morphine equivalents) than open RPLND patients.[11] In the same study examining health care quality of life (HCQOL) outcomes after RPLND, patients undergoing LRPNLD returned to within 80% of baseline activities as opposed to those undergoing open RPLND at 28.8 versus 50.5 days, respectively.[11]

Oncologic efficacy of L-RPLND has been encouraging in both diagnostic capacity and therapeutic capacity. From a diagnostic capacity, meta-analysis of the most recent comprehensive literature[7] shows no evidence of increased rates of recurrent disease in patients with negative nodes on staging compared with open RPLND. If staging had been inadequate, a higher rate of recurrences should be seen in pathologic stage N1 disease. The rate of positive nodes in comparably staged patients is 25% for both L-RPLND and open RPLND.[7]

For therapeutic value, no major series of L-RPLND has demonstrated recurrence within the template area of previous node dissection.[7] This result has held true for clinical stage 2 patients. In fact, when L-RPLND is compared with open RPLND, overall rate of retroperitoneal relapse (1.3% vs 1.4%), biochemical recurrence (0.9% vs 1.1%), and need for secondary retroperitoneal surgery (1.1% vs 1.5%) do not differ.[7]

COMPLICATIONS

The most feared and immediately life-threatening complication of L-RPLND is uncontrolled hemorrhage. This has higher incidence in postchemotherapy patients.[9] Given the large number of targeted lymph nodes around small branches off of the great vessels, minimal oozing can develop into uncontrolled hemorrhage very quickly if not properly controlled. If the bleeding cannot be quickly and effectively controlled laparoscopically, prompt conversion to open technique is necessary and easily accomplished through a midline vertical incision from the xyphoid process to the symphysis pubis, incorporating all of the port sites. Advanced laparocopic hemostatic agents and improved experience with laparoscopic technique have dropped open conversion rates to 1% to 5% in modern series.[7,12]

Laparoscopic control of hemorrhage can be accomplished in multiple ways. Arterial bleeding from small vessels can often be controlled using precise placement of metal clips. If the stump is very short off of the aorta, it may be necessary to suture the defect using a 5-0 vascular suture. Small vessels on the aorta can also be controlled with judicious use of the argon beam coagulator. Venous injury offers more options for control. Initial compression with a minilap sponge for minimum 5–10 minutes will control most venous bleeding. Once controlled, the addition of adjunctive hemostatic agents such as oxidized cellulose (Surgicel, Ethicon, Incorporated, Somerville, NJ, USA) or gelatin matrix (FloSeal, Baxter, Deerfield, IL, USA) can prevent rebleeding. Large injuries from the IVC or renal vein will often need to be repaired using 5-0 suture after initial compression.

Injury to the sympathetic trunk or nerve plexus is often unrecognized. Repair is usually not possible and not indicated. The only postoperative sign may be tachycardia, which may also result from reversible damage to the nerves. The most common persistent effect is retrograde ejaculation, present in up to 5% of patients even in high-volume, nerve-sparing centers.[13]

Ureteral injury is rare and certainly avoidable in cases where chemotherapy has not been administered. If unrecognized, this may develop into stricture. Injury or inadvertent ligation of accessory renal arteries may present as tachycardia, fever, and a leukocytosis. Long term, one may detect a slight decrease in glomerular filtration rate.

Bowel injury can occur at any time. It is important to place all trocars after the initial trocar under laparoscopic guidance to prevent this complication. In addition, after placing the initial trocar, the underlying bowel must be immediately inspected before rotation of the table moves it out of the field of view. During dissection, unrecognized bowel injury can occur by improperly grounded monopolar electrosurgical instruments (ie, the pin in laparoscopic scissors). These may manifest as delayed perforation and require emergent exploratory laparotomy and washout. If an injury is recognized and occurs in a cold, controlled fashion, laparoscopic repair of noncautery injuries can be performed using a double-layer silk suture technique. If persistent postoperative ileus occurs, urine leak, hematoma, abscess, lymphocele, chylous ascites, or pancreatitis should be ruled out.

Lymphatic leak can manifest in formation of a lymphocele or chylous ascities. Lymphocele can present with persistent postoperative flank pain. Hydronephrosis may develop due to ureteral compression. Initial management should be with percutaneous drainage when possible. In refractory cases, surgical marsupialization offers definitive therapy. Chylous ascites is rare (<3%).[1] This usually is the result of unrepaired damage to the cysterna chili. Presentation is usually in the early postoperative period and consists of any combination of prolonged ileus, ascites, chylous leakage from incisions, or pleural effusion. Initial treatment consisting of a low-fat, medium-chain triglyceride diet is often effective. If this fails, hyperalimentation can be used in conjunction with bowel rest. In recalcitrant cases, surgical exploration with ligation of lymphatics might be necessary.

In patients status postchemotherapy with bleomycin, significantly increased risk of atelectasis, pulmonary edema, and pneumonia exists.[8] The key to preventing complications is minimizing intraoperative fluids, watching concentration of inspired oxygen in the postoperative period, and aggressive pulmonary toilet. Care is supportive.

Rarely described complications including rhabdomyolysis, pulmonary embolus, and port-site metastasis (0.3%) have also been reported.

SUMMARY

L-RPLND is an effective staging and therapeutic procedure in patients with low-stage testicular cancer. It is an attractive alternative to the open approach, with faster recovery, improved cosmesis, and reduced post-operative morbidity driving its application. In experienced hands, it can be used in postchemotherapy patients. The transperitoneal technique offers replication of the conventional open RPLND and nerve-sparing approaches. Although rare, complications of uncontrolled hemorrhage and bowel injury may necessitate open conversion.

REFERENCES

1. Wein AJ, editor. Campbell-Walsh urology. 9th edition. Philadelphia: Elsevier; 2007.
2. Divrik RT, Akdogan B, Ozen H, et al. Outcomes of surveillance protocol of clinical stage I nonseminomatous germ cell tumors—is shift to risk adapted policy justified? J Urol 2006;176:1424.

3. Nelson JB, Chen RN, Bishoff JT, et al. Laparoscopic retroperitoneal lymph node dissection for clinical stage I nonseminomatous germ cell testicular tumors. Urology 1999;54:1064.

4. Amato RJ, Ro JY, Ayala AG, et al. Risk-adapted treatment for patients with clinical stage I nonseminomatous germ cell tumor of the testis. Urology 2004;63:144.

5. Bhayani SB, Ong A, Oh WK, et al. Laparoscopic retroperitoneal lymph node dissection for clinical stage I nonseminomatous germ cell testicular cancer: a long-term update. Urology 2003;62:324.

6. Janetschek G, Hobisch A, Holtl L, et al. Retroperitoneal lymphadenectomy for clinical stage I nonseminomatous testicular tumor: laparoscopy versus open surgery and impact of learning curve. J Urol 1996; 156:89.

7. Rassweiler JJ, Scheitlin W, Heidenreich A, et al. Laparoscopic retroperitoneal lymph node dissection: does it still have a role in the management of clinical stage I nonseminomatous testis cancer? A European perspective. Eur Urol 2008;54:1004.

8. Westermann DH, Studer UE. High-risk clinical stage I nonseminomatous germ cell tumors: the case for chemotherapy. World J Urol 2009;27:455.

9. Palese MA, Su LM, Kavoussi LR. Laparoscopic retroperitoneal lymph node dissection after chemotherapy. Urology 2002;60:130.

10. Schwartz MJ, Kavoussi LR. Controversial technology: the Chunnel and the laparoscopic retroperitoneal lymph node dissection (RPLND). BJU Int 2010;106:950.

11. Poulakis V, Skriapas K, de Vries R, et al. Quality of life after laparoscopic and open retroperitoneal lymph node dissection in clinical stage I nonseminomatous germ cell tumor: a comparison study. Urology 2006;68:154.

12. Beck SD, Peterson MD, Bihrle R, et al. Short-term morbidity of primary retroperitoneal lymph node dissection in a contemporary group of patients. J Urol 2007;178:504.

13. Morash C, Cagiannos I. High-risk clinical stage I NSGCT: the case for RPLND. World J Urol 2009; 27:449.

Lymphadenectomy in Penile Cancer

Simon Horenblas, MD, PhD

KEYWORDS

- Penile cancer • Lymphadenectomy • Surgical oncology
- Squamous cell carcinoma

Most penile cancers are squamous cell carcinomas (~95%), which typically show a stepwise lymphogenic spread before hematogenic dissemination. The primary draining lymph nodes are invariably located within the inguinal lymphatic region. Thereafter, dissemination usually continues to the pelvic nodes or distant sites. At initial presentation, distant metastases are present in only 1% to 2% of patients and are virtually always associated with clinically evident lymph node metastases.

The presence of nodal involvement is the single most important prognostic factor.[1–7] Because the currently available noninvasive staging modalities have a low sensitivity in detecting the regional lymph node status (ie, missing micrometastatic disease), the optimal management of patients who are clinically node negative (cN0) has been the subject of debate[1]; approximately 20% to 25% of these patients have occult metastasis. Some clinicians manage these patients with close surveillance, whereas others will perform an inguinal lymphadenectomy.

Other approaches are dynamic sentinel node biopsy, modified lymphadenectomy, and the concept of lymphadenectomy in those patients considered to be at risk for occult metastases, the so-called risk-adapted approach.[2] Although close surveillance may lead to an unintentional delay because of outgrowth of occult metastases in 20% to 25% of patients with cN0 disease, elective and risk-adapted inguinal lymphadenectomy is considered unnecessary in 75% to 80% of such cases because of the absence of metastases.[3] Furthermore, lymphadenectomy is associated with a high morbidity rate. Up to 35% to 70% of patients have short- or long-term complications.[8–11]

ANATOMY OF THE INGUINAL LYMPH NODES

The lymph nodes in the inguinal lymphatic region are the first draining nodes for the penis, and the anatomy has been described by various investigators.[12,13] Historically, the inguinal lymphatic region was divided into 2 groups: the superficial and deep lymph nodes. The superficial inguinal lymph nodes are located beneath the Camper fascia and above the fascia lata covering the muscles of the thigh. The deep inguinal nodes are located deep to the fascia lata and medial to the femoral vein. These nodes intercommunicate with each other and then drain into the pelvic nodes. From a clinical perspective, this anatomic distinction is not useful because the superficial nodes cannot be distinguished from the deep nodes by physical examination or imaging. Daseler and colleagues[12] divided the inguinal region into 5 sections by drawing a horizontal and a vertical line through the point where the saphenous vein drains into the femoral vein with one central zone directly overlying the junction. A recent lymphoscintigraphic study by Leijte and colleagues[14] showed that most of the first draining lymph nodes are located in Daseler's superomedial segment, although there is individual variation.

ASSESSMENT OF INGUINAL LYMPH NODES

The key issue in lymph node staging is the unreliability of the currently available modalities that detect occult nodal involvement. However, given

Department of Urology, The Netherlands Cancer Institute-Antoni van Leeuwenhoek Hospital, Plesmanlaan 121, 1066 CX Amsterdam, The Netherlands
E-mail address: s.horenblas@nki.nl

Urol Clin N Am 38 (2011) 459–469
doi:10.1016/j.ucl.2011.07.004
0094-0143/11/$ – see front matter © 2011 Elsevier Inc. All rights reserved.

that early resection of the inguinal lymph nodes is associated with a therapeutic benefit,[15-17] it is imperative that those patients with metastatic disease in the inguinal lymph nodes undergo an inguinal lymphadenectomy at the earliest possible time. Unfortunately, the high morbidity rate associated with performing an elective inguinal lymphadenectomy makes the operation unsuitable for every patient with penile cancer who does not have inguinal nodal involvement. Hence, there is uncertainty about the timing of lymphadenectomy and identifying those patients who would benefit. However, 3 clinical groups can be identified: those with cN0 groins, those with palpable inguinal lymph nodes (cN+), and those with immobile (fixed) inguinal lymph nodes.

CLINICAL EXAMINATION

Most patients diagnosed with penile cancer in Western countries present without any palpable abnormalities in the groins; only 20% present with palpable nodes.[18] Inguinal lymph nodes that become palpable during follow-up are due to metastasis in nearly 100% of cases.[19] Physical examination of the inguinal region is of limited value in accurate detection, especially of small metastases. Approximately 20% to 25% of patients with cN0 disease will harbor occult metastases. These occult metastases are, by definition, not detected by physical examination. In the patients with cN+ disease, approximately 70% will actually have metastatic inguinal nodal involvement.[4] The remainder will have enlarged inguinal nodes secondary to infection of the primary tumor. Traditionally, antibiotic treatment was advised for 6 weeks to treat the inflammation, with a further reassessment of the inguinal lymph nodes thereafter. However, to avoid a delay in diagnosis, this is no longer recommended. Patients with lymph node involvement should undergo inguinal lymphadenectomy.[20]

INVESTIGATIONS

The currently available noninvasive staging techniques that can be used to stage the groin besides physical examination include ultrasonography combined with fine-needle aspiration cytology (FNAC) of morphologically suspicious-looking nodes, computed tomography (CT) scanning, magnetic resonance (MR) imaging, and positron emission tomography (PET)/CT scanning. These modalities are especially useful in patients who are obese or those who are difficult to examine because additional imaging may identify metastases not found by physical examination.

ULTRASOUND WITH FINE-NEEDLE ASPIRATION CYTOLOGY

Ultrasound is noninvasive, quick, and inexpensive and can easily be combined with FNAC of morphologically suspicious-looking lymph nodes. In a series of 43 patients with 83 cN0 groins, ultrasound-guided FNAC had a sensitivity and specificity of 39% and 100%, respectively.[21] Ultrasound-guided FNAC has been used preoperatively to screen cN0 groins and to further analyze the groins of patients with palpable inguinal lymph nodes (cN+). In a series of 16 patients staged cN+ and not having antibiotic treatment, FNAC alone (without ultrasonography) showed a sensitivity and specificity of 93% and 91%, respectively.[22] False-negative rates for FNAC have been reported in up to 15%. If the clinician remains suspicious, repeat FNAC is indicated, and if it is still inconclusive, then excisional biopsy can be performed. Care must be taken when performing an open biopsy such that in the event of a malignant node, the site of the biopsy can be excised during the subsequent lymphadenectomy.

CT IMAGING

The role of CT in staging the inguinal lymph nodes is poorly understood because of a paucity of studies. One report published in 1991 described a small series of 14 patients who underwent preoperative CT scanning. A sensitivity and specificity of 36% and 100% were found, respectively. None of the occult metastases in the cN0 groins were identified. However, these results are a reflection of the CT technology available at the time of the study. Currently, with the use of multi-slice CT scanners and increased spatial resolution, results are probably better. Nevertheless, the problem of missing a small metastasis still remains. The diagnostic accuracy regarding the pelvic lymph nodes is poor, in accordance with the experience recently reported by other centers.[23] Therefore, CT imaging is not recommended as the initial staging tool for staging in patients with cN0 disease, although it is suitable in those who are difficult to examine (eg, patients who are obese). By contrast, CT scanning can be useful in patients with cN+ disease to determine the extent of disease, and this is discussed later.

MR IMAGING

MR imaging with lymphotropic nanoparticles (LN-MRI), such as coated ultrasmall particles of iron oxide and ferrumoxtran-10, has shown promising results in identifying occult metastasis in a study of 7 patients with penile cancer.[24] MR imaging was performed before and also 24 hours after intravenous ferumoxtran-10 administration. In this small series, LN-MRI has shown a sensitivity of 100% and a specificity of 97%. This imaging technique has also revealed high diagnostic accuracies in staging lymph nodes in prostate cancer and bladder cancer.[25] However, ferrumoxtran-10 is not approved by the Food and Drug Administration, hence, it is not commercially available. Furthermore, the manufacturer has withdrawn the application for marketing authorization for lymphotropic nanoparticles in Europe. In addition, conventional MR imaging is also limited by its spatial resolution. Thus, its use is also limited for staging the cN0 groin.

PET/CT SCAN

PET instrumentation detects subnanomolar concentrations of radioactive tracer in vivo. Following malignant transformation, a range of tumors can be characterized by elevated glucose metabolism and subsequent increased uptake of the intravenously injected radiolabelled glucose analog [F18]-fluorodeoxyglucose. PET combined with low-dose CT imaging (PET/CT) in a single scanner fuses the acquired data into 1 image containing both functional and anatomic information. The accuracy of the combined images is reported to be higher than separate PET and CT images.[26–28]

In 2005, Scher and colleagues[29] published the first results of PET/CT scanning in penile cancer.

They found promising results with a sensitivity of 80% and specificity of 100% on a per-patient basis, respectively. However, these results may be a little optimistic. The limitations of MR imaging regarding spatial resolution are also true for PET/CT. In a recent prospective study of 42 cN0 groins that underwent preoperative PET/CT scanning without pretreatment antibiotics, PET/CT missed 1 out of 5 occult metastases. In addition, 3 false-positive results were found among the 37 remaining groins, leading to a specificity of 92%.[30] The false-positive findings were associated with inflammatory responses within the lymph nodes.

MANAGEMENT OF THE INGUINAL LYMPH NODES IN PATIENTS WITH CN0 DISEASE

Several risk-adapted management approaches have been used and advocated during the last decades (**Table 1**). Basically, these management policies can be divided into noninvasive management (surveillance), minimally invasive staging (dynamic sentinel node biopsy/modified inguinal lymphadenectomy), or invasive staging techniques (complete inguinal lymphadenectomy). The fact that approximately 20% of the patients with cN0 disease have occult metastases indicates that inguinal lymphadenectomy is an unnecessary procedure in approximately 80% of patients. Furthermore, lymphadenectomy is associated with risks and prone to several complications that are discussed later. In general, a lymphadenectomy

Table 1
Available management approaches for patients with cN0 disease

	Advantages	Disadvantages
1. Close surveillance	No morbidity in patients without occult metastasis	Survival disadvantage compared with early dissection; some patients develop inoperable inguinal recurrences
2. Nomogram/risk-adapted lymphadenectomy	Reduction in number of inguinal node dissections and, hence, decreased overall morbidity	Significant overtreatment despite risk adaptation
3. Minimally invasive staging		
a) Modified inguinal lymphadenectomy	High incidence of detection of micrometastasis and lower risk of complications than radical surgery	Significant overtreatment (>80% of inguinal specimens will be benign)
b) Dynamic sentinel node biopsy	Patients are pathologic staged with minor morbidity. Only patients with pN+ disease suffer from (completion) lymph node dissection morbidity	In some patients, metastases are missed (ie, false negative) and develop inguinal recurrences. Some patients cannot be salvaged hereafter
4. Elective bilateral radical lymphadenectomy	No occult metastases are missed	Unnecessary in 80% of patients and severe short- and long-term morbidity

in all patients with cN0 disease (sometimes described as early, prophylactic, or preemptive) is not recommended.

Close Surveillance

The basis of close surveillance involves a regular clinical examination of patients proceeding to lymphadenectomy when lymph node metastases become clinically evident. This surveillance avoids the morbidity associated with lymphadenectomy and, therefore, patients with cN0 disease who subsequently are unlikely to develop inguinal lymph node metastases are not overtreated. Although this has been advocated in the past with seemingly good results, recent nonrandomized retrospective studies indicates that this approach is associated with a negative effect on survival rates.[15–17]

Predictive Nomogram for Occult Metastasis/ Risk-Adapted Lymphadenectomy

Another noninvasive approach is the use of a preoperative nomogram predictive of inguinal metastases.[31] In one nomogram, the following parameters were used for risk assessment: tumor thickness ($\leq$5 mm vs >5 mm), growth pattern (vertical vs horizontal), grade (well vs intermediate vs poor), lymphovascular invasion (absent vs present), corpora cavernosa infiltration (absent vs present), corpora spongiosum infiltration (absent vs present), urethral infiltration (absent vs present), cN status (cN0 vs cN+). In clinical practice, this particular nomogram may be a useful tool but still requires validation. It remains to the discretion of the doctor in collaboration with patients to determine at which cut-off point to embark on a lymphadenectomy.

The basis of risk-adapted approaches is risk assessment of lymph node metastases based on histopathologic factors of the primary tumor, such as tumor stage (T stage),[32,33] tumor grade (ie, grade [G] 1, 2, or 3),[33–35] presence of lymphovascular (LVI),[36,37] perineural invasion,[34,35] and depth of infiltration.[34] The European Association of Urology (EAU) guidelines have included tumor stage, grade, and absence or presence of LVI into a risk-adapted approach for the management of the inguinal regions. Three risk groups have been identified: low risk tumors (pTis, pTa, pT1G1), intermediate risk tumors (pT1G2, no LVI), and high-risk tumors (pT1G3, pT2-3G1-3, or presence of LVI).[32,38] If patients are considered suitable for surveillance, the 2009 EAU guidelines advise follow-up in patients with low-risk tumors only, and surgical staging in intermediate and high-risk patients with cN0 disease. In a prospective study

of 100 patients managed according to these EAU guidelines, none of the patients considered low risk developed lymph node metastases during a mean follow-up of 29 months. On the other hand, elective lymphadenectomy was unnecessary in 82% of the patients with high-risk features because no evidence of metastatic spread was found with histopathology.[5] In another series of 118 patients, it was estimated that 63% of the high-risk patients will be subjected to unnecessary lymphadenectomy.[39] Both studies indicate that current EAU high-risk stratification is not accurate enough to stratify these patients. It seems that the risk of occult nodal involvement in patients with cN0 disease with low risk (T1G1) is low and these patients can still be subjected to close surveillance with subsequently inguinal lymphadenectomy when metastases become clinically evident.

Minimally Invasive Staging Techniques

To circumvent the previously mentioned dilemmas of the timing of lymphadenectomy, minimally invasive staging techniques have been developed. The basis of these techniques is to limit the morbidity in patients with pathologic node-negative (pN0) groins and to identify occult metastases at the earliest moment. Only patients with proven lymphatic spread undergo a completion therapeutic lymphadenectomy. In the last 2 decades, 2 approaches have been introduced worldwide: modified inguinal lymphadenectomy (MIL) and dynamic sentinel node biopsy (DSNB).

Modified inguinal lymphadenectomy

Catalona[40] proposed the MIL in 1988 after being performed in 6 patients with invasive carcinoma of the penis or distal urethra. The aim of this approach is to remove all of the lymph nodes that are at the most probable location of first-line lymphatic invasion and excluding the regions lateral to the femoral artery and caudal to the fossa ovalis. The lymph node packet can be analyzed by frozen section, and if it confirms metastatic disease then a complete inguinal lymphadenectomy can be performed. The anatomic location of these lymph nodes was based on earlier lymphatic drainage studies. The medial margin of MIL was the adductor longus muscle, the lateral margin was the lateral border of the femoral artery, the superior margin was the external oblique muscle above the spermatic cord, and the inferior margin was the fascia lata just distal to the fossa ovalis. The advantages of this MIL are a smaller skin incision and a smaller node dissection resulting in reduced morbidity compared with standard lymphadenectomy. However, limiting the dissection field led to a high number of false-negative findings as reported by several other investigators.

Dynamic sentinel node biopsy

Cabañas[41] first reported sentinel node biopsy for penile cancer in 1977. This report was based on lymphangiograms of the penis and the lymph node medial to the superficial epigastric vein and was identified as being the first echelon lymph node or the so-called sentinel node. It was assumed that a negative sentinel node indicated the absence of further lymphatic spread and, therefore, no lymphadenectomy was indicated. Sentinel node surgery consisted of identification and removal of this lymph node with completion lymphadenectomy only in those with a tumor-positive lymph node. However, this initial static procedure, based on anatomic landmarks only, did not take into account individual drainage patterns. Several false-negative results were reported, and the technique was largely abandoned. The sentinel node procedure was revived by Morton and colleagues[42] in 1992 by using patent blue V or isosulfan blue dye as a tracer enabling individual lymphatic mapping. This technique, with the addition of a preoperative radioactive tracer (technetium-99m-labeled nanocolloid ^{99m}Tc), forms the basis of the modern sentinel node biopsy era and is also used in, for example, breast cancer and melanoma.

In 2001, Horenblas and colleagues[43] described the DSNB procedure for penile cancer in a report of 55 patients with T2 or greater tumors. With this dynamic approach, a sensitivity of 80% was reported. However, the false-negative rates raised concerns about its diagnostic accuracy. Furthermore, patients with negative sentinel nodes remained on rigid follow-up. During the years, the DSNB protocol has been modified after detailed analysis of the false-negative cases.[44] The initial procedure was extended by the pathologic examination of the sentinel node by serial sectioning and immunohistochemical staining instead of routine paraffin sections, and the addition of preoperative ultrasonography with FNAC to detect pathologically enlarged nodes, that fail to pick up radioactivity. Furthermore, exploration of groins with nonvisualization on preoperative lymphoscintigram (occurring in approximately 4%–6% of cN0 groins)[14,23,45] and intraoperative palpation of the wound have been introduced. The current modified procedure has evolved into a reliable minimally invasive staging technique with an associated sensitivity of 93% to 95% together with low morbidity[39,46] and is comparable with the results in breast cancer and melanoma. In a large prospective series of 323 patients from 2 tertiary referral hospitals that use essentially the same protocol, DSNB has shown to be a reliable method with a low complication rate.[47] The combined sensitivity of this procedure was 93% with a specificity of 100%. Complications occurred in less than 5% of explored groins and almost all were transient and could be managed conservatively.

MANAGEMENT OF THE GROIN IN PATIENTS WITH CN+ DISEASE

Surgery remains the cornerstone of treatment in patients with metastatic disease in the groin. Cure can be attained in approximately 80% of patients who have 1 or 2 involved inguinal nodes without extranodal extension.[1–7] Preoperatively, inguinal nodal involvement can be found with FNAC or excision biopsy. The author prefers FNAC because it is easily performed in an outpatient setting, it is noninvasive, and it does not interfere with the subsequent lymphadenectomy. Although the reported sensitivity of FNAC is higher in patients with cN+ disease compared with patients with cN0 disease, it is recommended to repeat the ultrasound with FNAC when clinical suspicion remains despite tumor-negative cytologic results. If doubt remains, an excision biopsy is advised. In removing the suspicious enlarged node, the surgeon should pay attention to the anatomic localization of the inguinal incision because the inguinal scar should be removed at the time of completion of the inguinal lymphadenectomy. Patients presenting with fixed inguinal nodes are candidates for neoadjuvant chemotherapy before undergoing surgery.[48]

INDICATION FOR INGUINAL LYMPHADENECTOMY

Ipsilateral inguinal lymphadenectomy is indicated when tumor-bearing lymph nodes are found with sentinel node biopsy, FNAC, or excision biopsy. Should a bilateral inguinal dissection be undertaken in all patients with unilateral inguinal involvement? At the author's institute, the timing of detection, the number of palpable nodes, and the number of positive nodes found in the resection specimen were considered initially indicative for a contralateral lymphadenectomy.[49] Patients who developed a unilateral inguinal recurrence during follow-up were managed by unilateral dissection assuming that bilateral nodal metastases develop at the same rate and that the absence of clinical nodal involvement of the contralateral side after observation suggested a tumor-free groin. Previous studies have suggested that the likelihood of bilateral involvement is related to the number of involved nodes in the unilateral resected inguinal specimen.[1,49] With 2 or more metastases, the probability of occult contralateral involvement is 30%, and this may warrant an early contralateral inguinal lymphadenectomy. Currently, ultrasound-guided FNAC and DSNB are used to solve the problem at the author's institute in those patients presenting initially with unilateral positive nodes. Contralateral groins with tumor-negative sentinel nodes are under close surveillance. Hence, nodal staging and management has emerged from treatment per patient to management per groin.

INDICATION FOR PELVIC LYMPHADENECTOMY

In general, 20% to 30% of patients with positive inguinal nodes have positive pelvic nodes.[1,4,50] Although patients with pelvic lymphadenopathy are considered to have a bleak outcome, pelvic lymphadenectomy can be curative in some patients; those with occult pelvic metastases may especially benefit. Several investigators have shown that the likelihood of pelvic nodal involvement is related to the number of positive nodes in the inguinal specimen and presence of extranodal extension.[1–7,50] Patients with 1 intranodal inguinal metastasis have a low probability of pelvic node involvement (<5%, Graafland NM and colleagues, unpublished data, 2010).[4,50] At the author's institute, a pelvic dissection is considered unnecessary in these patients. An ipsilateral pelvic lymphadenectomy of the affected site is performed in all other patients with 2 or more inguinal nodes involved or with extranodal extension. There is ample clinical and published evidence that crossover from the groin to the contralateral pelvic area does not occur.[4,49,50] Therefore, contralateral pelvic lymphadenectomy is not recommended in patients with unilateral nodal involvement. Patients with preoperative evidence of pelvic metastases are unlikely to be cured by surgery alone and are candidates for neoadjuvant chemotherapy before undergoing surgery.

SURGICAL ASPECTS OF INGUINAL LYMPHADENECTOMY

Several surgical approaches have been described to minimize the complications associated with the procedure. Patients are placed supine with the legs abducted and externally rotated. A variety of incisions can be used. For inguinal node dissection, the incisions can be divided into horizontal and vertical. The vascular supply to the skin of the inguinal area is such that horizontal incisions are preferred to vertical ones. Correct tissue handling and ensuring that the skin flaps are developed in the correct plane minimizes the morbidity following lymphadenectomy. No lymph nodes are found in the layer between the skin and subcutaneous fascia. At the author's institute, a parainguinal incision, a few centimeters below the groin crease, is the preferred type of incision. The skin should be incised until the subcutaneous fascia is identified. Then the proximal and distal skin flaps are developed. The boundaries of the dissection are as follows: the proximal boundary is the inguinal ligament; the distal boundary is the crossing of the sartorius muscle and the adductor longus muscle (also referred to as the entrance of the Hunter canal, where the femoral vessels go under the muscles of the leg); the medial boundary is the adductor muscle; and the lateral margin is the sartorius muscle. The floor of the dissection consists of the fascia lata, the femoral vessels, and the pectineus muscle. Because the femoral nerve is located beneath the fascia lata, it is not seen during standard lymphadenectomy. It is important to meticulously remove all of the lymphatic tissue because inguinal lymphadenectomy can be a curative procedure. There have been a series of modifications to the technique of inguinal lymphadenectomy to reduce the morbidity. Transposition of the sartorius muscle according to Baronofsky can be undertaken if patients are deemed at high risk for wound complications. The origin of the sartorius muscle at the anterior superior iliac spine is transected and the muscle together with its overlying fascia is sutured to the inferior margin of the inguinal ligament. Excellent coverage of the femoral vessels is achieved with no long-term sequelae. The saphenous vein can also be spared, if possible, to minimize postoperative lymphedema. After performing the dissection, the skin edges are carefully inspected; any area with doubtful viability should be excised. There are no comparative studies on the use of antibiotics, but it seems reasonable to give prophylactic antibiotics at the time of surgery because this type of surgery should be considered a contaminated procedure because of coexisting inflammatory reactions within the lymph nodes. Along with the general recommendations for prophylactic antibiotics, the author's group gives 1 dose at the start of anesthesia. Before closing the wound, suction drains are inserted to prevent lymphocele formation and also increase the chance of primary wound healing. Postoperative antibiotic use is variable among surgeons performing the procedure. Some centers continue antibiotics until the drain is removed. After 1 week, the vacuum is removed and spontaneous drainage observed. Drains are removed if the drainage is less than 50 mL/d, although some centers wait until it is less than 30 mL/d. Recently, some studies have investigated the use of fibrin sealant in melanoma and vulvar carcinoma to reduce the complication rate, including lymphedema. Preliminary results show that complications are not significantly reduced by applying the fibrin sealant. Ambulation is strongly advised immediately after surgery. Patients at the author's institution were advised until recently to use elastic stockings for at least 6 months following surgery. A prospective randomized trial comparing 2 groups of patients with and without elastic stockings showed no difference in the prevention of postoperative lymphedema (in press). Therefore, the standard use of elastic stockings was abandoned. At the author's institution, it is routine to give low molecular weight heparin as prophylaxis for thrombosis starting the evening before surgery.

Is it necessary to perform an en bloc dissection to remove the primary tumor with the regional lymph nodes as one continuous specimen? Young[51] first introduced this type of surgery in 1931. Although oncologically sound, clinical experience shows this to be unnecessary in most patients. The rationale is that lymphatic spread occurs through a process of embolism and not through continuous growth. On practical and theoretical grounds, it is advisable to stage the treatment of the primary tumor and the regional nodes. One reason is the elimination of the primary tumor as a focus of infection and the other is the deposition of in-transit metastases in the regional nodes, thus, eliminating the potential risk of metastatic outgrowth in the tract between the primary tumor and the groin. En bloc dissection is only indicated in patients with extensive primary or recurrent disease with bilateral nodal involvement. Skin closure following lymphadenectomy can be difficult in patients with extensive metastatic disease with overlying skin involvement. The skin involved should be excised, although, inevitably, this leaves a large defect. Various methods can be used to manage this surgical problem. After a sartorius transposition, the wound can heal by secondary intention. Healing can be improved and hastened by a split-skin graft on the granulation tissue. Another method is the so-called skin-stretch method[6]; by gradually increasing the pressure on the skin edges in a cyclic fashion, large skin defects are closed with no tension. Island flaps that can be useful for closure are the rectus abdominis pedicle, gracilis pedicle, and the tensor fascia lata pedicle. In cases of en bloc removal, using scrotal skin and mobilizing the abdominal wall can also be used to assist in the closure of the defect. The femoral vessels can be protected by transposition of the scrotal content and suturing the scrotal content to the inguinal ligament.

PELVIC LYMPHADENECTOMY

Pelvic lymphadenectomy can be undertaken simultaneously at the time of inguinal node dissection or as a separate procedure. In the first case, removal of the lymph nodes using 1 or 2 incisions has been described; most investigators prefer 2 separate incisions. A comparison of the various types of incisions has shown that the lowest complication rate occurs when 2 separate incisions are used.[9,10] The pelvic node dissection is undertaken either through a lower abdominal midline incision or a unilateral muscle splitting incision. The boundaries of the pelvic node dissection are as follows: the proximal boundary is the common iliac vessels, the distal boundary is the passage of lymphatic vessels to the groin, the lateral boundary is the ilioinguinal nerve, the medial boundary is the bladder and prostate, and the base is the deepest part of the obturator fossa. Care must be taken to completely remove the obturator fossa, especially the space behind the external iliac vessels, all the way to the sacrum (triangle of Marcille). A large node can usually be found there, and if left it is prone to recurrence with intractable pain because of neural ingrowth. After the dissection, suction drains are left in place and removed if the spontaneous drainage is less than 50 mL. Laparoscopic pelvic node dissection has not had a major role in pelvic node dissection for penile cancer at the author's institute thus far, although it is used in other centers. In view of the therapeutic potential of node dissection (with or without chemotherapy or radiotherapy), a complete dissection should be attempted.

COMPLICATIONS OF LYMPH NODE DISSECTION

Even in the most experienced hands, lymphadenectomy is not without complications. This factor accounts for the reluctance in offering lymphadenectomy to every patient presenting with penile cancer. The reported complication rate varies from 35% to 88% and seems to be lower when inguinal lymphadenectomy is performed in a prophylactic or therapeutic setting compared with a palliative dissection.[7] Furthermore, pelvic node dissection and radiotherapy have shown to increase the complication rates.[4,9] The most commonly cited complications are wound infection (skin necrosis with or without wound dehiscence; $14 \pm 50\%$); lymphocele/seroma ($10 \pm 10\%$); lymphedema ($27 \pm 30\%$); and other complications, including hemorrhage, thrombosis, and even death. A summary of the most frequent complications is listed in **Table 2**.

MANAGEMENT OF COMPLICATIONS

After removing the suction drains, a lymphocele can develop in 10% to 20% of patients. This complication can usually be managed by outpatient aspiration with a large needle and a large syringe. After natural resolution of the space where the lymphocele develops, the accumulation of lymphatic fluid stops. Large wound defects can be closed using a vacuum assisted closure system. A sponge is inserted in the wound and sealed with plastic, and a draining tube is attached to a low vacuum pump. Excellent results have been obtained, increasing the time to secondary healing. If the defect remains large, a split skin graft can be laid on top of the granulation tissue.

Lymphedema develops in approximately 10% of patients, especially those in whom extensive surgery together with radiation therapy was necessary because of the burden of disease. Supporting therapy includes lymph massage and compression therapy. Surgical therapy using lymphatic-venous anastomoses has not been entirely successful. Legs with lymphedema are infection prone, especially with streptococcus A bacteria, leading to erysipelas. At the author's institutions, antibiotic prophylaxis with monthly penicillin depots is strongly advised after 2 bouts of erysipelaslike infections.

PROGNOSIS AND ADJUVANT TREATMENT

The single most important prognostic factor in penile cancer is the presence of nodal involvement. The extent of nodal involvement also has a predictive value for cancer-specific outcome. As mentioned previously, patients with 1 or 2 inguinal lymph node metastases have a 5-year survival rate of approximately 80%.[1–7] Several studies have indicated that the number of inguinal nodes involved, extranodal extension, and pelvic nodal involvement are unfavorable parameters for disease-specific survival (**Table 3**).[1–7] Hence, the indication for adjuvant treatment is based upon the presence of these adverse prognostic indicators. At the author's institutions, no adjuvant treatment is indicated when histopathologic analysis of the removed inguinal dissected specimen shows one intranodal metastasis because cure alone by surgery can be obtained in these patients. Adjuvant ipsilateral radiotherapy to the inguinal lymphatic region is given when histopathologic analysis shows 2 or more inguinal nodes involved or extranodal extension. The rationale for this arises from studies in head and neck squamous cell carcinomas showing an improvement in regional control following adjuvant radiotherapy.[52] Adjuvant radiotherapy to the pelvic region is administrated additionally when pelvic nodes are involved. Prophylactic radiation to the groins in all patients with penile cancer is not advised for the following reasons: Firstly, some patients with nonpalpable nodes will not benefit because they have no occult metastasis, which is the case for elective lymphadenectomy. Secondly, all patients will be exposed to the complications of radiation therapy (eg, short-term complications, such as epidermolysis, and long-term effects, such as lymphedema and fibrosis). Finally, the follow-up is more complicated because of the fibrotic changes, making physical examination less reliable. Although Ravi and colleagues have indicated that patients with large (>4 cm) or fixed regional nodes may benefit from preoperative radiotherapy, the previously mentioned disadvantages outweigh the preoperative use. There are no studies available that have investigated the efficacy of radiotherapy versus standard lymphadenectomy in terms of local control, (cancer-specific) outcome, or complications.

Table 2 Complications of lymphadenectomy (%)					
Number of Dissections	Wound Infection	Skin Edge Necrosis	Seroma Formation	Lymph Edema	Death
101[38]	14	50	16	50	0
405[55]	17	62	7	27	1
200[8]	15	45	10	23	–
106[9]	10	8	10	23	2
102[10,a]	22	8	18	56	0

[a] Per patient.

Table 3
Cancer-specific survival by pathologic nodal factors after inguinal lymphadenectomy

Factors	Number of Patients with Factor	5-Year Cancer-Specific Survival Estimates (%)
Pathologic node-negative nodes	103[11] 140[12]	95 96
Pathologic node-positive nodes	118[13] 111[14] 102[15] 156[54]	53 35 51 61
Number of positive nodes		
1	5[16]	82
1–3	58[17] 69[18]	81 76
≤2	111[54]	74
≥3	41[54]	33
>3	10[19]	50
4–5	25[20]	8
>5	8[21]	0
Unilateral	43[22] 74[23] 93[54]	86 63 69
Bilateral	24[24] 25[25] 28[26] 63[54]	12 60 21 49
Extranodal extension	22[27] 17[28] 54[29] 79[54]	5 0 9 42
Pelvic nodal involvement	22[30] 30[31] 21[32] 13[56] 34[53]	0 0 0 30 21

Despite adjuvant radiotherapy, a previous study at the author's institution of 102 patients with metastatic penile carcinoma treated between 1956 and 2001 showed that extranodal extension and pelvic nodal involvement are independent predictors for survival.[53] These results have recently been confirmed in an updated series that has included 156 patients with metastatic penile cancer treated between 1988 and 2008.[54] This data suggest that more effective treatment is needed in this subgroup of patients with high-risk metastatic penile cancer. Whether induction chemotherapy before surgery is of any benefit in this high-risk subgroup warrants further clinical studies.

REFERENCES

1. Srinivas V, Morse MJ, Herr HW, et al. Penile cancer: relation of extent of nodal metastasis to survival. J Urol 1987;137:880.
2. Ravi R. Correlation between the extent of nodal involvement and survival following groin dissection for carcinoma of the penis. Br J Urol 1993;72:817.
3. Horenblas S, van Tinteren H. Squamous cell carcinoma of the penis. IV. Prognostic factors of survival: analysis of tumor, nodes and metastasis classification system. J Urol 1994;151:1239.
4. Lont AP, Kroon BK, Gallee MP, et al. Pelvic lymph node dissection for penile carcinoma: extent of inguinal lymph node involvement as an indicator for pelvic lymph node involvement and survival. J Urol 2007;177:947.
5. Sanchez-Ortiz RF, Pettaway CA. The role of lymphadenectomy in penile cancer. Urol Oncol 2004;22:236.
6. Pandey D, Mahajan V, Kannan RR. Prognostic factors in node-positive carcinoma of the penis. J Surg Oncol 2006;93:133.
7. Ornellas AA, Kinchin EW, Nobrega BL, et al. Surgical treatment of invasive squamous cell carcinoma of the penis: Brazilian National Cancer Institute long-term experience. J Surg Oncol 2008;97:487.
8. Johnson DE, Lo RK. Complications of groin dissection in penile cancer. Experience with 101 lymphadenectomies. Urology 1984;24:312.
9. Ravi R. Morbidity following groin dissection for penile carcinoma. Br J Urol 1993;72:941.
10. Ornellas AA, Seixas AL, de Moraes JR. Analyses of 200 lymphadenectomies in patients with penile carcinoma. J Urol 1991;146:330.
11. Bevan-Thomas R, Slaton JW, Pettaway CA. Contemporary morbidity from lymphadenectomy for penile squamous cell carcinoma: the M.D. Anderson Cancer Center experience. J Urol 2002;167:1638.
12. Daseler EH, Anson BJ, Reimann AF. Radical excision of the inguinal and iliac lymph glands; a study based upon 450 anatomical dissections and upon supportive clinical observations. Surg Gynecol Obstet 1948;87:679.
13. Dewire D, Lepor H. Anatomic considerations of the penis and its lymphatic drainage. Urol Clin North Am 1992;19:211.
14. Leijte JA, Valdes Olmos RA, Nieweg OE, et al. Anatomical mapping of lymphatic drainage in penile carcinoma with SPECT-CT: implications for the extent of inguinal lymph node dissection. Eur Urol 2008;54:885.
15. McDougal WS. Carcinoma of the penis: improved survival by early regional lymphadenectomy based on the histological grade and depth of invasion of the primary lesion. J Urol 1995;154:1364.

16. Lont AP, Horenblas S, Tanis PJ, et al. Management of clinically node negative penile carcinoma: improved survival after the introduction of dynamic sentinel node biopsy. J Urol 2003;170:783.

17. Kroon BK, Horenblas S, Lont AP, et al. Patients with penile carcinoma benefit from immediate resection of clinically occult lymph node metastases. J Urol 2005;173:816.

18. Persson B, Sjodin JG, Holmberg L, et al. The National Penile Cancer Register in Sweden 2000-2003. Scand J Urol Nephrol 2007;41:278.

19. Ornellas AA, Seixas AL, Marota A, et al. Surgical treatment of invasive squamous cell carcinoma of the penis: retrospective analysis of 350 cases. J Urol 1994;151:1244.

20. Pizzocaro G, Algaba F, Horenblas S, et al. EAU penile cancer guidelines 2009. Eur Urol 2010; 57(6):1002–12.

21. Kroon BK, Horenblas S, Deurloo EE, et al. Ultrasonography-guided fine-needle aspiration cytology before sentinel node biopsy in patients with penile carcinoma. BJU Int 2005;95:517.

22. Saisorn I, Lawrentschuk N, Leewansangtong S, et al. Fine-needle aspiration cytology predicts inguinal lymph node metastasis without antibiotic pretreatment in penile carcinoma. BJU Int 2006;97:1225.

23. Jensen JB, Jensen KM, Ulhoi BP, et al. Sentinel lymph-node biopsy in patients with squamous cell carcinoma of the penis. BJU Int 2009;103:1199.

24. Tabatabaei S, Harisinghani M, McDougal WS. Regional lymph node staging using lymphotropic nanoparticle enhanced magnetic resonance imaging with ferumoxtran-10 in patients with penile cancer. J Urol 2005;174:923.

25. Thoeny HC, Triantafyllou M, Birkhaeuser FD, et al. Combined ultrasmall superparamagnetic particles of iron oxide-enhanced and diffusion-weighted magnetic resonance imaging reliably detect pelvic lymph node metastases in normal-sized nodes of bladder and prostate cancer patients. Eur Urol 2009;55(4):761–9.

26. Lardinois D, Weder W, Hany TF, et al. Staging of non-small-cell lung cancer with integrated positron-emission tomography and computed tomography. N Engl J Med 2003;348:2500.

27. Antoch G, Saoudi N, Kuehl H, et al. Accuracy of whole-body dual-modality fluorine-18-2-fluoro-2-deoxy-D-glucose positron emission tomography and computed tomography (FDG-PET/CT) for tumor staging in solid tumors: comparison with CT and PET. J Clin Oncol 2004;22:4357.

28. Ng SH, Yen TC, Chang JT, et al. Prospective study of [18F]fluorodeoxyglucose positron emission tomography and computed tomography and magnetic resonance imaging in oral cavity squamous cell carcinoma with palpably negative neck. J Clin Oncol 2006;24:4371.

29. Scher B, Seitz M, Reiser M, et al. 18F-FDG PET/CT for staging of penile cancer. J Nucl Med 2005;46: 1460.

30. Leijte JA, Graafland NM, Valdes Olmos RA, et al. Prospective evaluation of hybrid (18)F-fluorodeoxyglucose positron emission tomography/computed tomography in staging clinically node-negative patients with penile carcinoma. BJU Int 2009; 104(5):640–4.

31. Ficarra V, Zattoni F, Artibani W, et al. Nomogram predictive of pathological inguinal lymph node involvement in patients with squamous cell carcinoma of the penis. J Urol 2006;175:1700.

32. Solsona E, Iborra I, Rubio J, et al. Prospective validation of the association of local tumor stage and grade as a predictive factor for occult lymph node micrometastasis in patients with penile carcinoma and clinically negative inguinal lymph nodes. J Urol 2001;165:1506.

33. Slaton JW, Morgenstern N, Levy DA, et al. Tumor stage, vascular invasion and the percentage of poorly differentiated cancer: independent prognosticators for inguinal lymph node metastasis in penile squamous cancer. J Urol 2001;165:1138.

34. Ornellas AA, Nobrega BL, Wei Kin Chin E, et al. Prognostic factors in invasive squamous cell carcinoma of the penis: analysis of 196 patients treated at the Brazilian National Cancer Institute. J Urol 2008;180(4):1354–9.

35. Velazquez EF, Ayala G, Liu H, et al. Histologic grade and perineural invasion are more important than tumor thickness as predictor of nodal metastasis in penile squamous cell carcinoma invading 5 to 10 mm. Am J Surg Pathol 2008;32:974.

36. Lopes A, Hidalgo GS, Kowalski LP, et al. Prognostic factors in carcinoma of the penis: multivariate analysis of 145 patients treated with amputation and lymphadenectomy. J Urol 1996;156:1637.

37. Ficarra V, Zattoni F, Cunico SC, et al. Lymphatic and vascular embolizations are independent predictive variables of inguinal lymph node involvement in patients with squamous cell carcinoma of the penis: Gruppo Uro-Oncologico del Nord Est (Northeast Uro-Oncological Group) Penile Cancer data base data. Cancer 2005;103:2507.

38. Solsona E, Algaba F, Horenblas S, et al. EAU guidelines on penile cancer. Eur Urol 2004;46:1.

39. Leijte JA, Kroon BK, Valdés Olmos RA, et al. Reliability and safety of current dynamic sentinel node biopsy for penile carcinoma. Eur Urol 2007; 52:170.

40. Catalona WJ. Modified inguinal lymphadenectomy for carcinoma of the penis with preservation of saphenous veins: technique and preliminary results. J Urol 1988;140:306.

41. Cabanas RM. An approach for the treatment of penile carcinoma. Cancer 1977;39:456.

42. Morton DL, Wen DR, Wong JH, et al. Technical details of intraoperative lymphatic mapping for early stage melanoma. Arch Surg 1992;127:392.

43. Horenblas S, Jansen L, Meinhardt W, et al. Detection of occult metastasis in squamous cell carcinoma of the penis using a dynamic sentinel node procedure. J Urol 2000;163:100.

44. Kroon BK, Horenblas S, Estourgie SH, et al. How to avoid false-negative dynamic sentinel node procedures in penile carcinoma. J Urol 2004;171: 2191.

45. Hadway P, Smith Y, Corbishley C, et al. Evaluation of dynamic lymphoscintigraphy and sentinel lymph-node biopsy for detecting occult metastases in patients with penile squamous cell carcinoma. BJU Int 2007;100:561.

46. Kroon BK, Lont AP, Valdés Olmos RA, et al. Morbidity of dynamic sentinel node biopsy in penile carcinoma. J Urol 2005;173:813.

47. Leijte JA, Hughes B, Graafland NM, et al. Two-center evaluation of dynamic sentinel node biopsy for squamous cell carcinoma of the penis. J Clin Oncol 2009;27:3325.

48. Leijte JA, Kerst JM, Bais E, et al. Neoadjuvant chemotherapy in advanced penile carcinoma. Eur Urol 2007;52:488.

49. Horenblas S, van Tinteren H, Delemarre JF, et al. Squamous cell carcinoma of the penis. III. Treatment of regional lymph nodes. J Urol 1993;149:492.

50. Zhu Y, Zhang SL, Ye DW, et al. Prospectively packaged ilioinguinal lymphadenectomy for penile cancer: the disseminative pattern of lymph node metastasis. J Urol 2009;181:2103.

51. Young HH. A radical operation for the cure of cancer of the penis. J Urol 1931;26:285–94.

52. Bartelink H, Breur K, Hart G, et al. The value of postoperative radiotherapy as an adjuvant to radical neck dissection. Cancer 1983;52:1008.

53. Wespes E. The management of regional lymph nodes in patients with penile carcinoma and reliability of sentinel node biopsy. Eur Urol 2007;52:15.

54. Graafland NM, van Boven HH, Van Werkhoven E, et al. Prognostic significance of extranodal extension in pathological node-positive patients with penile carcinoma. J Urol 2010;184(4):1347–53.

55. Hegarty PK, Kayes O, Freeman A, et al. A prospective study of 100 cases of penile cancer managed according to European Association of Urology guidelines. BJU Int 2006;98:526.

56. Lopes A, Bezerra AL, Serrano SV, et al. Iliac nodal metastases from carcinoma of the penis treated surgically. BJU Int 2000;86:690.

Novel Imaging Modalities for Lymph Node Imaging in Urologic Oncology

Victoria Chernyak, MD

KEYWORDS

• Urologic oncology • Lymph node • Imaging • Staging

Precise lymph node staging in genitourinary (GU) malignancies is crucial for planning an appropriate treatment and establishing an accurate prognosis.[1] Computed tomography (CT) is a widely used tool for initial evaluation of the nodal involvement. According to the accepted size criteria, any node with a short-axis diameter greater than 1 cm and any rounded node larger than 8 mm is concerning for malignancy.[2] However, as nodal evaluation on CT relies solely on nodal size rather than on nodal function and physiology, this method is limited in its accuracy, as small nodes may harbor micrometastases and enlarged lymph nodes may be reactive in nature.[3,4] Improvement in preoperative diagnosis of nodal metastases is crucial, as micrometastases may be present in up to 25% of patients with clinically organ-confound prostate cancer.[5] Multiple novel techniques are emerging to improve the accuracy of nodal involvement in GU malignancies.

POSITRON EMISSION TOMOGRAPHY

Positron emission tomography (PET) scanning using ^{18}F-fluoro-2-deoxyglucose (FDG) has been shown to be an effective tool for nodal detection of some malignancies, such as small cell lung cancer.[6] ^{18}F-FDG is phosphorylated to FDG-6-phosphate (FDG-6P) and is accumulated in cells with increased rates of glycolysis. Tissues with elevated metabolic rates accumulate FDG-6P, and thus can be detected on PET scanning. ^{18}F-FDG PET has been shown to be a useful tool in differentiating fibrotic residual mass in seminomatous germ cell tumors on restaging.[7] However, ^{18}F-FDG PET has a low sensitivity and accuracy in staging prostate cancer, likely due to the low rates of accumulation of the tracer in the prostate cancer cells.[8] In addition, as FDG is eliminated by kidneys, the excreted FDG activity accumulating in the ureters and bladder may limit the evaluation of adjacent structures such as the prostate and pelvic lymph nodes.[9]

As with prostate cancer, the use of ^{18}F-FDG PET for staging of bladder cancer is hindered by urinary excretion of the tracer. For instance, Heicappell and colleagues[10] demonstrated a 66.7% detection rate for local lymph node metastasis of bladder cancer; Lodde and colleagues[11] demonstrated sensitivity of 57%. Moreover, in a study of 51 patients with patients with nonmetastatic invasive bladder cancer (T2 or higher, M0) or recurrent high-risk superficial disease (T1G3 with or without Tis, M0), Swinnen and colleagues[12] found the accuracy, sensitivity, and specificity for the diagnosis of node-positive disease of ^{18}F-FDG PET/CT to be 84%, 46%, and 97%, respectively. Thus, the investigators concluded that FDG-PET/CT had no advantage over conventional CT, which in their study had an accuracy of 80%, sensitivity of 46%, and specificity of 92%.[12] Although the sensitivity of ^{18}F-FDG PET is suboptimal, multiple studies have demonstrated high specificity for detection of nodal involvement.

Disclosure: The author is a contracted member of the Speaker's Bureau of Lantheus Medical Imaging for Ablavar MR contrast. No part of the article deals with the Ablavar-related topics.

Department of Radiology, Albert Einstein College of Medicine, Montefiore Medical Center, 111 East 210th Street, Bronx, NY 10467, USA
E-mail address: vchernya@montefiore.org

Urol Clin N Am 38 (2011) 471–481
doi:10.1016/j.ucl.2011.07.002
0094-0143/11/$ – see front matter © 2011 Elsevier Inc. All rights reserved.

Similar to the high specificity (97%) demonstrated by Swinnen's group, Jensen and colleagues[13] found high specificity of 93.3% when evaluating ^{18}F-FDG PET for preoperative staging of bladder cancer. In attempts to improving ^{18}F-FDG PET performance for bladder cancer, Anjos and colleagues[14] added 1-hour delayed images after furosemide injection. While clearing the tracer from the urinary system allowed detection of recurrent bladder lesions in an additional 6 (35%) of 17 patients, additional metastatic lymph nodes on the delayed images were seen only in 2 (12%) of 17 patients.[14] Although sensitivity of ^{18}F-FDG PET for detecting nodal involvement in bladder cancer is somewhat disappointing, it still may be a useful prognostic study.[15] For instance, in 40 patients with bladder carcinoma evaluated by Drieskens and colleagues,[15] median survival time of patients with nodal and/or distant metastases on ^{18}F-FDG PET/CT was 13.5 months, compared with 32 months in the patients with negative ^{18}F-FDG PET/CT, with $P<.004$.

Addition of CT to the PET acquisition improves anatomic localization of abnormal PET activity, and the combination of ^{18}F-FDG PET and CT was shown to be very accurate in detecting pelvic nodal metastases in the setting of penile carcinoma, with reported sensitivity of 88.2% to 91%, specificity of 98.1% to 100%, positive predictive value of 93.8% to 100%, and negative predictive value of 94% to 96.3%.[16,17]

Similarly high performance of ^{18}F-FDG PET/CT has been shown in detection of testicular cancer metastases with reported sensitivity, specificity, positive predictive value, and negative predictive value of 93.3%, 97%, 93.3%, and 97%, respectively.[18] ^{18}F-FDG PET has also been shown to be a useful tool in evaluation of residual disease in patients with metastatic nonseminomatous germ cell tumors (GCT). Kollmannsberger and colleagues[19] compared the ability of ^{18}F-FDG PET to predict the viability of 85 residual masses in 45 patients with nonseminomatous GCT after chemotherapy with that of CT and tumor marker changes. The investigators found that ^{18}F-FDG PET had higher sensitivity for predicting a viable residual tumor (59%) than CT and tumor marker changes (sensitivities of 55% and 42%, respectively), and specificity higher than that of CT (92% vs 86%, respectively) but less than that of tumor marker changes (92% vs 100%, respectively).[19] Similar results were demonstrated by Pfannenberg and colleagues,[20] who evaluated 60 residual masses following high-dose chemotherapy in 28 patients with metastatic GCT. The investigators found no difference in sensitivity

for prediction of viability of residual masses between ^{18}F-FDG PET, CT/magnetic resonance imaging (MRI), and tumor marker levels (sensitivities of 70%, 62%, and 69%, respectively), but specificity of ^{18}F-FDG PET (83%) was higher than that of CT/MRI (72%) but lower than that of tumor marker levels (88%).[20] In addition, combination of all 3 modalities resulted in very high sensitivity (93%) and specificity (100%) for predicting viable residual disease.[20] The investigators concluded that positive ^{18}F-FDG PET results are highly correlated with the presence of viable residual tumor, but residual masses with negative PET findings still require resection. When tumor progression is established by CT and elevated tumor markers, additional ^{18}F-FDG PET seems to be of no significant benefit, but in patients with stable disease or partial remission in CT/MRI and normalized tumor markers as well as in marker-negative disease, ^{18}F-FDG PET is a useful diagnostic adjunct.[20]

In addition to being able to predict presence of a viable residual disease in patients with metastatic GCT, ^{18}F-FDG PET has been demonstrated to be a useful tool for early prediction of treatment response to high-dose salvage chemotherapy in patients with relapsed GCT.[21] The clinical course of disease after high-dose salvage chemotherapy was correctly predicted by ^{18}F-FDG PET during chemotherapy in 21 of 23 (91%) patients.[21] All 7 (100%) of patients who had a negative ^{18}F-FDG PET after initial part of treatment remained disease-free after completion of the full treatment regimen, whereas 14 of 16 (88%) patients with positive ^{18}F-FDG PET relapsed within 6 months following completion of chemotherapy regimen, or the histology of the resected residual mass after the chemotherapy still revealed the presence of viable carcinoma.[21] Thus, sensitivity and specificity of ^{18}F-FDG PET for the prediction of the overall failure of salvage chemotherapy were 100% and 78%, respectively, with the positive predictive and negative predictive values being 88% and 100%, respectively.[21]

[11]C-Choline is a radiopharmaceutical for PET imaging that may be a preferred tracer for prostate and bladder cancer, as it lacks the urinary radioactivity seen with ^{18}F-FDG.[22] Choline is one of the components of phosphatidylcholine, an essential element of phospholipids in the cell membrane.[23] Malignant tumors show a high proliferation and increased metabolism of cell membrane components that will lead to an increased uptake of choline.[23] de Jong and colleagues[23] calculated a sensitivity of ^{11}C-choline PET for staging metastatic lymph node disease in patients with prostate cancer of

80%, a specificity of 96%, and an accuracy of 93%. In addition, ^{11}C-choline PET detected solitary extraregional lymph node metastases in 5 of 12 patients with nodal metastases.[23] Similarly, in patients with bladder cancer, ^{11}C-choline PET was demonstrated to have a higher accuracy for detection of nodal metastases compared with contrast-enhanced CT (89% vs 82%, P<.01).[24]

While demonstrating high potential accuracy, the use of ^{11}C-choline tracer is limited because of its short half-life, requiring a cyclotron to be in close proximity to the hospital.[25] Labeling choline with the radioactive isotope ^{18}F could avoid this issue. ^{18}F-Choline accumulates in metabolically active cells and therefore can be detected on PET/CT (**Fig. 1**). In their study of 132 patients with prostate cancer, Beheshti and colleagues[26] found per-patient sensitivity and specificity of ^{18}F-choline PET/CT, in detection of malignant lymph nodes,

to be 45% and 96%, respectively. Positive and negative predictive values were 82% and 92%, respectively.[26]

SINGLE-PHOTON EMISSION COMPUTED TOMOGRAPHIC IMAGING

In addition to changes in metabolism, malignant cells express tumor-specific antigens. Single-photon emission computed tomographic (SPECT) imaging uses radioactive-labeled antibodies against such antigens. Indium-111 capromab pendetide (ProstaScint) is a radioactively labeled monoclonal antibody directed against the intracellular portion of the prostate-specific membrane antigen, a glycoprotein that is expressed by the prostate epithelium and is upregulated in (metastatic) prostate cancer.[25] Polascik and colleagues[27] reported ProstaScint scanning to detect 62% of pathologically proven metastatic

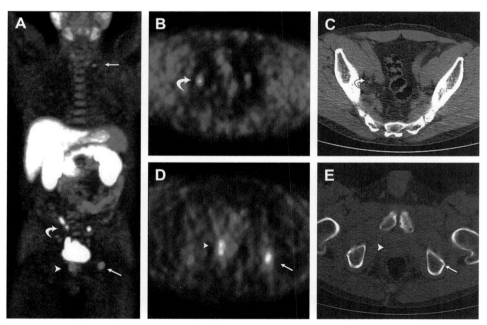

Fig. 1. Images obtained in a 71-year-old patient with prostate cancer that was upstaged at 18F-fluoromethylcholine (FCH) positron emission tomography (PET) (Gleason score, 7; prostate-specific antigen level, 4.7 ng/mL [4.7 mg/L]). (*A*) Maximum-intensity projection FCH PET image shows positive FCH uptake in the prostate (*arrowhead*), a right pelvic LN (*curved arrow*), and 2 bone metastases (*straight arrows*). (*B*) FCH PET image shows positive FCH uptake in a right external iliac LN metastasis (*curved arrow*). (*C*) The positive right pelvic LN seems to be unremarkable on the computed tomography (CT) portion of an FCH PET/CT image, with a 9 mm short-axis diameter (*arrow*). (*D*) FCH PET image shows positive FCH uptake in the right lobe of the prostate (*arrowhead*) and in the left acetabulum (*arrow*). (*E*) CT portion of an FCH PET/CT image shows no substantial morphologic change in the detected lesion in the left acetabulum (*arrow*), probably because of early bone marrow infiltration. The lesion detected at FCH PET was localized in the right prostate lobe (*arrowhead*). (*Reprinted from* Beheshti M, Imamovic L, Broinger G, et al. 18F choline PET/CT in the preoperative staging of prostate cancer in patients with intermediate or high risk of extracapsular disease: a prospective study of 130 patients. Radiology 2010; 254:932; Copyright RSNA 2010; with permission.)

lymph nodes. The investigators demonstrated that addition of a ProstaScint scan to the clinical predictive algorithms improves selection of candidates for definitive local therapy in men with clinically localized prostate carcinoma and significant risk of lymph node involvement.[27] In high-risk patients evaluated for risk of lymph node metastases prior to pelvic lymph node dissection, ProstaScint scan was found to have a sensitivity of 62%, specificity of 72%, positive predictive value of 62%, and negative predictive value of 72%.[28]

LYMPHOTROPIC NANOPARTICLE-ENHANCED MAGNETIC RESONANCE IMAGING

MRI is widely used when evaluating multiple primary neoplasms of the GU tract. MRI is particularly important in pretreatment evaluation of the prostate cancer.[29] Combination of various pulse sequences, each of which has its own strengths and weaknesses, has been demonstrated to yield an MRI examination that has a high sensitivity and specificity for detection of the prostate neoplasm as well as defining its extent.[29] High spatial and soft-tissue resolution of MRI as well as ability to obtain images in multiple planes allows for accurate assessment of local extent of the prostate cancer, including extension through the capsule and involvement of the seminal vesicles and/or neurovascular bundles (**Figs. 2** and **3**).[29] MR offers a superior soft-tissue resolution compared with CT, resulting in an improved ability to assess nodal morphology, signal-intensity changes, contrast enhancement with gadolinium, and central necrosis, all of which may be helpful in assessing malignant versus benign lymphadenopathy.[30] However, conventional MRI, as does CT, relies on nodal size and morphology for detection of nodal metastases (see **Fig. 2**), and thus demonstrates no improvement in accuracy over CT.[30]

Lymphotropic nanoparticle-enhanced MRI (LN-MRI) offers an accurate tool for lymph node staging in GU malignancies. This examination uses ultrasmall superparamagnetic iron oxide particles (USPIO), which are composed of a biodegradable monocrystalline, inverse spinel iron oxide core, and a polymer coating of low molecular weight dextran.[31] The iron oxide core measures 4.3 to 6.0 nm and the whole nanoparticle ranges in size from 30 to 50 nm, which is small enough to pass across capillary walls, drain via the lymphatic circulation, and localize in the lymph nodes where they allow for detailed characterization of these nodes independent of typically accepted size criterion.[31,32] The nanoparticles are packaged as a lyophilized powder, which is then reconstituted with normal saline and infused intravenously over 1 to 30 minutes at a dose of 2.6 mg per kg body weight.[31] The dextran coating of the nanoparticles aids in prolongation of their circulation time by preventing aggregation.[31] Once delivered to the lymph node, the nanoparticles are phagocytosed by macrophages of the reticuloendothelial system (RES), resulting in nanoparticle accumulation within the nodes.[30] Such accumulation results in shortening of T2* of the nodes and subsequent signal loss on T2-weighted and T2*-weighted images.[32] As metastatic lymph nodes lack normally functioning RES, their signal intensity remains intermediate to high on the T2-weighted and T2*-weighted sequences secondary to lack of USPIO accumulation (**Fig. 4**).[31,32]

LN-MRI has been shown to be effective in detection of nodal involvement with prostate cancer. Harisinghani and colleagues[33] reported 100% per-patient sensitivity, 95.7% per-patient specificity, and 97.5 per-patient accuracy of the LN-MRI. This result was a significant improvement over conventional MRI relying on size with per-patient sensitivity, specificity, and accuracy of 45.4%, 78.7%, and 65%, respectively.[33] In addition, LN-MRI was demonstrated to have high sensitivity, specificity, and accuracy of 96.4%, 99.3%, and 98.9%, respectively, for detection of metastases in lymph nodes with short axis of 5 to 10 mm.[33] Such nodal metastases would commonly be overlooked based on the size criteria of conventional MRI.

Heesakkers and colleagues[34] evaluated the value of LN-MRI in detecting lymph node metastases outside the routine surgical area. Of the examined 296 patients with prostate cancer and an intermediate to high risk for nodal metastases (prostate-specific antigen level >10 ng/mL, Gleason score >6, or stage T3 disease), 44 had pathologically proven nodal involvement.[34] In 18 of these 44 patients (41%), LN-MRI demonstrated metastatic nodes exclusively outside the routine dissection area (**Fig. 5**).[34] The investigators concluded that LN-MRI is a useful tool in guiding the area of extended pelvic lymph node dissection; in addition, LN-MRI helped in avoiding unnecessary radical prostatectomy in patients who might have otherwise been thought of as being free of nodal metastases.[34]

LN-MRI has been shown to improve nodal detection in the setting of bladder cancer.[35] Sensitivity and negative predictive value of the depiction of pelvic metastases improved significantly with USPIO administration compared with those of conventional MRI.[34] With the administration of USPIO, the sensitivity increased from 76% to 96% and specificity increased from 91% to 98%.[35] In addition, after USPIO administration,

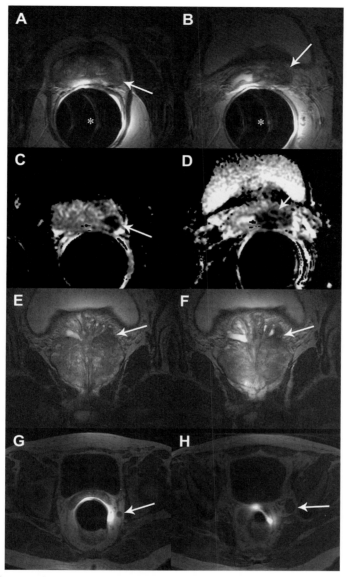

Fig. 2. Endorectal coil magnetic resonance imaging (MRI) in a 67-year-old man with biopsy-proven prostate cancer. (*A*) Axial T2-weighted image (repetition time [TR] in milliseconds, 4450/echo time [TE] in milliseconds, 82.4) demonstrates an area of low signal intensity in the left peripheral zone (*arrow*), consistent with a tumor. Asterisk denotes the endorectal probe. (*B*) Axial T2-weighted image (TR 4450/TE 82.4) superior to (*A*) demonstrates extension of the tumor into the left seminal vesicle (*arrow*). Asterisk denotes the endorectal probe. (*C, D*) Apparent diffusion coefficient (ADC) map at the levels similar to (*A*) and (*B*) demonstrate areas of restricted diffusion (*arrow*) corresponding to the areas of tumor involvement. (*E, F*) Coronal T2-weighted images (TR 3000/TE 88.5) at the level of the seminal vesicles demonstrate the tumor involvement of the left seminal vesicle (*arrows*). (*G, H*) Axial T1-weighted images (TR 400/TE 9.7) through the pelvis demonstrate metastatic left internal obturator (*G*) and internal iliac (*H*) lymph nodes (*arrows*). The left internal iliac lymph node (*H*) measures 1.4 cm in short axis, meeting the size criteria for lymphadenopathy. The left obturator lymph node (*G*), although measuring less than 1 cm in short axis, has an abnormally round configuration, raising suspicion for metastatic involvement.

metastases were prospectively found in 10 of 12 normal-sized nodes, with a short-axis diameter less than 10 mm, whereas these metastases were not detected on precontrast images.[35]

LN-MRI has been shown to improve sensitivity, specificity, and accuracy of nodal involvement detection in patients with testicular cancer in comparison with size criteria for detecting

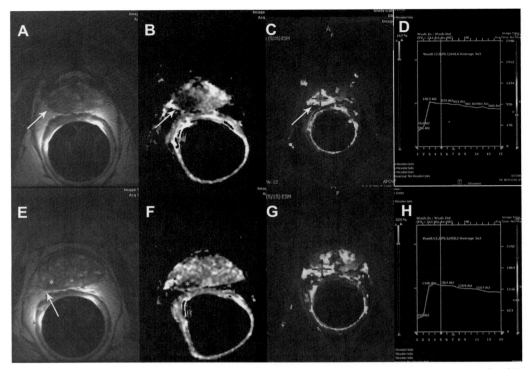

Fig. 3. Endorectal coil MRI in a 69-year-old man with biopsy-proven prostate cancer. (*A*) Axial T2-weighted image (TR 4450/TE 82.4), (*B*) ADC map, (*C*) perfusion map, and (*D*) wash-in/wash-out curve at the level of the superior prostate demonstrating a large neoplasm (*arrow*) with low signal intensity on T2-weighted sequences, restricted diffusion, and hypervascular pattern of enhancement. (*E*) Axial T2-weighted image (TR 4450/TE 82.4), (*F*) ADC map, (*G*) perfusion map, and (*H*) wash-in/wash-out curve at the level of neurovascular bundle demonstrate extension of the tumor (*asterisk*) though the capsule into the right neurovascular bundle (*arrow* in *A*).

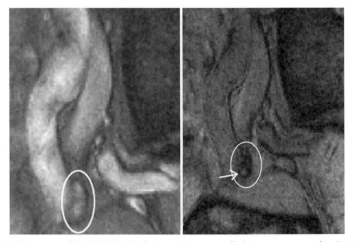

Fig. 4. T2*-weighted MR images (TR 800/TE 25.4) in a plane parallel to psoas muscle. Precontrast image (*left*) shows normal-sized (12 × 8 mm) node (*ellipse*). On postcontrast image (*right*), this same node shows signal intensity decrease with a small 2 mm area (*arrow*) of persistent high signal intensity. Histopathologic results confirmed small 2 mm metastases. (*Reprinted from* Deserno WM, Harisinghani MG, Taupitz M, et al. Urinary bladder cancer: preoperative nodal staging with ferumoxtran-10-enhanced MR imaging. Radiology 2004;233:453; Copyright RSNA 2004; with permission.)

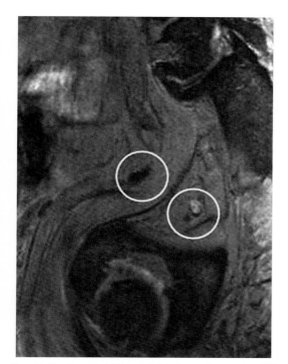

Fig. 5. Semisagittal T2*-weighted gradient-echo (TR 2200/TE 18) MR image obtained after the administration of ferumoxtran-10. The black lymph node (*top circle*) is normal, but the white node (*bottom circle*) is metastatic. This lymph node is located about 2 cm behind the obturator nerve and would not be removed during routine pelvic lymph node dissection. (*Reprinted from* Heesakkers RA, Jager GJ, Hövels AM. Prostate cancer: detection of lymph node metastases outside the routine surgical area with ferumoxtran-10-enhanced MR imaging. Radiology 2009;251:412; Copyright RSNA 2009; with permission.)

malignant nodes.[36] LN-MRI was found to have sensitivity of 88.2%, specificity of 92%, and accuracy of 90.4%, whereas conventional MRI had a sensitivity of 70.5%, specificity of 68%, and accuracy of 69%.[36] Similar promising results of LN-MRI have been demonstrated for the nodal detection in patients with penile cancer, with sensitivity, specificity, and positive and negative predictive values of 100%, 97%, 81.2%, and 100%, respectively.[37]

However promising as LN-MRI appears to be, it has some limitations. Interpretation of the images is time consuming because a node-by-node comparison must be made between two sets of images, before and after USPIO administration.[33,35] This comparison requires special expertise, which explains, at least in part, why USPIO has not yet received approval by the authorities, as the final approval by the Food and Drug Administration and the European Medicines Agency is still pending.[38]

DIFFUSION-WEIGHTED MAGNETIC RESONANCE IMAGING

Diffusion-weighted MRI (DW-MRI) relies on microscopic mobility of water molecules in the tissues. This mobility is classically called Brownian motion; it is caused by thermal motion and is highly influenced by the cellular environment of water. Thus, findings on DW-MRI can reflect biological abnormalities of the underlying tissues.[39] Apparent diffusion coefficient (ADC) values, derived from DW-MRI, are often used as a quantitative parameter to describe the microscopic water diffusibility. ADC values have been shown to be decreased in multiple primary genitourinary malignancies, including renal cell carcinoma, prostate carcinoma, and bladder cancer.[39] DW-MRI has proved to be crucial for detection of primary prostate cancer, increasing sensitivity and specificity of routine MRI (see **Fig. 3**).[40,41] While the value of DW-MRI in evaluating primary GU malignancies has been well established, its role in the detection of nodal metastases is still under investigation.[39] DW-MRI may have a role in the assessment of malignant lymph nodes from urogenital tumors, as malignant nodes are in theory expected to show impeded diffusion, resulting in low ADC values, because most primary malignant tumors show impeded diffusion caused by high cellularity.[39] Eiber and colleagues[42] compared the mean ADC values between benign and malignant lymph nodes in patients with prostate cancer and found a significant decrease in ADC values ($\times 10^{-3}$ mm^2/s) of malignant lymph nodes (1.07 $\pm$ 0.23) compared with those of the benign lymph nodes (1.54 $\pm$ 0.25). However, the role of DW-MRI in evaluation of nodal metastases is not fully researched. The use of DW-MR sequences with different parameters, on MRI scanners with different field strengths and/or from different manufacturers, may raise variability in the qualitative and quantitative assessment of DW-MRI.[39] This variation leads to lack of standardization in imaging technique and analysis, slightly hampers its use in clinical practice, and limits comparison between studies.[39]

The study conducted by Beer and colleagues[43] compared the information of functional MR imaging in DW-MRI with that of ^{11}C-choline PET/CT in patients with prostate cancer. In addition, the investigators compared the ADC values of benign and malignant lymph nodes to estimate whether DW-MRI might have the potential to be an ancillary tool for lymph node characterization in prostate cancer patients. This study demonstrated a moderate inverse correlation between ADC values and standard uptake value (SUV) on ^{11}C-choline PET/CT.[43] Diagnostic accuracies were similar between the two techniques, being 80.0% for DW-MRI and 85.4% for ^{11}C-choline PET/CT.[43]

Thoeny and colleagues[38] investigated the potential of combining LN-MRI and DW-MRI in patients with bladder and/or prostate cancer. As diffusion-weighted sequences are typically sensitive to T2* effect, normal lymph nodes accumulating USPIO are expected to significantly lose signal. On the other hand, the combination of reduced diffusion and relatively unchanged T2* after USPIO administration should result in preserved signal in the malignant lymph nodes on DW-MRI. The investigators demonstrated similar diagnostic accuracy between USPIO DW-MRI and LN-MRI. However, the former method resulted in significant reduction in interpretation times from an average of 80 minutes (range 45–180 minutes) to an average of 13 minutes (range 5–90 minutes).[38]

Whereas most studies report high diagnostic accuracy for both ^{11}C-choline PET/CT and DW-MRI, a recently published study by Budiharto and colleagues[44] seems to refute such results. The investigators evaluated 36 patients with histologically proven prostate cancer and no pelvic lymphadenopathy on contrast-enhanced CT. The patients had intermediate risk of lymph node metastases of between 10% and 35%; all of them had undergone ^{11}C-choline PET/CT and DW-MRI before radical prostatectomy with extended pelvic lymph node dissection.[44] The reported per-patient sensitivity, specificity, positive predictive value, and negative predictive value for ^{11}C-choline PET/CT were 18.8%, 95%, 75%, and 59.4%, respectively. For DW-MRI, the reported per-patient sensitivity, specificity, positive predictive value, and negative predictive value were 42.9%, 81.8%, 60%, and 69.2%, respectively.[44] In the 36 patients, 733 nodes were resected, and per-node sensitivity, specificity, positive predictive value, and negative predictive value for detection of nodal metastases were 9.4%, 99.7%, 75%, and 91.0%, respectively, in ^{11}C-choline PET/CT and 9.4%, 99.7%, 75%, 91.0%, respectively, for DW-MRI.[44] These results contradict most prior studies for both ^{11}C-choline PET/CT and DW-MRI, which the investigators in part attribute to a relatively high percentage (53.1%) of positive nodes containing micrometastases.[44] However, the investigators point out some flaws in the design of the older studies, stating that because such shortcomings were absent in their study, their results are more reliable and reflective of the true performance of the two studied modalities. Based on their results, Budiharto and colleagues[44] believe that ^{11}C-choline PET-CT and DW-MRI cannot be recommended for routine clinical use in nodal staging of high-risk prostate cancer patients before initial treatment. To date, only one article reports such poor performance of these imaging techniques. Further investigations are necessary to establish the optimal imaging modality for early nodal detection in patients with prostate cancer.

SENTINEL LYMPH NODE IMAGING

The lymphatic drainage pattern of a cancer determines the extent of lymph node dissection, allowing for less extensive surgery when appropriate and thus potentially decreasing the morbidity. Preoperative visualization of lymphatic drainage via lymphoscintigraphy involves injection of a radiopharmaceutical agent into the organ of interest followed by planar imaging and/or SPECT as well as intraoperative gamma probe. Sentinel node lymphadenectomy has been demonstrated to be accurate for lymph node staging in prostate cancer.[45] An advantage of sentinel node lymphadenectomy in prostate cancer is the fact that sentinel nodes outside of the routinely dissected area and possibly outside the extended pelvic lymphadenectomy region can also be localized and removed.[45] With the combination of SPECT and CT, the nodal tracer uptake detected by SPECT can be fused with CT, providing the surgeon with better information on the anatomic location of the sentinel node. Of the 46 patients with prostate cancer examined by Vermeeren and colleagues,[45] SPECT/CT revealed additional sentinel nodes not seen on planar imaging in 29 (63%). Definite advantage of detecting these additional nodes was observed in 63% of patients and presumable advantage in 24% of patients; only in 13% of patients did the additional findings of SPECT/CT have no clear advantage. Thirty-five percent of all patients had uncommon location of sentinel nodes outside the pelvic area, and 56% of these were seen only on SPECT/CT. In addition, of the 15 patients with positive sentinel nodes, 7 (47%) were present exclusively in the nodes detected by SPECT/CT only.[45]

In patients with squamous cell penile carcinoma, lymphoscintigraphy results in high rates of sentinel node visualization, ranging between 93% and 97%.[46,47] Lymphoscintigraphy using SPECT/CT has been successfully used in patients with penile cancer to define the extent of the required dissection field.[48] In patients with clinically node-negative penile squamous cell carcinoma, a sentinel node biopsy was able to detect nodal metastases in 79 (14%) of the 572 examined groins.[46] Sentinel node biopsy was shown to have a similar detection rate (12%) of metastatic involvement in clinically normal groin lymph nodes in patients with previous resection of the penile tumor.[47]

Lymphoscintigraphy has proved to be a useful technique in the staging of other urologic malignancies. Bex and colleagues[49] demonstrated feasibility for the use of SPECT/CT for localization and sampling of sentinel nodes in patients with renal cell carcinoma. Roth and colleagues[50] demonstrated that lymphoscintigraphy could also define the lymphatic drainage in patients with bladder cancer. In fact, the investigators were able to demonstrate that pelvic lymph node dissection limited to the ventral portion of the external iliac vessels and obturator fossa removed only about 50% of all primary lymphatic landing sites, whereas extension along the major pelvic vessels up to the ureteroiliac crossing removes about 90%.

SUMMARY

There are several novel techniques being developed to improve detection of nodal involvement in patients with GU malignancies. Continuing research with prospective design, using larger numbers of patients, will be necessary to establish which of the available techniques should be used as standard of care.

REFERENCES

1. Fleischmann A, Thalmann GN, Markwalder R, et al. Extracapsular extension of pelvic lymph node metastases from urothelial carcinoma of the bladder is an independent prognostic factor. J Clin Oncol 2005;23:2358–65.

2. Jager GJ, Barentsz JO, Oosterhof GO, et al. Pelvic adenopathy in prostatic and urinary bladder carcinoma: MR imaging with a three-dimensional TI-weighted magnetization prepared-rapid gradient-echo sequence. AJR Am J Roentgenol 1996;167:1503–7.

3. Tiguert R, Gheiler EL, Tefilli MV, et al. Lymph node size does not correlate with the presence of prostate cancer metastasis. Urology 1999;53:367–71.

4. Saksena MA, Kim JY, Harisinghani MG. Nodal staging in genitourinary cancers. Abdom Imaging 2006;31:644–51.

5. Bader P, Burkhard FC, Markwalder R, et al. Disease progression and survival of patients with positive lymph nodes after radical prostatectomy. Is there a chance of cure? J Urol 2003;169:849–54.

6. Pieterman RM, van Putten JW, Meuzelaar JJ, et al. Preoperative staging of non-small-cell lung cancer with positron-emission tomography. N Engl J Med 2000;343:254–61.

7. Spermon JR, De Geus-Oei LF, Kiemeney LA, et al. The role of [18]fluoro-2-deoxyglucose positron emission tomography in initial staging and re-staging after chemotherapy for testicular germ cell tumors. BJU Int 2002;89:549–56.

8. Liu IJ, Zafar MB, Lai YH, et al. Fluorodeoxyglucose positron emission tomography studies in diagnosis and staging of clinically organ-confined prostate cancer. Urology 2001;57:108–11.

9. Shvartz O, Han KR, Seltzer M, et al. Positron emission tomography in urologic oncology. Cancer Control 2002;9:335–42.

10. Heicappell R, Muller-Mattheis V, Reinhardt M, et al. Staging of pelvic lymph nodes in neoplasms of the bladder and prostate by positron emission tomography with 2-[(18)F]-2-deoxy-D-glucose. Eur Urol 1999;36:582–7.

11. Lodde M, Lacombe L, Friede J, et al. Evaluation of fluorodeoxyglucose positron-emission tomography with computed tomography for staging of urothelial carcinoma. BJU Int 2010;106(5):658–63.

12. Swinnen G, Maes A, Pottel H, et al. FDG-PET/CT for the preoperative lymph node staging of invasive bladder cancer. Eur Urol 2010;57:641–7.

13. Jensen TK, Holt P, Gerke O, et al. Preoperative lymph-node staging of invasive urothelial bladder cancer with (18)F-fluorodeoxyglucose positron emission tomography/computed axial tomography and magnetic resonance imaging: correlation with histopathology. Scand J Urol Nephrol 2011;45(2):122–8.

14. Anjos DA, Etchebehere EC, Ramos CD, et al. ^{18}F-FDG PET/CT delayed images after diuretic for re-staging invasive bladder cancer. J Nucl Med 2007;48:764–70.

15. Drieskens O, Oyen R, Van Poppel H, et al. FDG-PET for preoperative staging of bladder cancer. Eur J Nucl Med Mol Imaging 2005;32:1412–7.

16. Graafland NM, Leijte JA, Valdés Olmos RA, et al. Scanning with ^{18}F-FDG-PET/CT for detection of pelvic nodal involvement in inguinal node-positive penile carcinoma. Eur Urol 2009;56:339–45.

17. Schlenker B, Scher B, Tiling R, et al. Detection of inguinal lymph node involvement in penile squamous cell carcinoma by ^{18}F-fluorodeoxyglucose PET/CT: a prospective single-center study. Urol Oncol 2009. [Epub ahead of print].

18. Sterbis JR, Rice KR, Javitt MC, et al. Fusion imaging: a novel staging modality in testis cancer. J Cancer 2010;1:223–9.

19. Kollmannsberger C, Oechsle K, Dohmen BM, et al. Prospective comparison of [^{18}F]fluorodeoxyglucose positron emission tomography with conventional assessment by computed tomography scans and

serum tumor markers for the evaluation of residual masses in patients with nonseminomatous germ cell carcinoma. Cancer 2002;94:2353–62.

20. Pfannenberg AC, Oechsle K, Bokemeyer C, et al. The role of [(18)F] FDG-PET, CT/MRI and tumor marker kinetics in the evaluation of post chemotherapy residual masses in metastatic germ cell tumors–prospects for management. World J Urol 2004;22:132–9.

21. Bokemeyer C, Kollmannsberger C, Oechsle K, et al. Early prediction of treatment response to high-dose salvage chemotherapy in patients with relapsed germ cell cancer using [(18)F]FDG PET. Br J Cancer 2002;86:506–11.

22. Hara T, Kosaka N, Kishi H. PET imaging of prostate cancer using carbon-11-choline. J Nucl Med 1998; 39:990–5.

23. de Jong IJ, Pruim J, Elsinga PH, et al. ^{11}C-choline positron emission tomography for the evaluation after treatment of localized prostate cancer. Eur Urol 2003;44(1):32–8.

24. Picchio M, Treiber U, Beer AJ, et al. Value of ^{11}C-choline PET and contrast-enhanced CT for staging of bladder cancer: correlation with histopathologic findings. J Nucl Med 2006;47:938–44.

25. Pouliot F, Johnson M, Wu L. Non-invasive molecular imaging of prostate cancer lymph node metastasis. Trends Mol Med 2009;15:254–62.

26. Beheshti M, Imamovic L, Broinger G, et al. [18]F choline PET/CT in the preoperative staging of prostate cancer in patients with intermediate or high risk of extracapsular disease: a prospective study of 130 patients. Radiology 2010;254:925–33.

27. Polascik TJ, Manyak MJ, Haseman MK, et al. Comparison of clinical staging algorithms and 111-indium-capromab pendetide immunoscintigraphy in the prediction of lymph node involvement in high risk prostate carcinoma patients. Cancer 1999;85: 1586–92.

28. Rosenthal SA, Haseman MK, Polascik TJ. Utility of capromab pendetide (ProstaScint) imaging in the management of prostate cancer. Tech Urol 2001;7: 27–37.

29. Choi YJ, Kim JK, Kim N, et al. Functional MR imaging of prostate cancer. Radiographics 2007; 27:63–75.

30. Yang WT, Lam WW, Yu MY, et al. Comparison of dynamic helical CT and dynamic MR imaging in the evaluation of pelvic lymph nodes in cervical carcinoma. AJR Am J Roentgenol 2000;175: 759–66.

31. Feldman AS, McDougal WS, Harisinghani MG. The potential of nanoparticle-enhanced imaging. Seminars and Original Investigations. Urol Oncol 2008; 26:65–73.

32. Weissleder R, Elizondo G, Wittenberg J, et al. Ultra-small superparamagnetic iron oxide: an intravenous contrast agent for assessing lymph nodes with MR imaging. Radiology 1990;175:494–8.

33. Harisinghani MG, Barenztsz J, Hahn PF, et al. Noninvasive detection of clinically occult lymph-node metastases in prostate cancer. N Engl J Med 2003;348:2491–9.

34. Heesakkers RA, Jager GJ, Hövels AM, et al. Prostate cancer: detection of lymph node metastases outside the routine surgical area with ferumoxtran-10-enhanced MR imaging. Radiology 2009;251: 408–14.

35. Deserno WM, Harisinghani MG, Taupitz M, et al. Urinary bladder cancer: preoperative nodal staging with ferumoxtran-10-enhanced MR imaging. Radiology 2004;233:449–56.

36. Harisinghani MG, Saksena M, Ross R, et al. A pilot study of lymphotrophic nanoparticle-enhanced magnetic resonance imaging technique in early stage testicular cancer: a new method for noninvasive lymph node evaluation. Urology 2005;66:1066–71.

37. Tabatabaei S, Harisinghani M, McDougal WS. Regional lymph node staging using lymphotrophic nanoparticle enhanced magnetic resonance imaging with ferumoxtran-10 in patients with penile cancer. J Urol 2005;174:923–7.

38. Thoeny HC, Triantafyllou M, Birkhaeuser FD, et al. Combined ultrasmall superparamagnetic particles of iron oxide-enhanced and diffusion-weighted magnetic resonance imaging reliably detect pelvic lymph node metastases in normal-sized nodes of bladder and prostate cancer patients. Eur Urol 2009;55:761–9.

39. Petralia G, Thoeny HC. DW-MRI of the urogenital tract: applications in oncology. Cancer Imaging 2010;10:S112–23.

40. Haider MA, van der Kwast TH, Tanguay J, et al. Combined T2-weighted and diffusion-weighted MRI for localization of prostate cancer. AJR Am J Roentgenol 2007;189:323–8.

41. Yoshimitsu K, Kiyoshima K, Irie H, et al. Usefulness of apparent diffusion coefficient map in diagnosing prostate carcinoma: correlation with stepwise histopathology. J Magn Reson Imaging 2008;27:132–9.

42. Eiber M, Beer AJ, Holzapfel K, et al. Preliminary results for characterization of pelvic lymph nodes in patients with prostate cancer by diffusion-weighted MR-imaging. Invest Radiol 2010;45: 15–23.

43. Beer AJ, Eiber M, Souvatzoglou M, et al. Restricted water diffusibility as measured by diffusion-weighted MR imaging and choline uptake in (11)C-choline pet/ct are correlated in pelvic lymph nodes in patients with prostate cancer. Mol Imaging Biol 2011;13(2):352–61.

44. Budiharto T, Joniau S, Lerut E, et al. Prospective evaluation of (11)C-choline positron emission tomography/computed tomography and diffusion-weighted

magnetic resonance imaging for the nodal staging of prostate cancer with a high risk of lymph node metastases. Eur Urol 2011;60(1):125–30.

45. Vermeeren L, Valdés Olmos RA, Meinhardt W, et al. Value of SPECT/CT for detection and anatomic localization of sentinel lymph nodes before laparoscopic sentinel node lymphadenectomy in prostate carcinoma. J Nucl Med 2009;50:865–70.

46. Leijte JA, Hughes B, Graafland NM, et al. Two-center evaluation of dynamic sentinel node biopsy for squamous cell carcinoma of the penis. J Clin Oncol 2009;27:3325–9.

47. Graafland NM, Valdés Olmos RA, Meinhardt W, et al. Nodal staging in penile carcinoma by dynamic

sentinel node biopsy after previous therapeutic primary tumour resection. Eur Urol 2010;58:748–51.

48. Leijte JA, Valdés Olmos RA, Nieweg OE, et al. Anatomical mapping of lymphatic drainage in penile carcinoma with SPECT-CT: implications for the extent of inguinal lymph node dissection. Eur Urol 2008;54:885–92.

49. Bex A, Vermeeren L, de Windt G, et al. Feasibility of sentinel node detection in renal cell carcinoma: a pilot study. Eur J Nucl Med Mol Imaging 2010; 37:1117–23.

50. Roth B, Wissmeyer MP, Zehnder P, et al. A new multimodality technique accurately maps the primary lymphatic landing sites of the bladder. Eur Urol 2010;57:205–11.

Lymphadenectomy in Urologic Oncology: Pathologic Considerations

Riley E. Alexander, MD, MBA[a], Ming-Tse Sung, MD[b,c], Liang Cheng, MD[a,d],*

KEYWORDS

- Lymphadenectomy • Urothelial cancer • Urinary bladder
- Staging and classification • Sampling and reporting

Lymphadenectomy (LAD) in genitourinary (GU) cancer is an area in which close communication and understanding between the urologist and pathologist are required to ensure the procedure fulfills its potential to the patient. Although the primary histologic type of tumor varies between anatomic sites, lymph node status still plays a major role in the staging in all of these cases and is an integral part of the American Joint Committee on Cancer (AJCC) staging criteria (**Table 1**).[1]

This review discusses current recommendations on handling and submission protocols for the urologist and pathologist involving LAD specimens in GU oncologic surgery. To accomplish this goal, particular recommendations for the kidney, upper urinary tract, urinary bladder, prostate, penis, and testes, and their respective primary cancer types, are detailed. In addition, the use and appropriateness of intraoperative frozen sections are discussed. To conclude, how emerging molecular techniques are affecting the way pathologists report findings in LAD specimens is investigated. However, to begin an overview of the large similarities in specimen submission and pathologic evaluation is given.

SPECIMEN SUBMISSION AND PROCESSING

The initial step in determining if optimal conditions are met for lymph node assessment in LAD lies with the urologist. Of primary consideration is how the urologist submits the specimen, specifically en bloc or as separate/fragmented parts. The literature supports the submission of the LAD specimens in separate, properly labeled parts.[2-4] In doing so, the urologist is able to relay to the pathologist accurate, in vivo assessment of location and, in addition, maximize inspection by decreasing associated soft tissue. Submission of nodes en bloc was reported by Stein and colleagues[5] to reduce median total lymph nodes removed from 68 in the separately packaged group to 31 in the en bloc group. Because of this finding, the submission method directly affected important nodal prognostic indicators of total

Financial disclosures/Conflicts of interest: The authors have nothing to disclose.

[a] Department of Pathology and Laboratory Medicine, Indiana University School of Medicine, Room 4010, 350 West 11th Street, Indianapolis, IN 46202, USA

[b] Department of Pathology, Kaohsiung Chang Gung Memorial Hospital and Chang Gung University College of Medicine, 123 Ta Pei Road, Niao Sung District, Kaohsiung 833, Taiwan

[c] Department of Laboratory Medicine, Kaohsiung Chang Gung Memorial Hospital and Chang Gung University College of Medicine, 123 Ta Pei Road, Niao Sung District, Kaohsiung 833, Taiwan

[d] Department of Urology, Indiana University School of Medicine, 535 North Barnhill Drive, Indianapolis, IN 46202, USA

* Corresponding author. Department of Pathology and Laboratory Medicine, Indiana University School of Medicine, Room 4010, 350 West 11th Street, Indianapolis, IN 46202.

E-mail address: liang_cheng@yahoo.com

doi:10.1016/j.ucl.2011.07.001
0094-0143/11/$ – see front matter © 2011 Elsevier Inc. All rights reserved.

Table 1
Regional lymph node staging (AJCC Staging Manual, Seventh Edition)

Kidney

Stage	Stage Category Definitions
NX	Regional lymph nodes cannot be assessed
N0	No regional lymph node metastasis
N1	Regional lymph node metastasis

Renal pelvis and ureter

NX	Regional lymph nodes cannot be assessed
N0	No regional lymph node metastasis
N1	Metastasis in a single lymph node, 2 cm or less in greatest dimension
N2	Metastasis in a single lymph node, more than 2 cm but not more than 5 cm in greatest dimension; or multiple lymph nodes, none more than 5 cm in greatest dimension
N3	Metastasis in a lymph node, more than 5 cm in greatest dimension

Bladder

NX	Lymph nodes cannot be assessed
N0	No lymph node metastasis
N1	Single regional lymph node metastasis in the true pelvis (hypogastric, obturator, external iliac, or presacral lymph node)
N2	Multiple regional lymph node metastasis in the true pelvis (hypogastric, obturator, external iliac, or presacral lymph node metastasis)
N3	Lymph node metastasis to the common iliac nodes

Prostate

pNX	Regional lymph nodes not sampled
pN0	No positive regional nodes
pN1	Metastases in regional node(s)

Testes

NX	Regional lymph nodes cannot be assessed
N0	No regional lymph node metastasis
pN1	Metastasis with a lymph node mass 2 cm or less in greatest dimension and less than or equal to 5 nodes positive, none more than 2 cm in greatest dimension
pN2	Metastasis with a lymph node mass more than 2 cm but not more than 5 cm in greatest dimension; or more than 5 nodes positive, none more than 5 cm; or evidence of extranodal extension of tumor
pN3	Metastasis with a lymph node mass more than 5 cm in greatest dimension

Penis

pNX	Regional lymph nodes cannot be assessed
pN0	No regional lymph node metastasis
pN1	Metastasis in a single inguinal lymph node
pN2	Metastasis in multiple or bilateral inguinal lymph nodes
pN3	Extranodal extension of lymph node metastasis or pelvic lymph node(s) unilateral or bilateral

positive lymph nodes and the dependent figure of lymph node density.[5]

In addition, it is helpful to the pathologist if the urologist submits their assessment of nodes removed at the time of specimen submission.[6] Besides these intraoperative considerations, it is the responsibility of the urologist to ensure that the LAD specimens are placed as quickly as possible in fixative (10% buffered formalin) so that the tissue does not degrade before pathologic evaluation.[3,6–9]

Once these crucial initial steps have been fulfilled, it becomes the responsibility of the pathologist that the specimen is dissected and documented properly to obtain maximal diagnostic tissue for microscopic examination. Because LAD specimens are generally received with attached fatty soft tissue, careful palpation and sectioning through the specimen must be undertaken to identify all possible nodes.[3] Submission of 1 section of any grossly positive lymph node is allowed, but complete submission of all other nodes is required, along with documentation of any remarkable features (eg, calcification, hemorrhage, necrosis).[6,7] It is generally recommended to use 2-mm to 4-mm sections when sectioning the specimen.[10] Along with the number of nodes submitted, documentation of the size of grossly positive nodes, extranodal extension, the size of metastases present, and histologic grade of metastases present is required,[6,10,11] because this may affect prognosis and staging.[6,12]

Should examination of submitted tissue not reveal any or inadequate lymph nodes, placement in lymph node revealing solution (LNRS) is recommended to enhance lymph node yield (**Fig. 1**).[13] This procedure is particularly important when an institutional minimum node submission policy is in place because processing of the specimen

can occur without LNRS first and can then be used only in situations in which the minimum number is not met.[14] A subsequent examination after placement in LNRS that still yields no or inadequate lymph nodes warrants submission of all received adipose tissue labeled by the urologist as a submitted node or attached to the main specimen, if received en bloc.[15] The total number of nodes submitted is important and highlights one of the major site-specific discrepancies in pathology reporting of LAD specimens.

KIDNEY

LAD in the kidney in patients with renal cell carcinoma (RCC) is one of contentious debate. The low prevalence of nodal metastases has convinced some against broad use[16] of the procedure, whereas others have shown survival benefits to the procedure.[17,18] Recent evidence has shown that lymph node stage represented the most informative variable and achieved independent predictor status of cancer-specific survival.[19] This

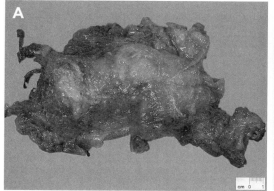
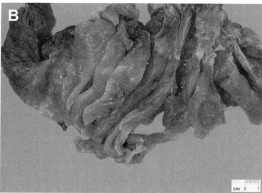
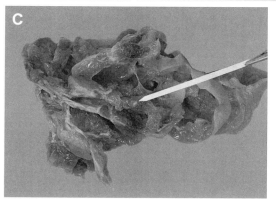

Fig. 1. Gross LAD specimen. (*A*) The appearance of a separated node packet removed during a radical cystectomy. This image was taken after formalin fixation. Note the fatty nature of the specimen and the lack of any easily identifiable lymph nodes. (*B*) The effects of LNRS (Carnoy solution, in this case) on the tissue after 12-hour fixation. Notice the lightening of the fatty tissue. (*C*) After thorough sectioning, a node is located (*arrow*) and identified by its brighter white color compared with adjacent fatty soft tissue.

finding has been shown to be especially true when there are no synchronous distant metastases; distant metastases diminish the prognostic impact of involved nodes when present.[20] Because of this situation, locoregional lymph node status may become an increasingly important staging/therapeutic procedure. However, detailed analysis of this controversial argument in RCC is beyond the scope of this review; until a consensus is reached, it is apparent that many urologists choose to perform LAD, and the pathologist must be aware of what is important to both the urologist and the patient.

Crispen and colleagues[21] advocate that when an LAD is performed in the setting of RCC, it should be performed from the crus of the diaphragm to the common iliac artery, involving the nodes of the ipsilateral great vessel and the interaortocaval region. It lies within the responsibilities of the pathologists to assess the specimen received and, if not received separately labeled, it may be necessary to contact the urologist to accurately judge anatomic geography of the specimen.

A consensus number on minimum nodes has not yet been established. However, the recent literature supports 13 as an accepted minimum.[21,22] Crispen and colleagues[21] showed a significantly greater percentage of nodal disease, 20.8% versus 10.2%, in similarly risk-stratified patients. Hence, if the pathologist is unable to locate 13 nodes during gross examination and no nodal disease is found on microscopic examination, more tissue needs to be submitted for possible nodes missed on the first examination or the urologist needs to be informed that the LAD is likely inadequate.

Recently, evaluations have taken place on the usefulness of frozen section diagnosis in patients with RCC as an adjunct to clinical and imaging risk stratification for nodal involvement. Ming and colleagues[23] reported that frozen section diagnosis had a sensitivity, specificity, concordance, and false-negative rate of 88.9%, 100%, 96.5%, and 11.1%, respectively. Furthermore, these investigators made the claim that many enlarged nodes turn out to be benign. Crispen and colleagues reported similar figures. However, others have claimed that if the low morbidity and benefit to staging and possible treatment preclude the value of frozen section and in patients at risk, LAD should proceed.[18] Communication between the urologist and pathologist is necessary so that an agreed procedure at their particular institution can be conducted until a consensus is reached.

As per the *AJCC Staging Manual, Seventh Edition*, the pathologist's report must also include other data that are considered prognostic factors.

These data include extranodal extension, size of metastasis in involved lymph nodes, and size of the largest tumor deposit in the lymph nodes.[1]

UPPER URINARY TRACT AND URINARY BLADDER

The literature strongly supports the role of LAD in the staging and treatment of upper tract urothelial carcinoma.[24,25] In addition, it has been shown to offer curative potential.[26] Despite the well-accepted nature of the practice, variation on extent and adequate number of nodes submitted/sampled still exists.

The studies described earlier reported a median lymph node range of 4 to 8, all showing benefit to the patient.[24–26] This small, but narrow, range of nodes submitted further emphasized the importance of close communications between urologists and pathologists. The pathologist can use LNRS to increase the yield of small nodes if correlation between estimated nodes submitted and nodes retrieved during gross examination is not achieved.[27]

LAD in the setting of urothelial carcinoma of the urinary bladder is well researched (**Fig. 2**). Standard nodal dissections have been shown to remove a mean of as high as 23 nodes,[28] but much discrepancy and controversy exist over the minimum number of nodes required for adequate LAD. Data from 9 of the largest series have shown an average number of lymph nodes removed to be 13.[10] Others have shown clinical benefit occurs only in patients with 16 nodes or more removed.[29,30] May and colleagues[29] specifically cited an increase in 5-year cancer-specific survival from 72% to 83% when 16 or more nodes are removed. Even higher goals are used by some.[31,32]

Of particular note in the studies collected in the review by Hurle and Naspro[10] is increased cancer-specific survival of patients with negative or independent node status when compared with those with positive nodes. For instance, in the report by Leissner and colleagues,[30] lymph node retrieval of 16 or more nodes showed a 5-year cancer-specific survival of 65% to 51% in those with less than 15 in the independent status group; this decreased to 35% and 23%, respectively, in those with positive node status. Similar 5-year results were obtained by Herr and colleagues[33] when comparing those with negative node status with 8 or more and less than 8 (82% and 41%, respectively) and those with positive node status with the 3-tiered nodes removed observation groups of more than 14, 9 to 14, and 1 to 8 nodes (50%, 38%, and 18%, respectively).

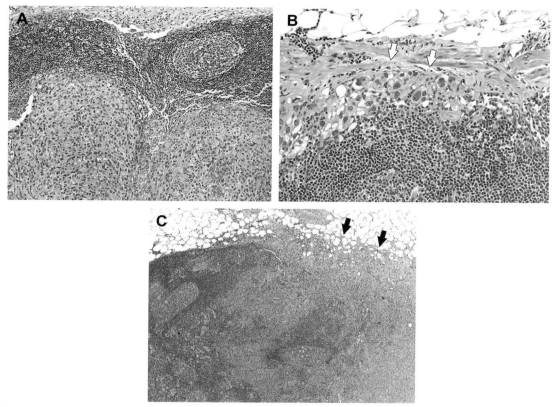

Fig. 2. Lymph node metastasis of bladder cancer. (*A*) Low-power microscopic view (hematoxylin and eosin) of a lymph node (*dark blue/purple staining area*) involved with metastatic urothelial cancer originating in the urinary bladder. (*B*) High-power view (hematoxylin and eosin) showing malignant urothelial cells (*open arrows*) adjacent to normal lymphoid cells. (*C*) Lymph node involved with metastatic urothelial cancer that is remarkable for the presence of extranodal extension (*solid arrows*) (hematoxylin and eosin).

The simple establishment of an institutional minimum number, which has been shown to increase sampling and diagnostic yield, may prove beneficial in its own right.[14] We recommend a minimum number of 8 nodes as an attainable and consistently achievable goal in standard LAD for urothelial cancer of the urinary bladder.[34]

An important consideration when interpreting these numbers is that they apply to standard pelvic LAD. When an extended LAD is performed by the urologist, reports have shown a mean yield of 51 nodes per patient.[27] Because of this large discrepancy, the urologist must communicate to the pathologist that an extended LAD has been performed to avoid misrepresenting nodal removal. To address this situation, Park and colleagues[35] propose that the number of lymph nodes removed has no impact on patient survival, but, instead, emphasize the adherence to the LAD template performed by the urologist and proper communication with the pathologist, allowing for optimum lymph node evaluation.

As a result of some of the controversy associated with lymph node numbers, the concept of lymph node density (positive lymph nodes per total number of lymph nodes) has been used and reported in numerous studies to show clinical significance.[36–38] The significant ratio seems to consistently be 20% nodal involvement. Five-year disease-free survival is reported to decrease from 54.6% in those with 20% or less versus 15.3% for those with more than 20%.[27] Furthermore, it has been proposed that lymph node density, rather than absolute number, may provide a better estimate of good surgical technique.[10]

However, lymph node density is a dependent variable with lymph node number. Therefore, when interpreting studies that show additional benefit with ever-increasing lymph node retrieval, it must be recognized that they are, in turn, decreasing lymph node density in those patients and placing those patients at a higher chance of entering the beneficial 20-node-or-less density category. However, Jeong and colleagues[39] have reported that in patients with 15 lymph nodes or more removed, lymph node density was the only predictor of cancer-specific survival after multivariate analysis.

An additional prognostic indicator from LAD is extranodal extension. Fleischmann and colleagues[28] reported that overall survival in the presence of extracapsular extension decreases from 60 months in those without extranodal extension to 12 months in those patients with extranodal extension identified.

The *AJCC Staging Manual, Seventh Edition* specifically cites reporting the number of nodes, the number of nodes involved by cancer, and the extent of location of positive nodes involved.[1] The use of intraoperative frozen sections for LAD for urinary bladder cancer is essentially limited to those cases in which the urologist is considering forgoing LAD if nodal disease is discovered.[40]

PROSTATE

In the modern era, evidence from the literature and widespread usage of nomograms that complements the concomitant increase in screening have reduced the overall frequency of LAD being routinely performed in the setting of radical prostatectomy for prostatic adenocarcinoma (**Fig. 3**).[12,41] Recent work has begun to show benefit in the procedure; however, it is likely that many urologists choose to perform the procedure in those patients they believe will benefit from the procedure.[42] Nomograms exist to assist the urologist in electing to proceed with LAD in only those patients whose benefit from the procedure will outweigh the associated surgical morbidity. These nomograms incorporate Gleason score, clinical stage, and prostate-specific antigen and, therefore, requires input from both the pathologist and urologist.[41]

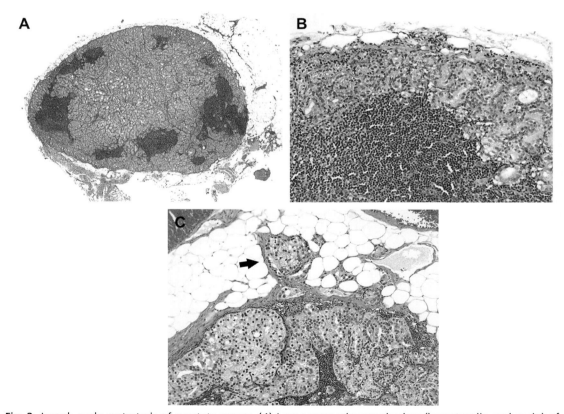

Fig. 3. Lymph node metastasis of prostate cancer. (*A*) Low-power microscopic view (hematoxylin and eosin) of a lymph node almost completely replaced by metastatic prostatic adenocarcinoma. (*B*) High-power view detailing metastatic prostatic adenocarcinoma cells (*lighter-stained cells*) adjacent to remaining lymphoid cells (*darker-stained cells*). (*C*) Focus of extranodal extension (*arrow*) shown in the perinodal fat just outside the capsule of the node. The node seems to be almost completely replaced by prostatic adenocarcinoma in this view (hematoxylin and eosin).

When LAD is performed, it is important for the urologist to label the location of nodal submissions appropriately because this reduces variability and increases harvest yield of nodes.[2,12] Furthermore, as evidence amasses in favor of extended node dissection providing clinical benefit in high-risk patients, separate submission ensures that the anticipated higher yield of nodes removed is detected in pathologic evaluation when there is currently no consensus minimum on node submission from prostatic LAD specimens.[2,42,43]

A consensus criterion on the minimum number of nodes submitted does not exist. Whereas some have reported that a minimum of 20 nodes is necessary to accurately assess nodal disease,[42] others have reported an acceptable median node retrieval of 16 and 13 nodes.[12,43] However, the International Society of Urological Pathology Consensus Conference on lymph node handling in radical prostatectomy specimens admits that this yield is rarely achieved and a minimum of 13 should be desired, but reporting of all detected nodes is an acceptable practice.[12] Montironi and colleagues[15] proposed that all adipose tissue from an LAD performed in concert with a radical prostatectomy be submitted, because 6.5% of cases revealed lymph node disease in nonrecognizable nodes at gross dissection. This finding is corroborated in Sung and Cheng's review.[44] Furthermore, analysis has shown that the rate of correctly predicting lymph node disease presence is near 0% when less than 10 nodes are removed or submitted and increases to near 100% when 30 or more nodes are removed or submitted.[45] This finding further emphasizes coordination between the urologist and pathologist in accurately assessing the nodes removed from LAD to achieve the greatest prognostic benefit to the patient.

Although much has been reported on the number of nodes removed in LAD for prostatic adenocarcinoma, evidence has shown that an absolute number of nodes removed may not provide any significant benefit to the patient.[46] However, significant benefit has been shown in patients with 2 positive nodes or less.[47,48] Briganti and colleagues[48] report that patients with 2 positive nodes or less had a 15-year cancer-specific survival of 84% compared with 64% in those with more than 2 positive nodes. In addition, Cheng and colleagues[49] have shown that patients with a single positive lymph node appeared to have a favorable clinical course. Specifically, these investigators cite that 5-year and 10-year cancer-specific survival rates in those with no lymph node metastases are 94% and 83% and 99% and 97% for those with a single positive node and those with no positive nodes, respectively.

As in urothelial bladder cancer, the concept of lymph node density has been receiving increasing attention in prostatic adenocarcinoma. A positive patient benefit has been reported when the number of nodes removed reduces the lymph node density to less than 15%.[47,50]

Further criteria for pathologic evaluation include extranodal extension and nodal Gleason score. The presence of extranodal extension has not been shown to decrease cancer-specific survival and has not been associated with distant metastases.[51,52] In the study by Cheng and colleagues,[52] nodal cancer volume was the only criterion examined that portended an adverse outcome after multivariate analysis. It has been shown in another study to be the most important nodal determinant of systemic progression.[53] This study calculated nodal cancer volume as a value based on all positive nodes and showed significant adverse outcome when 0.20 cm^3 or more of cancer tissue was present.

However, Boormans and colleagues[51] reported that, in addition to nodal cancer volume (described as diameter of largest metastasis in their study), nodal Gleason score of more than 7 is associated with an adverse outcome. Of important consideration when assessing Gleason score in lymph node metastases in prostate adenocarcinoma is the high rate of multifocal disease representing multiclonality.[54] Therefore, the Gleason score of the examined node may not represent the entire clinical picture for the patient.

Correlation of the Gleason score in the lymph node with the primary tumor is important; as Cheng and colleagues[55] have shown, dedifferentiation can occur in metastatic deposits in lymph nodes. Forty-five percent of these lymph nodes showed an increase in the Gleason score in the node compared with the primary. These investigators' report did show that dedifferentiation was not associated with disease progression when adjusted for the volume of metastatic deposit in the lymph node.[55]

Of special attention in the prostate is the focus given to the determination of micrometastases. Micrometastases are defined by single cells or small clusters of cells not more than 0.2 mm in greatest dimension.[15] Because of their small size, most reports promote the use of cytokeratin-containing immunohistochemical staining to aid the pathologist in the detection of micrometastases.[2,15,43] Specifically, Weckermann and colleagues[43] cited the use of immunohistochemistry in detecting 9 of 20 micrometastases in their study in samples that were negative for micrometastases with hematoxylin and eosin staining. Further reports have shown its benefit in increasing the sensitivity of detection of nodal involvement in high-risk patients.[56,57]

However, prospective studies validating the clinical usefulness and prognostic significance of these findings are lacking.[58] Current recommendations support reporting of these findings as N0.[15] In addition, evidence seems to indicate that size (diameter) of the largest metastasis carries more prognostic significance than the number of positive nodes alone.[12] Until further evidence accumulates, it is most likely that the urologist needs to request immunohistochemical evaluation of nodes, and only when macrometastases have not been found on routine hematoxylin and eosin staining.

The usefulness of frozen section in the setting of radical prostatectomy has been agreed on for years to be of little clinical value.[50,59] However, in the patient with a node suspicious of malignancy at the time of surgery or in a high-risk patient in whom a more aggressive LAD is being considered, the use of intraoperative frozen sections can be used to guide the approach and possibly spare the patient unnecessary morbidity when the frozen section is negative.[12]

The scope of the reportable findings listed earlier exceeds that currently used to stage and prognosticate patients via the *AJCC Staging Manual, Seventh Edition*.[1]

TESTES

LAD in the setting of germ cell neoplasm in the testes is performed for 3 primary indications: (1) a primary LAD for treatment and staging purposes; (2) removal of a residual mass status after chemotherapy and primary orchiectomy to evaluate response to treatment; and (3) removal of suspicious nodes in late recurrence.[7] Therefore, communication from the urologist to the pathologist must indicate the clinical and treatment status of the patient.

Once the resected specimen has been sent to the pathologist (once again, preferably labeled and separated), careful examination to assess the number of nodes present must take place.[7,60] This strategy is particularly important in posttreatment retroperitoneal LAD, in which assessment of residual tumor and histologic component of the nodes has an important prognostic implication. Of great importance is the identification of any differentiation into somatic malignancies because these carry a poor secondary treatment response.[7] Although the specific germ cell histology of the tumor in the diseased node does not carry prognostic information,[61] reporting of the histology may still be considered.

This point is further emphasized by the value of LAD in predicting the histology of residual disease outside the retroperitoneum. This finding has allowed for surveillance of pulmonary residua based on the findings in the retroperitoneal examination.[62] However, liver residua have been shown to be less concordant, only 49%, with retroperitoneal lymph node histology.[62]

A definitive minimum number of nodes has not been agreed, but Carver and colleagues[63] have reported that increasing nodes removed correlates with better relapse-free survival. These investigators' study reported a median amount of nodes in their sample of 248 patients to be 25. A 2-year relapse-free disease course reached 90% with as few as 10 nodes removed and increased to 97% only with 50 nodes removed.[63] However, Beck and colleagues[64] have proposed that both the number of nodes removed and the lymph node density of the specimen do not correlate with any benefit to disease-free survival. Although further studies are needed, the urologist should communicate estimates of the number of resected nodes to the receiving pathologist to ensure undersubmission does not take place.

The value of reporting extranodal extension has also been reviewed. It has been shown that extranodal extension carries no prognostic significance in those patients presenting for primary retroperitoneal LAD.[65] Further research is needed to assess any role this finding may play in recurrent disease.

In line with the *AJCC Staging Manual, Seventh Edition*, reporting the size of involved nodes is of greater importance to both the pathologic and clinical staging than the number of nodes involved.[1]

PENIS

LAD in the realm of penile squamous cell carcinoma (SCC) is a well-studied and accepted practice in the treatment and staging of the cancer.[66–70] However, unlike elsewhere in the realm of GU oncologic surgery, LAD in penile SCC relies on the use of sentinel node biopsy to guide LAD.[70,71] This procedure reduces postoperative morbidity from standard LAD from 88% to 8%, but it is limited to those patients deemed to be at risk of nodal disease, not to those with palpable lymph nodes.[67]

Because of the wide use of sentinel node evaluation, the use of intraoperative frozen section is an important aspect of penile SCC. Considering that sentinel node biopsy is indicated only in patients with clinically negative superficial nodes, the use of frozen section at the time of superficial LAD can be used to provide additional diagnostic evidence to the clinical node-negative status and allow the urologist to proceed with a more limited deep inguinal LAD with lower patient morbidity.[69]

Of particular importance in the pathologic examination of the sentinel node(s) is the documentation of the size of the metastasis. Kroon and colleagues have reported that sentinel nodes containing metastases of 2 mm or less had a low incidence of other involved lymph nodes.[66,72] Therefore, reporting of this finding to the urologist may spare the patient further lymph node dissection.

The number of lymph node metastases is an important feature in prognosticating the presence of contralateral involvement. When 2 or more nodes from a unilateral LAD are found, contralateral involvement has been reported at 30%.[69] The decision of the urologist to investigate this possibility represents another situation in which frozen sections are warranted. A limited contralateral LAD can be performed in concert with frozen section, thereby sparing the additional morbidity of a complete LAD if the frozen section results are negative.[67,69]

Once the nodes are obtained by the pathologist, the primary staging criteria as per the *AJCC Staging Manual, Seventh Edition* focuses on the number of nodes involved and whether they are in deep, pelvic, or superficial inguinal nodes, with deep and pelvic metastases carrying more dire prognostic implications.[1] However, Heyns and colleagues[67] noted that distinguishing between deep and superficial nodes both clinically and histopathologically presents a challenge. These investigators propose that the additional criteria of extracapsular extension and lymph node size should be reported and that both carry negative survival correlations.[67]

Because of the wide variability of LAD performed in penile SCC, a definitive number of nodes is dependent on the procedure performed. Communication between the urologist and the pathologist is crucial in ensuring that the estimated amount of nodes removed correlates with the nodes harvested at time of gross examination.

FUTURE CONSIDERATIONS

As mentioned earlier, a particular area of interest, primarily in prostatic carcinoma, is the issue of micrometastases.[58,73,74] Much of this interest has come about because of the development of new techniques such as molecular genetic assays, reverse-transcriptase polymerase chain reaction (RT-PCR), flow cytometry, and DNA analysis (**Box 1**).

Fujisawa and Miyake[58] reviewed many of these techniques and found that real-time RT-PCR was able to detect micrometastases in 143 additional

---

> **Box 1**
> **Principle techniques to evaluate micrometastases**
>
> Tissue-specific/organ-specific expression
>
> > RT-PCR
> >
> > Immunohistochemistry
> >
> > Flow cytometry sorting for tissue, liquid, and blood
> >
> > Immunomagnetic isolation for liquid and blood
> >
> > Others
>
> Tumor-specific gene alterations
>
> > RT-PCR
> >
> > PCR
> >
> > Immunohistochemistry
>
> Circulating tumor cells (CTCs)
>
> > CellSearch and others

---

lymph nodes in 32 patients in whom no pathologic evidence of lymph involvement was found. In addition, real-time PCR was shown to be superior to standard RT-PCR. These investigators also reported that, in their studies, evidence of micrometastases by real-time RT-PCR coincided with prognostic features of those with histopathologically positive lymph nodes. However, they assert that this finding is of limited usefulness and prospective studies are needed before the true benefit of this analysis is known.[58] Others agree with this assertion.[15,75]

In bladder urothelial cancer, it has been shown that qualitative RT-PCR to the *FXYD3* and *KRT20* genes detected positive nodes in 20.5% of patients who were deemed negative by histopathologic evaluation. Further investigation into the use of molecular markers has revealed increased predictive power when a combination of markers is used as opposed to an individual marker.[76] However, as per the reports of prostatic micrometastases discussed earlier, no correlation to clinical outcome was achieved.[77]

The role of immunohistochemistry in prostatic adenocarcinoma is described earlier as a measure to increase sensitivity in micrometastasis detection. However, Fujisawa and Miyake[58] compared this modality with real-time RT-PCR and reported that real-time RT-PCR is superior to immunohistochemistry in evaluating micrometastases. This finding insinuates that performance of real-time RT-PCR should be the method of choice when considering this type of evaluation.

Recently, the use of flow cytometry has also been assessed in evaluating nodal disease. Although Fujisawa and Miyake[58] reported this method is inferior to real-time RT-PCR in the evaluation of nodal tissue, they do admit that studies evaluating CTCs as a metric of disease have successfully used flow cytometry to conduct their analysis. Specifically, Moreno and colleagues[78] reported that through use of flow cytometry, the detection of 5 or more CTCs indicates poor survival in patients with metastatic prostate cancer. Additional work on mouse models has shown prognostic value in the setting of RCC.[79] Prospective studies are needed to validate the clinical significance of CTC analysis.

SUMMARY

LAD in GU oncologic surgery is of great prognostic and therapeutic benefit. However, for it to achieve full benefit, the procedure requires careful coordination and proper communication between urologist and pathologist. The vast differences in reporting, submission criteria, and expectations between anatomic site and cancer type reinforce this assertion. Moreover, in most of the examined sites, adhering strictly to defined staging criteria seems to be an inadequate level of reporting; the pathologist must work to include this critical information, and the urologist must be aware of it to expect it. Certain anatomic sites, specifically those of the bladder, are areas of contention as to the necessary submission and pathologic evaluation. Studies of a prospective nature are needed to determine a consensus. With the rapid advances in molecular techniques, a careful eye needs to be kept on any emerging clinical application of these procedures in the examination of LAD specimens for metastasis.

REFERENCES

1. Edge SB, Byrd DR, Compton CC, et al. AJCC cancer staging manual. 7th edition. New York: Springer; 2010.
2. Lattouf J, Beri A, Jeschke S, et al. Laparoscopic extended pelvic lymph node dissection for prostate cancer: description of the surgical technique and initial results. Eur Urol 2007;52:1347–57.
3. Algaba F, Trias I, Scarpelli M, et al. Handling and pathology reporting of renal tumor specimens. Eur Urol 2004;45:437–43.
4. Bochner BH, Herr HW, Reuter VE. Impact of separate versus en bloc pelvic lymph node dissection on the number of lymph nodes retrieved in cystectomy specimens. J Urol 2001;166:2295–6.
5. Stein JP, Penson DF, Cai J, et al. Radical cystectomy with extended lymphadenectomy: evaluating separate package versus en bloc submission for node positive bladder cancer. J Urol 2007;177(3):876–81 [discussion: 881–2].
6. Lopez-Beltran A, Bassi P, Pavone-Macaluso M, et al. Handling and pathology reporting of specimens with carcinoma of the urinary bladder, ureter, and renal pelvis. Eur Urol 2004;45:257–66.
7. Winstanley A, Mikuz G, Debruyne FR, et al. Handling and reporting of biopsy and surgical specimens of testicular cancer. Eur Urol 2004;45:564–73.
8. Mikuz G, Winstanley A, Schulman C, et al. Handling and pathology reporting of circumcision and penectomy specimens. Eur Urol 2004;46:434–9.
9. Boccon-Gibod L, van der Kwast TH, Montironi R, et al. Handling and pathology reporting of prostate biopsies. Eur Urol 2004;46:177–81.
10. Hurle R, Naspro R. Pelvic lymphadenectomy during radical cystectomy: a review of the literature. Surg Oncol 2010;19(4):208–20.
11. Chin J, Srigley J, Mayhew L, et al. Guideline for optimization of surgical and pathological quality performance for radical prostatectomy in prostate cancer management: evidentiary base. Can Urol Assoc J 2010;4(1):13–25.
12. Berney D, Wheeler T, Grignon D, et al. International Society of Urological Pathology (ISUP) Consensus Conference on Handling and Staging of Radical Prostatectomy Specimens. Working group 4: seminal vesicles and lymph nodes. Mod Pathol 2010; 24(1):39–47.
13. Koren R, Paz A, Lask D, et al. Lymph-node revealing solution: a new method for detecting minute lymph nodes in cystectomy specimens. Br J Urol 1997; 80:40–3.
14. Fang AC, Ahmad AE, Whitson JM, et al. Effect of a minimum lymph node policy in radical cystectomy and pelvic lymphadenectomy on lymph node yields, lymph node positivity rates, lymph node density, and survivorship in patients with bladder cancer. Cancer 2010;116(8):1901–8.
15. Montironi R, Van Der Kwast T, Boccon-Gibod L, et al. Handling and pathology reporting of radical prostatectomy specimens. Eur Urol 2003;44:626–36.
16. Blom J, Van Poppel H, Marechal JM, et al. Radical nephrectomy with and without lymph-node dissection: final results of European Organization for Research and Treatment of Cancer (EORTC) randomized phase 3 trial 30881. Eur Urol 2009;55: 28–34.
17. Leibovich BC, Blute ML. Lymph node dissection in the management of renal cell carcinoma. Urol Clin North Am 2008;35:673–8.
18. Van Poppel H. Lymph node dissection is not obsolete in clinically node-negative renal cell carcinoma patients. Eur Urol 2011;59:24–5.

19. Lughezzani G, Capitanio U, Jeldres C, et al. Prognostic significance of lymph node invasion in patients with metastatic renal cell carcinoma: a population-based perspective. Cancer 2009;115(24):5680–7.

20. Zubac DP, Bostad L, Seidal T, et al. The prognostic relevance of interactions between venous invasion, lymph node involvement and distant metastases in renal cell carcinoma after radical nephrectomy. BMC Urol 2008;8:19.

21. Crispen PL, Breau R, Allmer C, et al. Lymph node dissection at the time of radical nephrectomy for high-risk clear cell renal cell carcinoma: indications and recommendations for surgical templates. Eur Urol 2011;59:18–23.

22. Kirkali Z, Algaba F, Scarpelli M, et al. What does the urologist expect from the pathologist (and what can the pathologists give) in reporting on adult kidney tumour specimens? Eur Urol 2007;51:1104–201.

23. Ming X, Ningshu L, Hanzhong L, et al. Value of frozen section analysis of enlarged lymph nodes during radical nephrectomy for renal cell carcinoma. Urology 2009;74:364–9.

24. Secin FP, Koppie TM, Salamanca JI, et al. Evaluation of regional lymph node dissection in patients with upper urinary tract urothelial cancer. Int J Urol 2007;14:26–32.

25. Roscingo M, Shariat S, Margulis V, et al. The extent of lymphadenectomy seems to be associated with better survival in patients with nonmetastatic upper-tract urothelial carcinoma: how many lymph nodes should be removed? Eur Urol 2009; 56:512–8.

26. Brausi M, Gavioli M, De Luca G, et al. Retroperitoneal lymph node dissection (RPLD) in conjunction with nephroureterectomy in the treatment of infiltrative transitional cell carcinoma (TCC) of the upper urinary tract: impact on survival. Eur Urol 2007;52: 1414–20.

27. Karl A, Carroll P, Gschwend JE, et al. The impact of lymphadenectomy and lymph node metastasis on the outcomes of radical cystectomy for bladder cancer. Eur Urol 2009;55:826–35.

28. Fleischmann A, Thalmann GN, Markwalder R, et al. Extracapsular extension of pelvic lymph node metastases from urothelial carcinoma of the bladder is an independent prognostic factor. J Clin Oncol 2005;23:2358–65.

29. May M, Herrmann E, Bolenz C, et al. Association between the number of dissected lymph nodes during pelvic lymphadenectomy and cancer-specific survival in patients with lymph node-negative urothelial carcinoma of the bladder undergoing radical cystectomy. Ann Surg Oncol 2011;18(7):2018–25.

30. Leissner J, Hohenfellner R, Thüroff JW, et al. Lymphadenectomy in patients with transitional cell carcinoma of the urinary bladder; significance for staging and prognosis. BJU Int 2000;85(7):817–23.

31. Weingartner K, Ramaswamy A, Bittinger A, et al. Anatomical basis for pelvic lymphadenectomy in prostate cancer: results of an autopsy study and implications for the clinic. J Urol 1996;156:1969–71.

32. Fleischmann A, Thalmann GN, Markwalder R, et al. Prognostic implications of extracapsular extension of pelvic lymph node metastases in urothelial carcinoma of the bladder. Am J Surg Pathol 2005;29:89–95.

33. Herr HW, Bochner BH, Dalbagni G, et al. Impact of the number of lymph nodes retrieved on outcome in patients with muscle invasive bladder cancer. J Urol 2002;167:1295–8.

34. Cheng L, Montironi R, Davidson DD, et al. Staging and reporting of urothelial carcinoma of the urinary bladder. Mod Pathol 2009;22(Suppl 2):S70–95.

35. Park J, Kim S, Jeong IG, et al. Does the greater number of lymph nodes removed during standard lymph node dissection predict better patient survival following radical cystectomy? World J Urol 2011;29: 443–9.

36. Stein JP, Lieskovsky G, Cote R, et al. Radical cystectomy in the treatment of invasive bladder cancer: long-term results in 1,054 patients. J Clin Oncol 2001;19:666–75.

37. Herr HW. Superiority of ratio based lymph node staging for bladder cancer. J Urol 2003;169:943–5.

38. Ghoneim MA, Abol Enein H. Lymphadenectomy with cystectomy: is it necessary and what is its extent? Eur Urol 2004;46:457–61.

39. Jeong IG, Park J, Song K, et al. Comparison of 2002 TNM nodal status with lymph node density in node-positive patients after radical cystectomy for bladder cancer: analysis by the number of lymph nodes removed. Urol Oncol 2011;29(2):199–204.

40. Algaba F, Arce Y, Lopez-Beltran A, et al. Intraoperative frozen section diagnosis in urological oncology. Eur Urol 2005;47:129–36.

41. Bluestein D, Bostwick D, Bergstralh E, et al. Eliminating the need for bilateral pelvic lymphadenectomy in select patients with prostate cancer. J Urol 1994;151:1315–20.

42. Ordon M, Nam R. Lymph node assessment and lymphadenectomy in prostate cancer. J Surg Oncol 2009;99:215–24.

43. Weckermann D, Goppelt M, Dorn R, et al. Incidence of positive pelvic lymph nodes in patients with prostate cancer, a prostate-specific antigen (PSA) level of < or =10 ng/mL and biopsy Gleason score of < or = 6, and their influence on PSA progression-free survival after radical prostatectomy. BJU Int 2006;97:1173–8.

44. Sung MT, Cheng L. Contemporary approaches for processing and handling of radical prostactomy specimens. Histol Histopathol 2010;25(2):259–65.

45. Briganti A, Blute M, Eastham J, et al. Pelvic lymph node dissection in prostate cancer. Eur Urol 2009; 55:1251–65.

46. Boorjian SA, Thompson RH, Siddiqui S, et al. Long-term outcome after radical prostatectomy for patients with lymph node positive prostate cancer in the prostate specific antigen era. J Urol 2007; 178(3 Pt 1):864–70 [discussion: 870–1].

47. Palapattu GS, Singer EA, Messing EM. Controversies surrounding lymph node dissection for prostate cancer. Urol Clin North Am 2010;37(1):57–65.

48. Briganti A, Karnes JR, Da Pozzo LF, et al. Two positive nodes represent a significant cut-off value for cancer specific survival in patients with node positive prostate cancer. A new proposal based on a two-institution experience on 703 consecutive N+ patients treated with radical prostatectomy, extended pelvic lymph node dissection and adjuvant therapy. Eur Urol 2009;55(2):261–70.

49. Cheng L, Zincke H, Blute ML, et al. Risk of prostate carcinoma death in patients with lymph node metastasis. Cancer 2001;91:66–73.

50. Masterson TA, Bianco FJ Jr, Vickers AJ, et al. The association between total and positive lymph node counts, and disease progression in clinically localized prostate cancer. J Urol 2006;175(4):1320–4 [discussion: 1324–5].

51. Boormans J, Wildhagen M, Bangma C, et al. Histopathological characteristics of lymph node metastases predict cancer-specific survival in node-positive prostate cancer. BJU Int 2008;102: 1589–93.

52. Cheng L, Pisansky TM, Ramnani DM, et al. Extranodal extension in lymph node-positive prostate cancer. Mod Pathol 2000;13:113–8.

53. Cheng L, Bergstralh EJ, Cheville JC, et al. Cancer volume of lymph node metastasis predicts progression in prostate cancer. Am J Surg Pathol 1998;22: 1491–500.

54. Andreoiu M, Cheng L. Multifocal prostate cancer: biologic, prognostic, and therapeutic implications. Hum Pathol 2010;41(6):781–93.

55. Cheng L, Bergstralh EJ, Slezak J, et al. Dedifferentiation in metastatic progression of prostate cancer. Cancer 1999;86:657–63.

56. Palapattu GS, Allaf ME, Trock BJ, et al. Prostate specific antigen progression in men with lymph node metastases following radical prostatectomy: results of long-term followup. J Urol 2004;172(5 Pt 1):1860–4.

57. Wawroschek F, Wagner T, Hamm M, et al. The influence of serial sections, immunohistochemistry, and extension of pelvic lymph node dissection on the lymph node status in clinically localized prostate cancer. Eur Urol 2003;43(2):132–6 [discussion: 137].

58. Fujisawa M, Miyake H. Significance of micrometastases in prostate cancer. Surg Oncol 2008;17: 247–52.

59. Epstein JI, Oesterling JE, Eggleston JC, et al. Frozen section detection of lymph node metastases in prostatic carcinoma: accuracy in grossly uninvolved pelvic lymphadenectomy specimens. J Urol 1986; 136:1234–7.

60. Parkinson MC, Harland S, Harnden P, et al. The role of the histopathologist in the management of testicular germ cell tumour in adults. Histopathology 2001;38:183–94.

61. Beck SD, Foster RS, Bihrle R, et al. Does the histology of nodal metastasis predict systemic relapse after retroperitoneal lymph node dissection in pathological stage B1 germ cell tumors? J Urol 2005;174(4 Pt 1):1287–90 [discussion: 1290].

62. Jacobsen NE, Beck SD, Jacobson LE, et al. Is retroperitoneal histology predictive of liver histology at concurrent post-chemotherapy retroperitoneal lymph node dissection and hepatic resection? J Urol 2010; 184(3):949–53.

63. Carver B, Cronin AM, Eggener S, et al. The total number of retroperitoneal lymph nodes resected impacts clinical outcome after chemotherapy for metastatic testicular cancer. Urology 2010;75:1431–5.

64. Beck SD, Foster RS, Bihrle R, et al. Impact of the number of positive lymph nodes on disease-free survival in patients with pathological stage B1 nonseminomatous germ cell tumor. J Urol 2005;174(1): 143–5.

65. Beck SD, Cheng L, Bihrle R, et al. Does the presence of extranodal extension in pathological stage B1 nonseminomatous germ cell tumor necessitate adjuvant chemotherapy? J Urol 2007;177(3):944–6.

66. Leijte J, Kroon B, Valdes Olmos R, et al. Reliability and safety of current dynamic sentinel node biopsy for penile carcinoma. Eur Urol 2007;52:170–7.

67. Heyns C, Mendoza-Valdes A, Pompeo A. Diagnosis and staging of penile cancer. Urology 2010; 76(Suppl 2A):S15–23.

68. Hughes B, Leijte J, Shabbir M, et al. Non-invasive and minimally invasive staging of regional lymph nodes in penile cancer. World J Urol 2009;27:197–203.

69. Heyns C, Fleshner N, Sangar V, et al. Management of the lymph nodes in penile cancer. Urology 2010; 76(Suppl 2A):S43–57.

70. Pizzocaro G, Algaba F, Horenblas S, et al. EAU penile cancer guidelines 2009. Eur Urol 2010;57: 1002–12.

71. Jensen J, Jensen K, Ulhoi B, et al. Sentinel lymph-node biopsy in patients with squamous cell carcinoma of the penis. BJU Int 2009;103:1199–203.

72. Kroon B, Nieweg O, Van Boven H, et al. Size of metastasis in the sentinel node predicts additional nodal involvement in penile carcinoma. J Urol 2006;176:105–8.

73. Hering F, Rist M, Roth J, et al. Does microinvasion of the capsule and/or micrometastases in regional lymph nodes influence disease-free survival after radical prostatectomy? Br J Urol 1990;66:177–81.

74. Thiounn N, Saporta F, Flam TA, et al. Positive prostate-specific antigen circulating cells detected

by reverse transcriptase-polymerase chain reaction does not imply the presence of prostatic micrometastases. Urology 1997;50:245–50.

75. Martinez-Pineiro L, Rios E, Martinez-Gomariz M, et al. Molecular staging of prostatic cancer with RT-PCR assay for prostate-specific antigen in peripheral blood and lymph nodes: comparison with standard histological staging and immunohistochemical assessment of occult regional lymph node metastases. Eur Urol 2003;43:342–50.

76. Shariat SF, Chade DC, Karakiewicz PI, et al. Combination of multiple molecular markers can improve prognostication in patients with locally advanced and lymph node positive bladder cancer. J Urol 2010;183(1):68–75.

77. Marin-Aguilera M, Mengual L, Burset M, et al. Molecular lymph node staging in bladder urothelial carcinoma: impact on survival. Eur Urol 2008;54: 1363–72.

78. Moreno JG, Miller MC, Gross S, et al. Circulating tumor cells predict survival in patients with metastatic prostate cancer. Urology 2005;65:713–8.

79. Namdarian B, Tan KV, Fankhauser MJ, et al. Circulating endothelial cells and progenitors: potential biomarkers of renal cell carcinoma. BJU Int 2010; 106(7):1081–7.

Role of Radiation Therapy for the Treatment of Lymph Nodes in Urologic Malignancies

Thomas J. Pugh, MD*, Andrew K. Lee, MD

KEYWORDS

- Pelvis lymph node • Radiation • Genitourinary cancer

Radiation therapy (RT) represents an important therapeutic component in the management of many genitourinary (GU) malignancies. RT has been used to treat patients with proven involvement of the regional lymph nodes or delivered electively to patients at risk for occult regional lymph node metastases. Lymphatic basins at risk in GU malignancies include the presacral, external iliac, internal iliac, common iliac, para-aortic, and inguinal lymph node chains. The specific nodal basin and degree of risk is dependent on the primary cancer site, local extent of disease, and other prognostic factors. An overview of the modalities, indications, and techniques of RT for treatment of the lymphatic basins in GU malignancies is reviewed here.

BASIC PRINCIPLES OF RADIATION THERAPY
External Beam Radiation Therapy

External beam radiation therapy (EBRT) is a form of RT delivered from a source outside of the body. EBRT can be delivered in the form of photons (x-rays), charged particles (electrons or protons), neutrons, or heavy ions. Photons are the most common modality for delivery of nodal radiation in GU malignancies based on widespread availability, depth of tissue penetration, and dose-distribution properties.

The implementation of computed tomography (CT)-based EBRT planning and sophisticated dose-modeling software has revolutionized the field of radiation oncology. Conventional EBRT (2DXRT) is planned using 2-dimensional radiographs. Soft tissue structures are poorly visualized on these images; therefore, beam arrangements are designed in reference to bone landmarks to target an area of interest for treatment. This technique is well established, efficient, and reliable; however, 2DXRT lacks the dose modeling and conformity capabilities of more modern treatment-planning techniques. With the development of CT, 3-dimensional conformal radiation therapy (3DCRT) has become the most widely used method of treatment planning and delivery (**Fig. 1**). CT simulation provides the radiation oncologist with the ability to reconstruct the tumor and normal structures in 3 dimensions. In addition, multiple beam arrangements conform to the shape of the target area with consideration of individual patient anatomy and normal tissue tolerance of radiation dose.

The treatment-planning process begins with a CT scan of the patient in a reproducible position to create a virtual simulation of 3-dimensional daily treatment. With the aid of computer software and

The authors have nothing to disclose.
Statement of Originality: This article is the original work of the authors.
Division of Radiation Oncology, The University of Texas M.D. Anderson Cancer Center, 1840 Old Spanish Trail, Unit 0097, Houston, TX 77054, USA
* Corresponding author.
E-mail address: tpugh@mdanderson.org

Urol Clin N Am 38 (2011) 497–506
doi:10.1016/j.ucl.2011.07.006

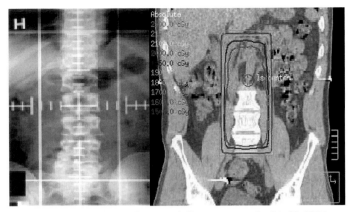

Fig. 1. CT-based treatment planning improves dose modeling compared with 2D XRT.

treatment-planning stations, the radiation oncologist selects the beam arrangement that optimizes dose distribution to the area at risk while minimizing the dose to surrounding normal tissue, thereby enhancing the therapeutic ratio.

Intensity-Modulated Radiation Therapy

Intensity-modulated radiation therapy (IMRT) is a specialized form of 3DCRT. Compared with most other treatment techniques, IMRT can achieve a more conformal radiation plan than with standard 3DCRT, thus further reducing dose and toxicity to normal tissue. The advantages of IMRT are particularly evident when the target volumes have complex shapes or concave regions. IMRT treatment planning is similar to 3DCRT; however, whereas 3DCRT delivers a uniform dose from each RT beam, IMRT has the added capability of varying the RT intensity within each beam. This allows the radiation oncologist to define the clinical target volume and set dose constraints to surrounding normal structures. Computer algorithms are used to modulate the intensity of the radiation beams to optimize the treatment plan (**Fig. 2**). Furthermore, varying the dose administered within each beam enables IMRT to simultaneously treat multiple areas within the target to different dose levels, thus providing a simultaneous integrated boost (SIB). Tight conformity of dose distributions to target structures allows IMRT to better preserve surrounding normal structures within the pelvis/abdomen from high-dose radiation, thereby limiting treatment-related toxicity.[1,2] For GU malignancies, IMRT allows for dose escalation to sites of gross disease or nodal involvement while reducing the radiation dose to the small bowel, rectum, and bladder.[3–7] Patient immobilization, positioning, and limitation of organ motion are essential for daily reproducibility when delivering highly conformal treatments. IMRT offers potential

advantages in the management of specific GU malignancies; these are addressed later in this article.

Charged Particles

Electrons and protons are charged particles that penetrate a certain distance into the body before depositing their energy. Electrons penetrate a short distance into tissue; therefore, electrons can be useful for treatment of superficial targets, such as the inguinal lymph nodes. Protons can penetrate much deeper into tissue than electrons. Protons also possess a more predictable range of energy deposition. Proton therapy provides an ability to more precisely localize the radiation dose at a depth in tissue similar to that achieved with photon therapy. These properties have made proton therapy an area of interest for

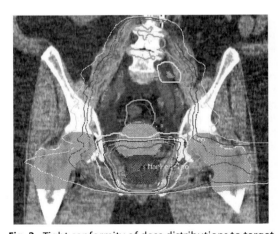

Fig. 2. Tight conformity of dose distributions to target structures allows IMRT to better preserve surrounding normal structures within the pelvis/abdomen from high-dose radiation, thereby limiting treatment-related toxicity.

treatment of regional lymphatics in GU and other pelvic malignancies.[8,9]

Target Volume and Dose

The dose of radiation required to treat solid tumors with definitive EBRT ranges from approximately 60 to 80 Gy. For sterilization of microscopic disease, as is often the case for elective lymph node coverage, the dose ranges from 45 to 60 Gy. The total dose is typically fractionated or spread out over time. Standard EBRT is delivered in once-daily fractions, typically 1.8 to 2.0 Gy, 5 days a week, for several weeks until the total prescribed dose is achieved. Fractionation decreases the amount of toxicity to healthy tissues by exploiting their capacity for sublethal damage repair and re-population compared with malignant tissue. Throughout the course of treatment, tumor cells undergo reoxygenation and reassortment into more sensitive phases of the cell cycle. Both of these processes increase their sensitivity to frac-tionated regimens.

Treatment-Related Toxicity

The incidence and severity of RT side effects depend on multiple factors, including the site and volume of tissue exposed, radiation dose, type of radiation, and fractionation pattern. Other modi-fying factors can influence RT-related toxicity, such as previous surgery, concomitant chemo-therapy, and comorbid medical conditions. Acute and subacute side effects occur during or within the first several months following completion of treatment. Acute and subacute side effects asso-ciated with treatment of GU cancer regional lymph nodes include injury to the skin and mucosal surfaces, fatigue, and diarrhea. Late effects are side effects occurring several months or years after RT. These effects can include fibrosis/bowel obstruction, stricture, fistula, radiation enteritis/proctitis, intestinal malabsorption, lymphedema, or secondary malignancies. The primary organ of concern when administering RT to regional lymph nodes for patients with GU malignancies is the small bowel. Although normal small bowel motion helps to reduce exposure to pelvic radiation, it can be at risk for late toxicity if excessive bowel is within the radiation field. An example of this is when adhesions from previous surgeries immobi-lize the small bowel within the pelvis. As part of the recent Quantitative Analyses of Normal Tissue Effects in the Clinic (QUANTEC) project, limiting the small bowel volume receiving more than 45 Gy to less than 195 mL substantially reduces the risk of acute grade 3 or greater gastrointestinal

toxicity. These dose/volume constraints are likely to translate to reduced late toxicity as well.[10]

SITE-SPECIFIC DISCUSSION
Prostate Cancer

Elective coverage of regional nodes
The pathologic status of the regional lymph nodes is typically unknown in men with clinically localized prostate cancer managed with RT. Risk of pelvic nodal metastasis for prostate cancer was initially established through pelvic lymph node dissection: generally, limited pelvic lymphadenectomies. Optimal RT for prostate cancer requires the accu-rate assessment of risk factors predicting patho-logic stage and prognosis. The current standard is to characterize the risk of biochemical failure and prostate cancer–specific mortality according to a patient's clinical (TNM) stage, Gleason grade, and serum prostate-specific antigen (PSA) level. Certain nomograms, equations, and tables have been developed by combining prognostic factors to predict pathologic stage, extracapsular spread, seminal vesicle involvement, and pelvic nodal metastasis.[11–13] Roach and colleagues[14] derived a simple equation to estimate the risk of pathologic pelvic lymph node involvement: positive lymph node % = (2/3) PSA × ([Gleason score – 6] × 10). Recent application of the Roach formula to popula-tion datasets suggests this simple equation may overestimate the true risk of pelvic lymph node disease in contemporary patients.[15] Although advanced T-stage tumors are seen less frequently in the era of PSA screening,[16] clinical T3–T4 disease also predicts a high risk for pelvic nodal metastasis and is notably absent from the Roach formula.[17] Regardless, the Roach formula is one of the many tools commonly used to estimate the likelihood of regional lymph node involvement and thus select patients for whole-pelvis RT (WPRT).

Patients with a less than 10% risk of lymph node metastases do not routinely require radiographic staging of the regional lymph nodes before cura-tive treatment[18]; however, improved methods to identify occult disease are greatly needed for patients with intermediate or high risk of nodal metastasis. Currently, CT scan and/or magnetic resonance imaging (MRI) scans are routinely used for pelvic nodal staging of prostate cancer. The limitations of CT imaging are such that a normal CT does not rule out the presence of nodal disease.[19] Although MRI is superior to CT scan in identifying the local extent of prostate tumors, it does not appear to provide any signifi-cant benefit in identifying nodal metastasis.[20,21] Both of these modalities are currently dependent on identification of lymph node enlargement.

Alternative imaging techniques independent of anatomic distortion would be useful for lymph node staging. This topic is covered in the article by Chernyak and colleagues elsewhere in this issue of *Urology Clinics*.

Regardless of the method of detection, regional therapy to involved nodal disease or areas at high risk of lymph node involvement seems reasonable, considering sterilization of all microscopic disease is a prerequisite for cure. If WPRT is effective at sterilizing microscopic disease, then progression-free survival (PFS) and overall survival (OS) should improve in patients with significant risk for regional nodal involvement. This rationale has been validated in other adenocarcinomas in which EBRT to regional lymph nodes is routine.[22,23]

The role of WPRT for men with intermediate-risk or high-risk prostate cancer remains uncertain. Some continue to advocate WPRT for men with an estimated risk of regional lymph node involvement of 15% or more.[24] Others have recommended WPRT be restricted to the investigational setting.[25] Two randomized trials have addressed the role of WPRT compared with prostate-only RT. Although both of these trials have failed to show an advantage of WPRT compared with prostate-only treatment, criticisms of both trials have allowed the issue of elective lymph node coverage in intermediate-risk to high-risk prostate cancer to remain unresolved.

In the Radiation Therapy Oncology Group (RTOG) 9413 trial, 1323 men with clinically localized prostate cancer and an estimated risk of nodal metastases of 15% or more were randomly assigned to WPRT (50.4 Gy to the pelvis and 70.2 Gy to the prostate using conventional techniques) or prostate-only RT (70.2 Gy).[14,26,27] Patients were further randomized, using a 2 × 2 factorial design, to neoadjuvant plus concurrent androgen deprivation therapy (ADT) administered for 2 months before and during RT, or adjuvant ADT given for the same length of time, but starting after the completion of RT. Most enrolled men had intermediate-risk or high-risk disease. The initial report of this trial suggested WPRT plus neoadjuvant plus concurrent ADT improved PFS compared with any of the 3 other treatment combinations.[27] The long-term analysis of this study showed no significant differences in PFS or OS when men treated with WPRT were compared with prostate-only RT.[26] Within the group that received WPRT, there was a trend toward better PFS and OS with neoadjuvant plus concurrent as compared with adjuvant-only ADT. The study was insufficiently powered to show a statistically significant difference between these 2 treatment arms. An unplanned subset analysis of RTOG 9413 was performed to determine whether RT field size significantly influenced PFS.[28] The analysis was limited to patients receiving neoadjuvant and concurrent hormone therapy to control for the interaction of ADT timing. The median and 7-year PFS improved with increased field size. However, late grade 3 gastrointestinal complications correlated with increasing field size as well. A complicated and unanticipated interaction between the timing of hormone therapy and radiation field size complicates interpretation of RTOG 9413. Furthermore, the use of WPRT with ADT in predecessor trials allows proponents of this approach to suggest WPRT should remain the standard in the setting of equivocal results.[29–33]

The results of a second trial support the long-term results of RTOG 9413. In a trial by the Genitourinary Study Group (Groupe d'Etude des Tumeurs Uro-Génitales), GETUG-01, 446 men were randomly assigned to WPRT or prostate-only RT.[34] ADT was allowed for high-risk patients at the treating physician's discretion. Use of ADT was balanced between the 2 groups. At a median follow-up of 42 months, the 5-year PFS and OS were not significantly different between the 2 treatments. This trial has been criticized for including men with more favorable disease (more than 50% of men with estimated risk of pelvic lymph node involvement <15%), relatively low RT dose delivery, smaller RT field size for WPRT, and using an antiquated definition of biochemical failure. Despite their limitations, there are now 2 randomized trials showing no significant differences in PFS or OS between prostate-only and elective pelvic lymph node treatment for men with clinically localized prostate cancer. Further study and longer follow-up of these issues are warranted before a standard of care can be recommended. Based on the available results, WPRT can be considered in cases where the risk of lymph node involvement is greater than 15%; however, WPRT should be used judiciously considering the potential for worse gastrointestinal toxicity with larger field size.

Postoperative RT

The use of RT alone for men with node-positive disease has been associated with high rates of local and distant recurrence.[35–38] RT alone has been used primarily for palliation for men with known lymph node involvement. The natural history of node-positive prostate cancer treated with RT alone is best illustrated by a subset analysis of RTOG 7506.[38] In a total of 90 men with regional node-positive prostate cancer, the 10-year survival rate was 29%. Only 5 patients were progression free at 10 years. Three of the 5 patients without progression were not assessed by PSA.

There are only limited data on combining radical prostatectomy with postoperative RT in men with lymph node–positive prostate cancer. There are several nonrandomized series suggesting a benefit of postoperative adjuvant RT in select men with pathologically positive regional lymph nodes.[39–41] Men with a lower burden of regional lymphatic disease may be the population of patients who benefit most from postoperative RT.[42,43] Briganti and colleagues[44] conducted a recent matched-pair analysis of 703 consecutively treated patients with documented lymph node metastases (pN+). Comparisons were made between patients treated with adjuvant ADT alone versus adjuvant ADT plus WPRT. Patients were matched for age at surgery, pathologic T stage, Gleason score, number of nodes removed, surgical margin status, and length of follow-up. Patients treated with adjuvant WPRT plus ADT had significantly higher 10-year prostate cancer–specific survival (86% vs 70%; $P = .004$) and OS (74% vs 55%; $P<.001$) compared with patients treated with ADT alone. Similar improvements were seen when patients were stratified according to the extent of nodal invasion (≤ 2 vs >2 positive nodes; $P = .006$). These results reinforce the benefits of a multimodality approach in the treatment of node-positive prostate cancer.

The efficacy of RT as a primary treatment modality for localized prostate cancer suggests a role for postoperative RT in men with node-negative disease who have a high likelihood of residual cancer in either the prostate bed or regional lymph nodes. To realize a benefit using this approach, certain presumptions must be true. First, any residual disease must be confined to a definable treatment volume. Second, the toxicity from additional local therapy must be low and manageable. RT can be integrated into the postoperative management of prostate cancer either by delivery soon after surgery to those at high risk for relapse with an undetectable PSA (adjuvant RT) or delayed delivery until evidence of PSA relapse (salvage RT). The former approach has the advantage of treating a potentially lower disease burden, although unnecessarily treating a preponderance of men who were not actually destined for PSA relapse.

Historically, postoperative RT for men with node-negative disease has been limited to the prostate bed and has not included elective treatment of the pelvic lymph nodes. There are 3 published randomized controlled trials comparing adjuvant RT with no planned additional treatment for patients at high risk of local failure following prostatectomy.[45–47] All of these trials showed that adjuvant RT is effective at reducing progression with indications for adjuvant therapy including pT3 disease or positive surgical margin. The target volume in all of these trials included the prostatic fossa without specific targeting of the regional lymphatics. RTOG 96-01 compared adjuvant RT with or without an antiandrogen.[48] This trial also did not allow for inclusion of the regional lymph nodes as a radiation target. In part because of the lack of clarity regarding elective lymph node treatment in the intact prostate setting, the RTOG initiated a trial to evaluate elective regional lymphatic coverage and the use of ADT in men with a rising PSA following prostatectomy. RTOG 0534 includes 3 arms: prostate bed–only RT; prostate bed RT plus ADT; and WPRT plus ADT. RTOG 0534 is currently in the active phase and results are not anticipated for several years.

Bladder Cancer

The implementation of effective radiosensitizing chemotherapy agents has allowed chemoradiation to become an integral component of a bladder-conserving approach for select patients with muscle-invasive bladder cancer.[49–51] In this setting, EBRT is delivered using a conventional 4-field treatment technique targeting the bladder and first-echelon lymph nodes. The lymphatic drainage of the urinary bladder includes the external iliac, obturator, and other internal iliac chain lymph nodes situated along the pelvic sidewall medial to the acetabulum. The superior border of the pelvic field is placed at the bifurcation of the common iliac arteries (approximately mid-sacroiliac joint) creating a "mini-pelvis" field (Fig. 3). After a dose of approximately 40 to 45 Gy is delivered to the pelvis with concurrent chemotherapy, the response to treatment is assessed through cystoscopy with directed biopsies and urine cytology. If a complete response is obtained in the primary tumor, an additional 20 to 28 Gy is delivered to the bladder/primary tumor before transurethral resection of bladder tumor. Improvements in the delivery of radiation therapy with improved conformal techniques, including IMRT,[52] proton beam therapy,[53] and the use of image guidance,[54] will likely further improve outcomes of bladder-preserving treatments and allow conformal dose-escalation to the regional lymph nodes. Such improvements may also reduce the volume of normal tissues exposed to higher doses and thereby are likely to decrease the morbidity of therapy, especially when combined with radiosensitizing systemic agents.

Testicular Cancer

Regional lymph node RT for men with testicular cancer is primarily confined to men with early-stage

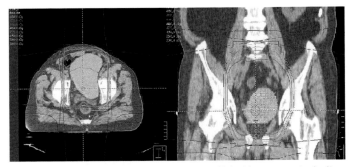

Fig. 3. Sagittal and axial images from 3D conformal treatment of bladder cancer including regional lymph nodes in a patient receiving bladder-preserving therapy.

seminoma and is slightly different from RT for other GU malignancies. First, the dose required to sterilize microscopic disease or gross nodal disease for seminoma is markedly lower than for other solid tumors (20–30 Gy and 30–40 Gy, respectively). Second, the retroperitoneal lymph nodes are considered first-echelon lymph nodes because of the specific lymphatic drainage of the testicles. EBRT effectively prevents relapse in most patients with clinical stage I and nonbulky stage II seminoma. Although most patients experience no serious adverse treatment effects, impaired fertility, second malignancies, and bowel effects have raised concerns about adjuvant EBRT in this setting. These concerns led to the evaluation of active surveillance and adjuvant chemotherapy as alternative treatments in men with stage I seminoma. Nevertheless, adjuvant RT remains an important option in carefully selected patients.

The technique for adjuvant infradiaphragmatic RT has evolved over the past several decades to include a smaller RT target area with less radiation dose.

Target for adjuvant radiation

Excellent results have been reported using a "dog-leg" RT field.[55,56] This field includes the ipsilateral renal hilum/pelvic lymph nodes and the bilateral para-aortic nodes. Considering the PA lymph nodes are the first-echelon nodes for testicular tumors, a prospective trial by the Medical Research Council (MRC) Testicular Tumor Working Group directly compared PA-only RT to a classic "dog-leg" RT field following inguinal orchiectomy.[57] In this trial, 478 men with stage I testicular seminoma were randomly assigned to one of the adjuvant RT treatments. The short-term side effects of RT were improved and the incidence of azospermia was significantly decreased in patients receiving PA-only RT. The number of pelvic relapses was higher in the group receiving PA-only RT, but the total number of relapses were similar. Three-year

survival was equivalent (>99%). As a result, PA-only RT is considered the standard treatment for men with stage I seminoma receiving adjuvant RT. Inclusion of the ipsilateral pelvic lymph nodes may be considered when there is risk of aberrant nodal drainage based on prior history and is considered standard adjuvant therapy for men with nonbulky clinical stage II seminoma following orchiectomy.[58]

Radiation dose

Owing to the radiosensitivity of seminoma, the required doses for sterilization of microscopic or macroscopic disease are some of the lowest used in therapeutic radiation. The MRC conducted a multinational trial where 625 men with seminoma were randomly assigned to 20 Gy delivered in 10 fractions, or 30 Gy delivered in 15 fractions following orchiectomy.[59] There was no difference in disease-free survival (approximately 98%). Men treated with higher-dose radiation had significantly more lethargy (20% vs 5%) and inability to work (46% vs 28%) measured 1 month after treatment. These differences disappeared by 3 months after RT. Alternative dose regimens using a lower dose per fraction to a slightly higher, but biologically equivalent, dose are common in the United States (ie, 25.5 Gy delivered in daily 1.5-Gy fractions). For areas with gross nodal involvement, a smaller "boost" field is used to bring the total dose to 36 Gy.

Penile Cancer

The inguinal lymph nodes are the primary lymphatic basin at risk in men with penile cancer. Elective RT to the inguinal lymph nodes is not recommended for patients without cytologically or histologically proven lymph node metastases or in those men with microscopic lymph node metastases treated with inguinal lymph node dissection. This contention is because of the potential for treatment-related morbidity (dermatitis, impaired wound healing, lymphedema) without a clearly defined benefit of RT versus surveillance alone in this population.[60,61] Inguinal RT might improve local control for men with multiple positive lymph nodes, bulky disease (>4 cm), or extranodal extension.[62–64] The possible morbidity of an uncontrolled inguinal recurrence must be weighed against the risk of treatment-related toxicity. The evidence for treatment of the regional lymph nodes in patients with high-risk factors for nodal recurrence is primarily supported though small retrospective series and extrapolations from other disease sites (vulvar and head/neck squamous cell carcinoma) where postoperative treatment of the regional lymph nodes in select patients seems to provide a therapeutic gain.[65,66] Prospective trials are needed to better define the role of regional lymph node radiation in men with penile cancer who have high-risk features for recurrence.

SUMMARY

RT plays an important and evolving role as definitive and adjuvant therapy for GU malignancies, including the treatment of the regional lymphatics. Defining the patient population most likely to benefit from regional treatment is paramount for all of these heterogeneous diseases.

Advances in treatment planning and delivery of EBRT, 3DCRT, IMRT, proton beam therapy, and image-guided RT provide the technology to precisely plan, target, and deliver RT with the goal of optimizing the radiation dose to the target while sparing normal tissue. Continued investigation and standardization of these techniques are needed to continue to improve the therapeutic ratio.

REFERENCES

1. Zelefsky MJ, Levin EJ, Hunt M, et al. Incidence of late rectal and urinary toxicities after three-dimensional conformal radiotherapy and intensity-modulated radiotherapy for localized prostate cancer. Int J Radiat Oncol Biol Phys 2008;70(4):1124–9.
2. Sanguineti G, Cavey ML, Endres EJ, et al. Does treatment of the pelvic nodes with IMRT increase late rectal toxicity over conformal prostate-only radiotherapy to 76 Gy? Strahlenther Onkol 2006;182(9):543–9.
3. Lips I, Dehnad H, Kruger AB, et al. Health-related quality of life in patients with locally advanced prostate cancer after 76 Gy intensity-modulated radiotherapy vs. 70 Gy conformal radiotherapy in a prospective and longitudinal study. Int J Radiat Oncol Biol Phys 2007;69(3):656–61.
4. Vora SA, Wong WW, Schild SE, et al. Analysis of biochemical control and prognostic factors in patients treated with either low-dose three-dimensional conformal radiation therapy or high-dose intensity-modulated radiotherapy for localized prostate cancer. Int J Radiat Oncol Biol Phys 2007;68(4):1053–8.
5. Yoshimura K, Kamoto T, Nakamura E, et al. Health-related quality-of-life after external beam radiation therapy for localized prostate cancer: intensity-modulated radiation therapy versus conformal radiation therapy. Prostate Cancer Prostatic Dis 2007;10(3):288–92.
6. Shu HK, Lee TT, Vigneauly E, et al. Toxicity following high-dose three-dimensional conformal and intensity-modulated radiation therapy for clinically localized prostate cancer. Urology 2001;57(1):102–7.
7. Ashman JB, Zelefsky MJ, Hunt MS, et al. Whole pelvic radiotherapy for prostate cancer using 3D conformal and intensity-modulated radiotherapy. Int J Radiat Oncol Biol Phys 2005;63(3):765–71.
8. Chera BS, Vargas C, Morris CG, et al. Dosimetric study of pelvic proton radiotherapy for high-risk prostate cancer. Int J Radiat Oncol Biol Phys 2009;75(4):994–1002.
9. Georg D, Georg P, Hillbrand M, et al. Assessment of improved organ at risk sparing for advanced cervix carcinoma utilizing precision radiotherapy techniques. Strahlenther Onkol 2008;184(11):586–91.
10. Kavanagh BD, Pan CC, Dawson LA, et al. Radiation dose-volume effects in the stomach and small bowel. Int J Radiat Oncol Biol Phys 2010;76(Suppl 3):S101–7.
11. Partin AW, Kattan MW, Subong EN, et al. Combination of prostate-specific antigen, clinical stage, and Gleason score to predict pathological stage of localized prostate cancer. A multi-institutional update. JAMA 1997;277(18):1445–51.
12. Partin AW, Mangold LA, Lamm DM, et al. Contemporary update of prostate cancer staging nomograms (Partin Tables) for the new millennium. Urology 2001;58(6):843–8.
13. Partin AW, Yoo J, Carter HB, et al. The use of prostate specific antigen, clinical stage and Gleason score to predict pathological stage in men with localized prostate cancer. J Urol 1993;150(1):110–4.
14. Roach M, Marquez C, Yuo HS, et al. Predicting the risk of lymph node involvement using the pre-treatment prostate specific antigen and Gleason score in men with clinically localized prostate cancer. Int J Radiat Oncol Biol Phys 1994;28(1):33–7.
15. Nguyen PL, Chen M, Hoffman KE, et al. Predicting the risk of pelvic node involvement among men with prostate cancer in the contemporary era. Int J Radiat Oncol Biol Phys 2009;74(1):104–9.

16. Cooperberg MR, Moul JW, Carroll PR. The changing face of prostate cancer. J Clin Oncol 2005;23(32): 8146–51.

17. Ward JF, Slezak JM, Blute ML, et al. Radical prosta-tectomy for clinically advanced (cT3) prostate cancer since the advent of prostate-specific antigen testing: 15-year outcome. BJU Int 2005;95(6):751–6.

18. Lee N, Newhouse JH, Olsson CA, et al. Which patients with newly diagnosed prostate cancer need a computed tomography scan of the abdomen and pelvis? An analysis based on 588 patients. Urology 1999;54(3):490–4.

19. Abuzallouf S, Dayes I, Lukka H. Baseline staging of newly diagnosed prostate cancer: a summary of the literature. J Urol 2004;171(6 Pt 1):2122–7.

20. Wolf JS, Cher M, Dall'era M, et al. The use and accu-racy of cross-sectional imaging and fine needle aspiration cytology for detection of pelvic lymph node metastases before radical prostatectomy. J Urol 1995;153(3 Pt 2):993–9.

21. Villeirs GM, L Verstraete K, De Neve WJ, et al. Magnetic resonance imaging anatomy of the pros-tate and periprostatic area: a guide for radiothera-pists. Radiother Oncol 2005;76(1):99–106.

22. Krook JE, Moertel CG, Gunderson LL, et al. Effective surgical adjuvant therapy for high-risk rectal carci-noma. N Engl J Med 1991;324(11):709–15.

23. Overgaard M, Hansen PS, Overgaard J, et al. Postop-erative radiotherapy in high-risk premenopausal women with breast cancer who receive adjuvant chemotherapy. Danish Breast Cancer Cooperative Group 82b Trial. N Engl J Med 1997;337(14):949–55.

24. Roach M. Targeting pelvic lymph nodes in men with intermediate- and high-risk prostate cancer, and confusion about the results of the randomized trials. J Clin Oncol 2008;26(22):3816–7 [author reply: 3817–8].

25. Nguyen PL, D'Amico AV. Targeting pelvic lymph nodes in men with intermediate- and high-risk prostate cancer despite two negative randomized trials. J Clin Oncol 2008;26(12):2055–6 [author reply: 2056–7].

26. Lawton CA, DeSilvio M, Roach M, et al. An update of the phase III trial comparing whole pelvic to prostate only radiotherapy and neoadjuvant to adjuvant total androgen suppression: updated analysis of RTOG 94-13, with emphasis on unexpected hormone/radi-ation interactions. Int J Radiat Oncol Biol Phys 2007; 69(3):646–55.

27. Roach M, DeSilvio M, Lawton C, et al. Phase III trial comparing whole-pelvic versus prostate-only radio-therapy and neoadjuvant versus adjuvant combined androgen suppression: Radiation Therapy Oncology Group 9413. J Clin Oncol 2003;21(10):1904–11.

28. Roach M, DeSilvio M, Valicenti R, et al. Whole-pelvis, "mini-pelvis," or prostate-only external beam radio-therapy after neoadjuvant and concurrent hormonal

therapy in patients treated in the Radiation Therapy Oncology Group 9413 trial. Int J Radiat Oncol Biol Phys 2006;66(3):647–53.

29. Pilepich MV, Winter K, Lawton CA, et al. Androgen suppression adjuvant to definitive radiotherapy in prostate carcinoma—long-term results of phase III RTOG 85-31. Int J Radiat Oncol Biol Phys 2005; 61(5):1285–90.

30. Lawton CA, Winter K, Grignon D, et al. Androgen suppression plus radiation versus radiation alone for patients with stage D1/pathologic node-positive adenocarcinoma of the prostate: updated results based on national prospective randomized trial Radiation Therapy Oncology Group 85-31. J Clin Oncol 2005;23(4):800–7.

31. Bolla M, Collette L, Blank L, et al. Long-term results with immediate androgen suppression and external irradiation in patients with locally advanced prostate cancer (an EORTC study): a phase III randomised trial. Lancet 2002;360(9327):103–6.

32. Pilepich MV, Winter K, John MJ, et al. Phase III radia-tion therapy oncology group (RTOG) trial 86-10 of androgen deprivation adjuvant to definitive radio-therapy in locally advanced carcinoma of the pros-tate. Int J Radiat Oncol Biol Phys 2001;50(5):1243–52.

33. Hanks GE, Pajak TF, Porter A, et al. Phase III trial of long-term adjuvant androgen deprivation after neo-adjuvant hormonal cytoreduction and radiotherapy in locally advanced carcinoma of the prostate: the radiation therapy oncology group protocol 92-02. J Clin Oncol 2003;21(21):3972–8.

34. Pommier P, Chabaud S, Lagrange JL, et al. Is there a role for pelvic irradiation in localized prostate adenocarcinoma? Preliminary results of GETUG-01. J Clin Oncol 2007;25(34):5366–73.

35. Smith JA, Haynes TH, Middleton RG. Impact of external irradiation on local symptoms and survival free of disease in patients with pelvic lymph node metastasis from adenocarcinoma of the prostate. J Urol 1984;131(4):705–7.

36. Lawton CA, Cox JD, Glisch C, et al. Is long-term survival possible with external beam irradiation for stage D1 adenocarcinoma of the prostate? Cancer 1992;69(11):2761–6.

37. Lee RJ, Sause WT. Surgically staged patients with prostatic carcinoma treated with definitive radio-therapy: fifteen-year results. Urology 1994;43(5): 640–4.

38. Hanks GE, Buzydlowski J, Sause WT, et al. Ten-year outcomes for pathologic node-positive patients treated in RTOG 75-06. Int J Radiat Oncol Biol Phys 1998;40(4):765–8.

39. Zagars GK, Sands ME, Pollack A, et al. Early androgen ablation for stage D1 (N1 to N3, M0) pros-tate cancer: prognostic variables and outcome. J Urol 1994;151(5):1330–3.

40. Sands ME, Pollack A, Zagars GK. Influence of radiotherapy on node-positive prostate cancer treated with androgen ablation. Int J Radiat Oncol Biol Phys 1995;31(1):13–9.

41. Whittington R, Malkowicz SB, Machtay M, et al. The use of combined radiation therapy and hormonal therapy in the management of lymph node-positive prostate cancer. Int J Radiat Oncol Biol Phys 1997; 39(3):673–80.

42. Anscher MS, Prosnitz LR. Prognostic significance of extent of nodal involvement in stage D1 prostate cancer treated with radiotherapy. Urology 1992; 39(1):39–43.

43. Schmid HP, Mihatsch MJ, Hering F, et al. Impact of minimal lymph node metastasis on long-term prognosis after radical prostatectomy. Eur Urol 1997; 31(1):11–6.

44. Briganti A, Karnes RJ, Pozzo LF, et al. Combination of adjuvant hormonal and radiation therapy significantly prolongs survival of patients with pT2-4 pN+ prostate cancer: results of a matched analysis. Eur Urol 2011;59(5):832–40.

45. Thompson IM, Tangen CM, Paradelo J, et al. Adjuvant radiotherapy for pathologically advanced prostate cancer: a randomized clinical trial. JAMA 2006; 296(19):2329–35.

46. Wiegel T, Bottke D, Steiner U, et al. Phase III postoperative adjuvant radiotherapy after radical prostatectomy compared with radical prostatectomy alone in pT3 prostate cancer with postoperative undetectable prostate-specific antigen: ARO 96-02/AUO AP 09/95. J Clin Oncol 2009;27(18):2924–30.

47. Bolla M, van Poppel H, Collette L, et al. Postoperative radiotherapy after radical prostatectomy: a randomised controlled trial (EORTC trial 22911). Lancet 2005;366(9485):572–8.

48. Shipley W, Hunt D, Lukka H, et al. Initial report of RTOG 9601: a phase III trial in prostate cancer: anti-androgen therapy (AAT) with bicalutamide during and after radiation therapy (RT) improves freedom from progression and reduces the incidence of metastatic disease in patients following radical prostatectomy (RP) with pT2-3, no disease, and elevated PSA levels. Int J Radiat Oncol Biol Phys 2010;78(3 Suppl 1):S27.

49. Rödel C, Grabenbauer GG, Kühn R, et al. Combined-modality treatment and selective organ preservation in invasive bladder cancer: long-term results. J Clin Oncol 2002;20(14):3061–71.

50. Shipley WU, Winter KA, Kaufman DS, et al. Phase III trial of neoadjuvant chemotherapy in patients with invasive bladder cancer treated with selective bladder preservation by combined radiation therapy and chemotherapy: initial results of Radiation Therapy Oncology Group 89-03. J Clin Oncol 1998;16(11):3576–83.

51. Shipley WU, Kaufman DS, Zehr E, et al. Selective bladder preservation by combined modality protocol treatment: long-term outcomes of 190 patients with invasive bladder cancer. Urology 2002;60(1):62–7 [discussion: 67–8].

52. Søndergaard J, Høyer M, Petersen JB, et al. The normal tissue sparing obtained with simultaneous treatment of pelvic lymph nodes and bladder using intensity-modulated radiotherapy. Acta Oncol 2009; 48(2):238–44.

53. Hata M, Miyanaga N, Tokuuye K, et al. Proton beam therapy for invasive bladder cancer: a prospective study of bladder-preserving therapy with combined radiotherapy and intra-arterial chemotherapy. Int J Radiat Oncol Biol Phys 2006;64(5):1371–9.

54. Vestergaard A, Søndergaard J, Petersen JB, et al. A comparison of three different adaptive strategies in image-guided radiotherapy of bladder cancer. Acta Oncol 2010;49(7):1069–76.

55. Dosoretz DE, Shipley WU, Blitzer PH, et al. Megavoltage irradiation for pure testicular seminoma: results and patterns of failure. Cancer 1981;48(10): 2184–90.

56. Fosså SD, Aass N, Kaalhus O. Radiotherapy for testicular seminoma stage I: treatment results and long-term post-irradiation morbidity in 365 patients. Int J Radiat Oncol Biol Phys 1989;16(2):383–8.

57. Fosså SD, Horwich A, Russell JM, et al. Optimal planning target volume for stage I testicular seminoma: a medical research council randomized trial. Medical Research Council Testicular Tumor Working Group. J Clin Oncol 1999;17(4):1146.

58. Schmoll HJ, Souchon R, Krege S, et al. European consensus on diagnosis and treatment of germ cell cancer: a report of the European Germ Cell Cancer Consensus Group (EGCCCG). Ann Oncol 2004;15(9):1377–99.

59. Jones WG, Fossa SD, Mead GM, et al. Randomized trial of 30 versus 20 Gy in the adjuvant treatment of stage I testicular seminoma: a report on Medical Research Council Trial TE18, European Organisation for the Research and Treatment of Cancer Trial 30942 (ISRCTN18525328). J Clin Oncol 2005;23(6):1200–8.

60. Ravi R. Morbidity following groin dissection for penile carcinoma. Br J Urol 1993;72(6):941–5.

61. Horenblas S. Lymphadenectomy for squamous cell carcinoma of the penis. Part 2: the role and technique of lymph node dissection. BJU Int 2001; 88(5):473–83.

62. Chen M, Chen W, Wu C, et al. Contemporary management of penile cancer including surgery and adjuvant radiotherapy: an experience in Taiwan. World J Urol 2004;22(1):60–6.

63. Ravi R, Chaturvedi HK, Sastry DV. Role of radiation therapy in the treatment of carcinoma of the penis. Br J Urol 1994;74(5):646–51.

64. Langsenlehner T, Mayer R, Quehenberger F, et al. The role of radiation therapy after incomplete resection of penile cancer. Strahlenther Onkol 2008; 184(7):359–63.

65. Katz A, Eifel PJ, Jhingran A, et al. The role of radiation therapy in preventing regional recurrences of invasive squamous cell carcinoma of the vulva. Int J Radiat Oncol Biol Phys 2003; 57(2):409–18.

66. Cooper JS, Pajak TF, Forastiere AA, et al. Postoperative concurrent radiotherapy and chemotherapy for high-risk squamous-cell carcinoma of the head and neck. N Engl J Med 2004;350(19): 1937–44.

Complications of Lymphadenectomy in Urologic Surgery

Steve K. Williams, MD[a], Farhang Rabbani, MD[a,b],*

KEYWORDS

• Lymphadenectomy • Urology • Surgery • Complications

Lymphadenectomy is the surgical removal of local and regional lymph nodes draining a malignant tumor. In urologic oncology, lymphadenectomy provides important staging information that may determine the need for further adjuvant therapies and, for some tumors, it may prove therapeutic. As with all surgical interventions, lymph node dissection has the potential for adverse side effects. This article describes the complications associated with lymph node dissection for genitourinary malignancies and outlines strategies that may be helpful in preventing or treating these complications.

INGUINAL LYMPHADENECTOMY

Squamous cell carcinoma of the penis accounts for 0.4% to 0.6% of all malignancies in men. Surgical therapy includes treatment of the primary tumor, of locoregional disease (ie, inguinal and pelvic lymph nodes), and more aggressive resections such as hemipelvectomy and hemicorporectomy. Penile cancer usually has a predictable stepwise pattern of spread. At first, regional inguinal lymph node metastasis occurs, followed by pelvic nodal metastasis and then distant spread. The presence and extent of this metastasis to the regional lymph nodes are the key predictors for survival, even more so than grade or morphohistologic determinants.[1] Tumor stage and grade are also important predictors of lymph node metastases, with a reported incidence of 19% to 29% for grade I, 46% to 65% for grade II, and 82% to 85% for grade III penile squamous cell cancer (SCC).[2] Less than 3% of patients present with distant metastases.[3]

Five-year cancer-specific survival decreases from 90% to 100% in patients with node-negative squamous cell carcinoma of the penis to approximately 60% in patients with resected inguinal nodal metastases.[4] Survival among lymph node-positive patients depends on the number of nodes involved, lymph node density, size of largest nodal deposit, presence of extranodal tumor extension, bilateral groin metastases, and involvement of the pelvic lymph nodes.[4,5] The evidence suggests that patients with minimal nodal involvement (ie, 2 or fewer lymph nodes involved and with no evidence of extranodal extension or pelvic disease) derive the most benefit from curative inguinal lymph node dissection, with 5-year cancer-specific survival approaching 80%. In a prospective study, the 3-year disease-specific survival of men with pathologic N0 disease was 100%.[5] Men found to have a single lymph node involved (N1 disease) had a 100% 3-year disease-specific survival without any adjuvant therapy.

The management of clinically negative nodes in squamous cell carcinoma of the penis involves the accurate identification of patients at high risk of harboring occult inguinal nodal metastases, and the sparing of the morbidity of inguinal node dissection in patients destined to have pathologically negative nodes. This management is based on risk stratification based on the primary tumor characteristics such as pathologic primary tumor stage, tumor grade, and presence of lymphovascular invasion (LVI), which have been shown to correlate with the probability of lymph node metastasis.[6,7] The current European Association of Urology (EAU) guidelines stratify patients into

a Department of Urology, Albert Einstein College of Medicine, Bronx, NY, USA
b Montefiore Medical Center, 111 East 210th Street, Bronx, NY 10467, USA
* Corresponding author. Montefiore Medical Center, 111 East 210th Street, Bronx, NY 10467.
E-mail address: frabbani@montefiore.org

Urol Clin N Am 38 (2011) 507–518
doi:10.1016/j.ucl.2011.07.013
0094-0143/11/$ – see front matter © 2011 Elsevier Inc. All rights reserved.

3 risk groups according to their probability of harboring metastatic lymphadenopathy. These groups are based on stage and grade of the primary tumor: low risk groups are pTis, pTa grade 1 to 2, and pT1 grade 1 tumors; intermediate-risk groups are pT1 grade 2 tumors; high-risk groups are pT2 or higher or grade 3 tumors.[6] EAU guidelines recommend modified inguinal lymph node dissection for patients in intermediate-risk and high-risk categories.

A therapeutic groin dissection is indicated for men with overtly palpable adenopathy. Approximately 85% of patients with squamous cell carcinoma of the penis with palpable, but not fixed, inguinal lymph nodes at the time of initial presentation harbor metastatic nodal disease.[8] A 4-week to 6-week course of antibiotic therapy is usually administered before groin dissection to treat any associated infection and this helps reduce the risk of wound sepsis from an infected primary tumor. A classic inguinal lymph node dissection of the involved, grossly positive, and contralateral groins is usually performed, followed by bilateral pelvic lymphadenectomy. Select patients with bulky groin metastases benefit from induction systemic therapy, followed by a palliative bilateral inguinal and pelvic lymph node dissection (PLND) with or without adjuvant radiotherapy based on the extent of residual disease. Close collaboration with reconstructive surgeons is essential because large portions of involved inguinal skin may be resected en bloc, necessitating myocutaneous flaps for reconstruction.

Relevant Surgical Anatomy

The regional lymph nodes of the penis are located in the inguinal region and have been traditionally divided into the superficial and the deep groups. The superficial nodes are located under the subcutaneous fascia in the deep membranous layer of the superficial fascia of the thigh above the fascia lata. The superficial nodes have been divided into 5 anatomic groups: the central nodes around the saphenofemoral junction, superolateral nodes around the superficial circumflex vein, inferolateral nodes around the lateral femoral cutaneous and superficial circumflex veins, superomedial nodes around the superficial external pudendal and superficial epigastric veins, and inferomedial nodes around the greater saphenous vein.[4] The deep inguinal nodes lie in the region of the fossa ovalis where the greater saphenous vein drains into the femoral vein through an opening in the fascia lata. The node of Cloquet is the most cephalad of this deep group and is situated between the femoral vein and the lacunar ligament.

Superficial and deep inguinal nodes are considered to be the first draining nodes of the penis; from there, lymphatic drainage is to the second-line regional nodes, which are those in the pelvis around the iliac vessels and in the obturator fossa.

Complications of Inguinal Lymphadenectomy

Surgical morbidity is a significant problem after radical inguinal lymphadenectomy (ILND). Historically, ILND has been associated with a high complication rate of between 80% and 100%).[9] However, more recent surgical series report an overall complication rate of between 42% and 57% for patients undergoing ILND as part of the management for penile cancer.[10,11] Complications reported in groin dissection series are generally related to disruption of the lymphatics draining the lower extremities and damage to the overlying skin flaps from devascularization. Reported complications include flap necrosis/skin edge necrosis in 2.5% to 64%; wound breakdown in 38% to 61%; seroma in 5% to 87%; lymphorrhea in 33%; wound infection in 3% to 70%; lymphocele in 2.5% to 87%; leg lymphedema in 5% to 100%; deep vein thrombosis/thrombophlebitis in 6% to 9%; myocardial infarction in 9%; femoral neuropraxia in 2%; death in 1.3% to 3%; and an overall complication rate of 24% to 100%.[12]

Wound Infection

Reported rates of wound infections following ILND are between 14% and 17%.[9,13] Inguinal colonization together with its moist environment predisposes the inguinal region to infection after ILND. Gram-negative rods, Staphylococcus species, diphtheroids, and Peptostreptococcus microorganisms are the organisms most commonly isolated.[14] The use of broad-spectrum antibiotics (eg, ampicillin/gentamicin or ampicillin/ciprofloxacin) before surgery decreases wound colonization before lymphadenectomy. Meticulous hemostasis further reduces the risk of hematoma formation, which could potentially become infected.

Lymphedema

The incidence of lymphedema after ILND is as high as 50%, with severe lymphedema occurring in 35% of patients.[15] Clinically, the affected limb is swollen with enhanced skin creases, increased dermal turgor, hyperkeratosis, and papillomatosis. Lymphedema is traditionally described as nonpitting but, in early cases, pitting may be present. Disabilities from lymphedema include pain, limb heaviness, reduced mobility, impaired function, and recurrent bouts of cellulitis induced by lymphostasis. The surgical removal of lymph nodes and disruption of lymphatic channels during dissection of the inguinal region clearly contribute, but there are other variables that play a role, including treatment-related variables such as use of adjuvant radiation therapy, and patient-related variables. Radiation therapy can promote development of lymphedema by blocking lymph vessels or by compressing lymph vessels through radiation fibrosis.[16] Some of the most frequently reported patient-related variables are increasing age, higher body mass index, weight gain, and infection.

Lymphadenectomy associated with saphenous vein preservation has been shown to reduce lymphedema. In 1988, Catalona[17] published results regarding a modified ILND that targeted the superior medial quadrant, where the highest percentage of positive nodes is found. This modified approach decreased the length of the incision, allowed deeper skin flaps, preserved the saphenous vein, and did not transpose the sartorius muscle, thus decreasing the morbidity associated with the standard groin dissection. In his initial 6 patients, the modified technique did not compromise cancer control, although it was stressed that this method should be used only with clinically negative or minimally positive nodes, and pointed out that preserving the saphenous vein could decrease postoperative complications during ILND. Zhang and colleagues[18] completed a randomized prospective trial of ILND for vulvar cancer comparing saphenous vein sparing ILND with ILND without sparing the vein. Short-term lower extremity lymphedema occurred in 43% in the sparing group and 67% patients in the excision group (P<.01). However, sparing the saphenous vein is not always possible, particularly in patients with a large burden of metastatic disease.

Following the completion of the ILND, it is recommended that a closed suction drain be placed within the inguinal wound to avoid the development of a postoperative fluid collection (ie, lymphocele, seroma, or hematoma). The drain is usually removed when there is minimal drainage (typically <30 to 50 mL per 24 hours). The avoidance of infection is paramount because this promotes increased wound fibrosis and decreased limb drainage. The use of compression stockings, sequential compression devices, early ambulation after 8 hours of bed rest, avoidance of subcutaneous heparin, and physical therapy has been recommended as a method of reducing the incidence and impact of postoperative lymphedema.[19] Early ambulation decreases the risk of deep vein thrombosis (DVT) formation and also assists in moving the patient to a status that is consistent with the level of ambulation required for discharge. Heparin may be avoided because

of the concern for an increased risk of lymphocele formation. Strict leg elevation may be maintained in the hospital when the patients are not ambulating.

Skin Flap Necrosis

Skin flap necrosis remains a frequent complication of groin dissection. The blood supply to the skin of the inguinal region is from the superficial branches of the inferior epigastric, external pudendal, and circumflex iliac arteries and these vessels are ligated during groin node dissection. The viability of the skin edge is therefore reliant on anastomotic vessels running in the superficial fatty layer of the Camper fascia parallel to the inguinal ligament.

Several surgical modifications have been developed to minimize skin flap necrosis. Because lymphatic drainage of the penis to the groin is beneath the Camper fascia, this layer can be preserved and left attached to the overlying skin when the skin flaps are fashioned. Straight vertical and S-shaped incisions cut across the anastomotic vessels in the Camper fascia, and postoperative swelling puts traction on these incisions. Smaller operative fields and thick vascular flaps have resulted in decreased skin edge necrosis in patients undergoing prophylactic dissections. Generous use of well-vascularized myocutaneous flaps has decreased skin edge necrosis among patients undergoing therapeutic and palliative dissections. Ornellas and colleagues[8] noted that a Gibson approach provided good exposure to the iliac and inguinal lymph nodes while minimizing morbidity (flap necrosis in 5%) compared with the S-shaped or bi-iliac incisions (72%–82%, respectively). Ravi[13] reported a 0% incidence of skin flap necrosis in a later cohort of 30 patients undergoing therapeutic dissection with myocutaneous flap reconstruction compared with an earlier cohort of patients undergoing lymphadenectomy without flap reconstruction (skin edge necrosis was 61%–78%). Meticulous atraumatic handling of the tissues throughout, limitation of the extent of flap mobilization (superior to the inguinal ligament and inferior to the tip of the femoral triangle) are also helpful in preserving flap viability.

PREVENTING COMPLICATIONS
Antibiotics

Antibiotic therapy with broad-spectrum antibiotics for 4 to 6 weeks after treatment of the primary tumor as discussed previously has traditionally been administered to allow resolution of septic lymphadenitis before ILND. In patients with active infection, bacterial cultures should be obtained, and culture-specific antibiotics should be given before surgery. Prophylactic antibiotics are administered at the time of lymphadenectomy and are usually continued for 1 week after surgery or until the wound drains have been removed.[20] The microorganisms isolated from septic ILND wounds have included gram-negative rods, *Staphylococcus* species, diphtheroids, and *Peptostreptococcus*.

DVT Prophylaxis

Venous thromboembolism is a serious complication that should be aggressively prevented when possible. Some studies have indicated that the perioperative use of low-dose heparin may be associated with an increased risk of wound hematoma and lymph drainage without reducing the incidence of DVT.[19,21] It has been suggested that, in patients with a remote history of DVT, perioperative heparin should be continued until postoperative day 28. With a history of DVT or pulmonary embolism in the preceding 6 months, a therapeutic dose of heparin should be restarted when the risk of postoperative hemorrhage is minimal, with subsequent conversion to oral warfarin.[22] The use of antiembolic stockings or intermittent compression devices immediately before anesthetic induction to prevent DVT has also been recommended.

PLND

The role of PLND has progressively been defined from tumor staging to potentially curative. In urologic oncology, it is performed frequently at the time of radical surgery for penile, prostate, and bladder cancer. Although potentially curative in bladder cancer, the role of pelvic lymphadenectomy is not yet clearly defined. This article discusses the indications of PLND for prostate and bladder cancer before reviewing the literature on reported complications. Penile cancer has been previously discussed.

Radical Prostatectomy

Pelvic lymphadenectomy is frequently performed simultaneously with radical prostatectomy to determine lymph node status. Current radical retropubic prostatectomy series indicate that the incidence of lymph node metastasis is less than 10%. The presence of lymph node metastasis in men diagnosed with clinically localized prostate cancer is a poor prognostic finding and has important implications on the initiation of adjuvant therapy. The original staging lymphadenectomy approach was transperitoneal with biopsies of the para-aortic, common iliac, hypogastric, external iliac, and obturator lymph nodal basins

guided by pedal lymphangiography.[23] This approach provided excellent exposure, although it increased perioperative morbidity compared with an extraperitoneal approach. For PLND in prostate cancer, the anatomic boundaries (ie, extent) of dissection remain controversial because of a lack of standardization. Currently standard pelvic lymphadenectomy involves the dissection and removal of lymphatic tissue from the level of the external iliac vein to the obturator nerve, extending proximally to the common iliac artery bifurcation and distally to the proximal femoral canal to include the node of Cloquet. An extended lymphadenectomy is the extension of resection to include the lymphatic tissue surrounding the internal iliac vein and presacral region.

The therapeutic benefit of pelvic lymphadenectomy for disease clearance in the era of prostate cancer stage migration and lymph node micrometastasis is still largely unknown. Bhatta-Dar and colleagues[24] retrospectively examined the role of pelvic lymphadenectomy in 336 men who underwent radical prostatectomy. Patients had a prostate-specific antigen (PSA) level of less than 10 ng/mL, Gleason score of less than 7, and clinical stage T1 or T2 disease. Only 140 men underwent pelvic lymphadenectomy, according to the discretion of the operating surgeon who performed the radical prostatectomy. Both groups were matched in terms of age, family history of prostate cancer, race, clinical stage, and PSA level. The pelvic lymphadenectomy boundaries included the external iliac vein, pelvic side wall, obturator nerve, bifurcation of the common iliac artery, and the inguinal ligament.

The pelvic lymphadenectomy group had a 0.7% metastasis rate. The results showed no statistically significant difference in biochemical relapse rates after 60 months. On multivariate analysis, pelvic lymphadenectomy also did not seem to be an independent predictor of outcome. The 6-year biochemical relapse-free survival did not show any statistical significance between the 2 groups.

The advent of PSA screening has led to considerable stage migration and a low incidence of lymph node involvement in contemporary radical prostatectomy series. The incidence of lymph node metastasis has decreased in the last decade from 20% to 40% in the 1970s and 1980s to the present rate of about 6%.[25] Some investigators have suggested that PLND may be omitted in patients deemed to be at low risk for lymph node metastasis. The Partin tables, Memorial Sloan-Kettering Cancer Center Prostate Nomogram, and the Hamburg Algorithm have been developed as methods of identifying patients who are at increased risk of lymph node metastasis before surgery.[26] These tools have proved to be useful guides in clinical decision making, and their performance has been established.

Radical cystectomy

In 2010, bladder cancer was the fourth most common tumor in men and the 11th most common in women in the United States, with 90% of cases being urothelial carcinoma.[27] Approximately 30% of patients present with a muscle-invasive disease at the time of diagnosis. Currently, radical cystectomy (RC) accompanied by PLND is the gold standard surgical treatment of muscle-invasive bladder cancer. Approximately 25% of patients with stages T1 to T4 N0 M0 bladder cancer who undergo RC and PLND are found to have lymph node metastases. The incidence of lymph node tumor involvement correlates with increasing tumor stage, including 5% with nonmuscle invasive primary bladder tumors (P0, Pa, Pis, P1); 18% with superficial muscle-invasive tumors (P2a); 27% with deep muscle-invasive tumors (P2b); 45% with extravesical tumors (P3); and 45% with P4 primary bladder tumors.[28,29] Lymph node metastases are associated with an increased risk of local recurrence and disease progression and a decreased chance of survival. Skinner[30] reported a 36% improvement of 5-year survival in patients with bladder cancer with limited nodal disease undergoing bilateral PLND at the time of cystectomy and concluded that a meticulous PLND could provide cure and control of pelvic disease in some patients with regional lymph node metastases without increasing morbidity.

Anatomy of Lymphatic Drainage of the Bladder

The anatomy of bladder lymphatic drainage has traditionally been divided into 6 distinct areas: (1) the visceral lymphatic plexus within the bladder wall, originating inside the submucosa and extending into the muscular layer of the organ; (2) the intercalated lymph nodes, which are juxtavesical lymph nodes located within the perivesical fat arranged into anterior, lateral, and posterior groups; (3) the pelvic collecting trunks, which are lymph nodes medial to the external iliac and hypogastric lymph nodes; (4) regional pelvic lymph nodes, which include the external iliac, hypogastric, and presacral lymph node groups; (5) lymphatic trunks leading from the regional pelvic lymph nodes; and (6) common iliac lymph nodes on the common iliac vessels.[31] The primary drainage starts from the external and internal iliac and obturator sites, secondary drainage is from the common iliac sites, and tertiary drainage is from the trigone and posterior bladder wall is to the presacral nodes.

Pelvic Lymphadenectomy in Bladder Cancer

Presence or absence of lymph node involvement has been shown to be predictive of outcome in patients who undergo RC and PLND. Present guidelines for the pretreatment assessment of lymph node status are mainly based on cross-sectional imaging techniques like computed tomography (CT) and magnetic resonance imaging (MRI) with contrast enhancement.[32] The assessment of nodal status based simply on size is limited by the inability of both CT and MRI to identify metastases in normal-sized or minimally enlarged nodes. The overall sensitivity for detection of lymph node metastases is low and ranges from 48% to 87%. Specificities are also low because nodal enlargement may be caused by benign conditions. Pelvic nodes greater than 8 mm and abdominal nodes greater than 10 mm in maximum short-axis diameter (MSAD) should be regarded as enlarged on CT and MRI.

The curative value of lymph node dissection is still unknown and a standardized lymph node dissection has yet to be defined. Standard PLND includes the whole primary lymphatic drainage of the bladder.[33] The standard PLND has been defined as having the following boundaries: common iliac bifurcation (cephalad extent), genitofemoral nerve (lateral), circumflex caudal iliac vein and lymph node of Cloquet (distal), and hypogastric vessels (posterior), including the obturator fossa. Extended PLND has been defined to include nodes in the boundaries of the aortic bifurcation and common iliac vessels (proximal/cephalad), genitofemoral nerve (lateral), circumflex (distal) and caudal iliac vein and lymph node of Cloquet, hypogastric vessels (posterior), including the obturator fossa, presacral lymph nodes anterior to the sacral promontory. In some cases, an extended dissection may extend more superiorly to the level of the inferior mesenteric artery and include paracaval and para-aortic areas.[30]

Pelvic Lymphadenectomy in Bladder Cancer and Survival

Herr and Donat[34] analyzed the outcome of patients with grossly node-positive bladder cancer after PLND and RC. Included in this study were 83 patients treated with surgery alone (no neoadjuvant or adjuvant chemotherapy), presenting with N2 to 3 disease, and with a follow-up of up to 10 years. Twenty patients (24%) survived, and 64 patients (76%) died of the disease. This finding would suggest that some patients with grossly node-positive bladder cancer have a chance of cure with RC through PLND. In a multivariate analysis, the extent of the lymph node dissection, number of lymph nodes removed, and number of cases performed by the individual surgeon were found to be the most significant factors influencing survival in patients undergoing cystectomy for bladder cancer.[35] In this prospective trial, 270 patients underwent cystectomy, and half were randomized to receive neoadjuvant chemotherapy. In a separate analysis of this trial, various surgical factors were analyzed. In this cohort of patients, 24 had undergone no lymph node dissection, 98 had undergone a limited dissection (obturator lymph nodes only), and 146 underwent a standard (not extended) PLND. The 5-year survival rates for these groups were 33%, 46%, and 60%, respectively. The median number of lymph nodes removed for the cohort was 10. The survival rate for patients with less than 10 lymph nodes removed was significantly lower compared with patients with more than 10 lymph nodes removed (44% vs 61%, respectively).

COMPLICATIONS OF PELVIC LYMPHADENECTOMY

Generally, PLND is well tolerated, with complication rates between 4.1% and 10.6%.[36] Laparoscopic and robotic-assisted PLND seem to show similar rates of complications. The most commonly reported complications include symptomatic lymphocele, deep vein thrombosis, ureteral injury, nerve injury, vascular injury, and lower extremity edema. Most studies suggest that morbidity associated with PLND may be associated with the extent of dissection. Lymphoceles, nerve injures, and ureteral injuries are discussed here. Lymphedema has been discussed in detail earlier.

Lymphoceles

A lymphocele is defined as a collection of lymphatic fluid without distinct epithelial lining, resulting from the transection of afferent lymphatic channels, and is the most frequent postoperative complication related to pelvic lymphadenectomy.[37] Although the incidence of any lymphocele detected by ultrasound or radiograph ranges from 27% to 61%, only a few become symptomatic.[38] A greater rate was suggested for patients undergoing extraperitoneal PLND.[39] Symptomatic patients may present with ileus, fever, abdominal pain, lower extremity edema, gastrointestinal symptoms, or lower urinary tract symptoms from mass effect on adjacent organs.[40] In a recent series, the incidences of symptoms related to symptomatic lymphoceles were fever in 47%, abdominal pain in 40%, lower

extremity swelling in 37%, genital swelling in 25%, groin pain in 22%, abdominal swelling in 9%, and back and flank pain in 6% and 5%, respectively.[41] In addition, compression of the pelvic veins by the lymphocele increases the risk of thromboembolic events. The correlation between lymphocele formation and deep vein thrombosis and/or pulmonary embolism has been shown by several investigators.[39,42] Physical examination may reveal a fluctuant mass in the lower abdomen and the diagnosis may be confirmed by radiological imaging. On ultrasound imaging, lymphoceles appear as anechoic cystic structures that may contain thin septations and debris. On CT scan, lymphoceles are seen as thin-walled hypodense lesions with negative Hounsfield unit values. A finding of a thickened wall with regional enhancement suggests the presence of infection.

Various factors have been identified that may increase the risk of lymphocele after PLND. Naselli and colleagues[43] reviewed prognostic factors of symptomatic lymphocele after pelvic lymphadenectomy in 359 patients during radical prostatectomy. After adjusting for covariates, logistic regression analysis revealed that only the number of nodes was significantly associated with the onset of a symptomatic lymphocele. The risk of lymphocele seemed to increase linearly with the number of nodes retrieved. Other investigators have shown that excessive use of diathermy, the presence of metastatic lymph nodes, the long-term use of steroids or diuretics, prior radiation therapy, and subcutaneous heparin can contribute to lymphocele risk.[41,44] Kropfl and colleagues[45] showed that the risk of lymphocele formation was considerably reduced when the heparin was injected into an upper limb as opposed to the lower abdomen or thigh. Drainage fluid from all patients who had heparin injected into the thigh was found to contain high levels of heparin, but fluid from patients who had heparin injected into the arm lacked heparin. Paucity of clotting factors and lack of platelets are believed to render the lymphatic fluid more vulnerable to the effect of anticoagulants than is blood.

Treatment of lymphoceles varies depending on the degree of symptoms. Small asymptomatic lymphoceles are typically observed but, for larger collections, initial management involves placement of a percutaneous drain. Fluid obtained by percutaneous aspiration is evaluated for bacterial culture and analysis of creatinine to exclude urine leak. Reported success rates with the drainage tube are approaching 80%, with a mean drainage duration ranging from a few days to several months.[39] A major disadvantage of this technique, particularly when prolonged treatment is required, is the need for frequent tube exchanges as a result of clogging of the small-caliber side holes. If percutaneous drainage fails, sclerosing agents such as 96% ethanol, 10% povidone-iodine, and tetracycline have been used.[37] Surgical options include marsupialization into the peritoneal cavity, which may be performed using an open or laparoscopic approach.[46] Open external drainage is generally reserved primarily for loculated, infected lymphoceles that fail to respond to percutaneous drainage and antibiotic therapy.

Ureteral Injury

The ureters lie in the retroperitoneum and enter the pelvis in the region of the bifurcation of the common iliac artery. After crossing these vessels, they course along the inferior lateral pelvis into the bladder. The ureters are rarely injured during PLND; this occurs in less than 1% of cases.[39] As the ureter courses over the iliac vessels to enter the pelvis, it may be injured by inadvertent clip placement or aggressive dissection.

Nerve Injury

The close anatomic relationship between the pelvic lymph node chains and pelvic nerves puts these nerves at risk for injury during PLND. The reported incidence of nerve injuries after PLND is approximately 3.2%.[37] There are 3 general categories of nerve injury. Neuropraxia, which is a nerve contusion, is a functional injury. It is caused by nerve compression or traction and results in a conduction block without overt axonal degeneration. Recovery from neurapraxia is expected to occur within 6 weeks. Axonotmesis is a more severe injury caused by prolonged compression or excessive traction. In this case, neural elements distal to the injury sites degenerate, although the supporting structures of epineurium, perineurium, and endoneurium remain undisturbed. The supporting neuronal structures allow for nerve regeneration, and function recovers slowly in 6 months to 1 year. The most severe of injuries is termed neurotmesis and denotes complete division of the nerve. In this case, both neural elements and supporting structures are disrupted and recovery is not expected.

Nerves that may be injured during PLND include the obturator, femoral, and genitofemoral nerves. Obturator nerve injuries are the most frequent type of nerve injury associated with PLND.[40] This is reported in 0% to 1.8% of recent series, with a higher frequency observed in several early series of laparoscopic PLND.[47] The obturator nerve is an important landmark during PLNDs. While performing pelvic lymphadenectomy, the obturator nerve is used as the inferior extent of dissection. The nerve enters the pelvis behind the iliac arteries, runs laterally along the pelvic sidewall, and exits via the obturator foramen. It provides sensory innervations to the skin on the medial aspect of the thigh, as well as motor innervation of the adductor muscles in the thigh, and may be injured by excessive traction, cautery, clip, or inadvertent transaction. Cautery and clip placement may result in neurapraxia affecting the sensory innervation to the medial aspect of the thigh as well as the motor adductors of the thigh. A neurapraxia typically resolves after several weeks and physical therapy.

A clinical indicator of obturator nerve injury may be either sensory or motor. Clinically, the Howship-Romberg sign has been shown to be suggestive of injury to the obturator nerve. It is represented by pain down the medial thigh into the knee, and occasionally into the hip, and is exacerbated by extension and abduction or inward thigh rotation. Frank transection that is recognized intraoperatively should be repaired primarily with 6-0 nonabsorbable suture. It is crucial that a sound knowledge of the anatomic course of the nerve be known to reduce the risk of injury. Complete exposure of the nerve is facilitated by its careful dissection laterally away from the accompanying obturator vessels and nodes. Node packet division, proximal and distal, should be performed only after the nerve can be visualized throughout its entire course within the obturator fossa.

The genitofemoral nerve is a mixed motor and sensory nerve with a preponderance of sensory fibers. It originates from the L1 to L2 nerve roots, then travels obliquely between the 2 bellies of the psoas muscle, perforating the psoas major descending along its anterior belly. The nerve commonly lies adjacent to the common iliac vessels, in the groove between the vessels and the medial aspect of the psoas muscle. It then descends caudal and lateral to the external iliac vessels and, at a variable distance above the inguinal ligaments, divides into its terminal branches, which are the genital and the femoral branches. The genital branch receives sensory input from the skin of the scrotum in men and the mons pubis in women and innervates the cremasteric muscle. Genitofemoral nerve injury occurs infrequently during an extended PLND, when it may occur where the nerve courses lateral to the iliac artery during dissection of the common and external iliac lymph nodes. Injury may present with neurapraxia of the medial aspect of the ipsilateral groin and thigh. Typically, these paresthesias are self-limiting.[37]

Postoperative femoral neuropathy is a well-documented complication of pelvic and perineal surgical procedures in urology. Most cases of femoral neuropathy following pelvic lymphadenectomy result from direct compression injury from the placement of self-retaining retractors and indirect compression from retracting the psoas muscle laterally while pressing on the nerve against the pelvic sidewall. The severity of the injury is usually related to the duration of retraction and positioning of the patient.

The femoral nerve originates in the lumbar plexus from branches of the posterior division of the L2, L3, and L4 roots. The nerve emerges from the psoas major muscle at its lateral border, passes caudally between the psoas and iliac muscles, and then courses posterior to the femoral artery. It innervates the iliac, sartorius, and quadriceps muscles. It receives sensory innervation from the anterior thigh (via the anterior femoral cutaneous nerve) and the medial foreleg (via the saphenous nerve). Femoral nerve injury usually produces weakness of knee extension secondary to quadriceps paresis.

After surgery, femoral neuropathy is managed by physical therapy to prevent muscle wasting. Chronic neurogenic pain may be treated with non-narcotic analgesics. Drugs such as carbamazepine and amitriptyline are useful adjuncts to analgesics. Femoral nerve compression almost invariably resolves spontaneously; however, the time to resolution remains variable.[37]

RETROPERITONEAL LYMPHADENECTOMY

Each year, approximately 8000 new cases and almost 400 deaths caused by testicular cancer are expected. The development of effective cisplatin-based chemotherapy regimens, the identification of reliable serum tumor markers, as well as the appropriate integration of systemic chemotherapy and surgery has led to an overall survival for patients with testicular cancer of greater than 90%.[27] Germ cell tumors of the testes have a predictable and systematic pattern of metastatic spread from the primary site to the retroperitoneal lymph nodes and subsequently to distant sites (most commonly the lung and posterior mediastinum). Anatomic studies and detailed mapping studies of retroperitoneal lymph node dissections (RPLNDs) have identified the first echelon of lymph nodes draining the right testis to the interaortocaval region, followed by the precaval and preaortic nodes. For left-sided testicular tumors, the primary landing zone includes the preaortic and para-aortic lymph nodes, followed by the interaortocaval nodes.[48] There are 4 to 8 lymphatic vessels that

accompany the spermatic vessels through the internal ring into the retroperitoneum. At the point where the spermatic vessels cross ventral to the ureter, lymph channels fan out medially in relation to the aorta and inferior vena cava (IVC) and drain into the retroperitoneal lymph node chain extending from approximately L5 to T11. Contralateral lymphatic flow is often seen, particularly for right-sided lymphatics.[49]

A RPLND in patients is essential because the retroperitoneum is the initial (and often solitary) site of metastatic spread in 75% to 90% of patients with GCT.[50] A properly performed RPLND is also essential for accurate clinical staging of the retroperitoneum, which is supported by studies reporting a 20% to 30% incidence of pathologic upstaging to stage II disease in patients with clinical stage I.[51] Further, there is a 20% incidence of teratoma and/or viable carcinoma in resected masses of patients with radiographically normal CT scans after chemotherapy. RPLND has an established role for the resection of residual masses given the risk of residual viable malignancy and/or teratoma.[52]

Perioperative morbidity of RPLND is generally related to surgeon experience, the complexity of the surgical procedure and to prior exposure to chemotherapy. A large retroperitoneal tumor burden with a desmoplastic reaction observed after chemotherapy makes postchemotherapy RPLND technically more challenging than primary RPLND. The reported complication rates associated with postchemotherapy RPLND have been reported to be greater than those for primary RPLND. Early published reports of the overall complication rates associated with open postchemotherapy RPLND ranged from 20.7% to 35%.[53] Improvements in surgical technique, such as the introduction of modified templates and nerve sparing, have significantly decreased the intraoperative complications, as well as the occurrence postoperative complications such as retrograde ejaculation.

Vascular Complications

Vascular injury is a rarely reported complication after RPLND. It is more commonly reported after postchemotherapy RPLND and in those patients with bulky suprahilar disease.[54] The split-and-roll technique with division of the lumbar arteries and veins is commonly used in RPLND for circumferential removal of the tumor and lymphatic tissues surrounding the great vessels down to the level of the anterior spinal ligament. In postchemotherapy RPLND, because of the considerable desmoplastic reaction, dissection of the tumor may lead to the creation of a subadventitial plane, which renders the major retroperitoneal blood vessels susceptible to injury. In bulky tumors that extend into the suprarenal hilar region, special care must be taken to avoid injury to the superior mesenteric and celiac artery. To avoid vascular complications, it is also essential that the operating surgeon be familiar with the vascular anomalies that may be encountered, including persistence of a retroaortic or circumaortic left renal vein, ascending lumbar veins, caval duplication, and, rarely, a transposed left-sided vena cava. Preoperative imaging can help in recognizing these vascular anomalies and planning for the appropriate surgical approach.

On rare occasions during an RPLND, particularly for left-sided dissections, an adjunctive nephrectomy may be required[55] because the lymphatic drainage on the left side is immediately inferior to the renal hilum, whereas on the right side it is more remote. The proximity of lymphatic tissue to the left renal pedicle makes safe dissection of the left renal artery challenging, especially in patients with a large mass in the para-aortic region. During RPLND, injury to the renal veins or IVC may result in substantial morbidity. The left renal vein is particularly susceptible to damage because of its longer course and multiple tributaries. To avoid nephrectomy, primary repair of the vein should be preformed. The incidence of involvement of the IVC by tumor necessitating resection is 7% to 11%.[56] Resection of the IVC usually results in significant morbidity caused by venous congestion of the lower extremities and continued extravasation of lymphatic drainage into the peritoneal cavity and accumulation of chylous ascites.

Bowel Complications of RPLND

Direct injury of the bowel during RPLND is rare during primary surgery, and most commonly occurs to the duodenum usually during surgery after chemotherapy. This condition results in duodenal leak or an often-fatal aortoduodenal fistula. Mobilization and retraction of the duodenum may result in transient pancreatitis with increased serum levels of amylase and lipase. Postoperative paralytic ileus is reported in approximately 0.2% of patients undergoing primary transabdominal RPLND and in 2% of those undergoing the procedure after chemotherapy.[57] Ligation of the inferior mesenteric artery during RPLND is usually well tolerated in young patients because the blood supply to the distal colon can be maintained via the marginal artery of the colon. However, in elderly patients with preexisting atheromatous narrowing of the mesenteric vessels, vascular compromise of the colon can occur. This condition may present acutely as postoperative sepsis, secondary to a necrotic colon, or late as a colonic stricture with an associated colocutaneous fistula.[55,57]

Ejaculatory Dysfunction

Normal antegrade ejaculation is a coordinated, sequential process of seminal emission and ejaculation proper. A complete discussion of the physiology of ejaculation is beyond the scope of this article. Briefly, for normal ejaculation to ensue, 3 separate events must occur, namely closure of the bladder neck, seminal emission, and ejaculation. During ejaculation proper, the semen is ejected through the penile urethra. Ejaculation is prompted by the rhythmical contractions of the bulbocavernosus and ischiocavernosus muscles coupled with complete bladder neck closure and relaxation of the external urethral sphincter and urogenital diaphragm. The ejaculatory phase is controlled by a somatic spinal reflex at the S2 to S4 level, whereas seminal emission and bladder neck closure are governed by the sympathetic nervous system and are most vulnerable to damage during RPLND.

Loss of antegrade ejaculation caused by damage of sympathetic nerve fibers is a source of significant long-term morbidity after standard bilateral RPLND.[58] The incidence of this complication is related to the extent of the retroperitoneal dissection. Sympathetic fibers from the thoracolumbar outflow tract decussating around the aortic bifurcation are responsible for seminal emission into the posterior urethra. Preservation of these fibers is crucial to maintain antegrade ejaculation.[59] An improved understanding of the neuroanatomy of seminal emission and ejaculation, anatomic studies of the distribution of retroperitoneal metastasis for right-sided and left-sided tumors, and surgical mapping studies have resulted in the development of a modified-template RPLND and, more recently, nerve-sparing dissections using nerve-sparing techniques in an effort to reduce the incidence of ejaculatory dysfunction. Nerve-sparing techniques rely on precise dissection and preservation of vital neuroanatomic structures. A selective or unilateral nerve-sparing technique may be performed in patients with limited residual retroperitoneal disease but is more difficult after chemotherapy. A modified dissection template limits the extent of dissection to anatomic regions likely to be at increased risk of metastatic disease. Combining nerve-sparing techniques with modified templates has resulted in postoperative ejaculation rates of 84% to 98%.[37]

Lymphatic Complications of RPLND

The main lymphatic channels in the retroperitoneum travel posterior and parallel to the aorta and IVC and are formed by the coalescence of the common iliac lymph vessels. Typically, both lymphatic trunks merge posterior and medial to the aorta to form the cisterna chyli. The cisterna chyli is commonly situated behind the left crus of the diaphragm. Transection of major lymphatics, particularly those that drain directly into the cisterna chyli, may result in formation of chylous ascites in around 2% of patients undergoing RPLND.[60] Risk factors include resection of the IVC and dissection above the level of the renal vessels, an area of abundant lymphatic vessels that also contains the cisterna chyli.[57] Abdominal distention, enlarging girth, and disproportionate weight gain are among the most common clinical features of chylous ascites.

The diagnosis of chylous ascites is generally made by diagnostic paracentesis. The fluid aspirated appears milky, is odorless, and has a high content of protein (>3 g/dL) and triglycerides (twofold to eightfold higher than that of plasma). Most patients are treated successfully by dietary treatment, including restriction of fat, administration of medium-chain triglyceride and diuretics, and administration of a somatostatin analogue, with the occasional need for intravenous hyperalimentation. The somatostatin analogue octreotide greatly reduces the lymphatic output through the fistula within 24 to 72 hours after initiating therapy and should be attempted early in the course of treatment. Rarely, patients require more invasive treatments, such as the placement of peritoneovenous shunts or surgical intervention.

REFERENCES

1. Horenblas S, van Tinteren H, Delemarre JF, et al. Squamous cell carcinoma of the penis. III. Treatment of regional lymph nodes. J Urol 1993;149(3):492–7.
2. Solsona E, Iborra I, Rubio J, et al. Prospective validation of the association of local tumor stage and grade as a predictive factor for occult lymph node micrometastasis in patients with penile carcinoma and clinically negative inguinal lymph nodes. J Urol 2001;165(5):1506–9.
3. el-Demiry MI, Oliver RT, Hope-Stone HF, et al. Reappraisal of the role of radiotherapy and surgery in the management of carcinoma of the penis. Br J Urol 1984;56(6):724–8.
4. Wein AJ, Kavoussi LR, Novick AC. Tumors of the penis. In: Wein AJ, Kavoussi LR, Novick AC, editors. Campbell-Walsh urology. Philadelphia: Saunders; 2007. p. 959–92.
5. Hegarty PK, Kayes O, Freeman A, et al. A prospective study of 100 cases of penile cancer managed according to European Association of Urology guidelines. BJU Int 2006;98(3):526–31.
6. Solsona E, Algaba F, Horenblas S, et al, European Association of Urology. EAU guidelines on penile cancer. Eur Urol 2004;46(1):1–8.
7. Slaton JW, Morgenstern N, Levy DA, et al. Tumor stage, vascular invasion and the percentage of poorly differentiated cancer: independent prognosticators for inguinal lymph node metastasis in penile squamous cancer. J Urol 2001;165(4):1138–42.
8. Ornellas AA, Kinchin EW, Nobrega BL, et al. Surgical treatment of invasive squamous cell carcinoma of the penis: Brazilian National Cancer Institute long-term experience. J Surg Oncol 2008; 97(6):487–95.
9. Johnson DE, Lo RK. Complications of groin dissection in penile cancer. Experience with 101 lymphadenectomies. Urology 1984;24(4):312–4.
10. Coblentz TR, Theodorescu D. Morbidity of modified prophylactic inguinal lymphadenectomy for squamous cell carcinoma of the penis. J Urol 2002; 168(4 Pt 1):1386–9.
11. Milathianakis C, Bogdanos J, Karamanolakis D. Morbidity of prophylactic inguinal lymphadenectomy with saphenous vein preservation for squamous cell penile carcinoma. Int J Urol 2005;12(8): 776–8.
12. Heyns CF, Fleshner N, Sangar V, et al. Management of the lymph nodes in penile cancer. Urology 2010; 76(2 Suppl 1):S43–57.
13. Ravi R. Morbidity following groin dissection for penile carcinoma. Br J Urol 1993;72(6):941–5.
14. Josephs LG, Cordts PR, DiEdwardo CL, et al. Do infected inguinal lymph nodes increase the incidence of postoperative groin wound infection? J Vasc Surg 1993;17(6):1077–80 [discussion: 1080–2].
15. Johnson DE, Lo RK. Management of regional lymph nodes in penile carcinoma. Five-year results following therapeutic groin dissections. Urology 1984;24(4):308–11.
16. Brismar B, Ljungdahl I. Postoperative lymphoedema after treatment of breast cancer. Acta Chir Scand 1983;149(7):687–9.
17. Catalona WJ. Modified inguinal lymphadenectomy for carcinoma of the penis with preservation of saphenous veins: technique and preliminary results. J Urol 1988;140(2):306–10.
18. Zhang XL, Sheng XG, Li HQ, et al. [Preservation of the saphenous vein during inguinal lymphadenectomy for vulval malignancies]. Ai Zheng 2007; 26(3):290–3 [in Chinese].
19. Nelson BA, Cookson MS, Smith JA Jr, et al. Complications of inguinal and pelvic lymphadenectomy for squamous cell carcinoma of the penis: a contemporary series. J Urol 2004;172(2):494–7.

20. Horenblas S. Lymphadenectomy for squamous cell carcinoma of the penis. Part 2: the role and technique of lymph node dissection. BJU Int 2001;88(5):473–83.

21. Catalona WJ. Role of lymphadenectomy in carcinoma of the penis. Urol Clin North Am 1980;7(3):785–92.

22. Spiess PE, Hernandez MS, Pettaway CA. Contemporary inguinal lymph node dissection: minimizing complications. World J Urol 2009;27(2):205–12.

23. Freiha FS, Salzman J. Surgical staging of prostatic cancer: transperitoneal versus extraperitoneal lymphadenectomy. J Urol 1977;118(4):616–7.

24. Bhatta-Dhar N, Reuther AM, Zippe C, et al. No difference in six-year biochemical failure rates with or without pelvic lymph node dissection during radical prostatectomy in low-risk patients with localized prostate cancer. Urology 2004;63(3):528–31.

25. Partin AW, Kattan MW, Subong EN, et al. Combination of prostate-specific antigen, clinical stage, and Gleason score to predict pathological stage of localized prostate cancer. A multi-institutional update. JAMA 1997;277(18):1445–51.

26. Sivalingam S, Oxley J, Probert JL, et al. Role of pelvic lymphadenectomy in prostate cancer management. Urology 2007;69(2):203–9.

27. Jemal A, Siegel R, Xu J, et al. Cancer statistics, 2010. CA Cancer J Clin 2010;60(5):277–300.

28. Leissner J, Hohenfellner R, Thuroff JW, et al. Lymphadenectomy in patients with transitional cell carcinoma of the urinary bladder; significance for staging and prognosis. BJU Int 2000;85(7):817–23.

29. Vazina A, Dugi D, Shariat SF, et al. Stage specific lymph node metastasis mapping in radical cystectomy specimens. J Urol 2004;171(5):1830–4.

30. Skinner DG. Management of invasive bladder cancer: a meticulous pelvic node dissection can make a difference. J Urol 1982;128(1):34–6.

31. Leadbetter WF, Cooper JF. Regional gland dissection for carcinoma of the bladder; a technique for one-stage cystectomy, gland dissection, and bilateral uretero-enterostomy. J Urol 1950;63(2):242–60.

32. Stenzl A, Cowan NC, De Santis M, et al. The updated EAU guidelines on muscle-invasive and metastatic bladder cancer. Eur Urol 2009;55(4):815–25.

33. Bochner BH, Cho D, Herr HW, et al. Prospectively packaged lymph node dissections with radical cystectomy: evaluation of node count variability and node mapping. J Urol 2004;172(4 Pt 1):1286–90.

34. Herr HW, Donat SM. Outcome of patients with grossly node positive bladder cancer after pelvic lymph node dissection and radical cystectomy. J Urol 2001;165(1):62–4 [discussion: 64].

35. Herr HW. Surgical factors in bladder cancer: more (nodes) + more (pathology) = less (mortality). BJU Int 2003;92(3):187–8.

36. Briganti A, Blute ML, Eastham JH, et al. Pelvic lymph node dissection in prostate cancer. Eur Urol 2009; 55(6):1251–65.

37. Patel A. Complications of urologic surgery- prevention and management. 3rd edition. Philadelphia: Saunders; 2001. p. 370–85.

38. Solberg A, Angelsen A, Bergan U, et al. Frequency of lymphoceles after open and laparoscopic pelvic lymph node dissection in patients with prostate cancer. Scand J Urol Nephrol 2003;37(3):218–21.

39. Musch M, Klevecka V, Roggenbuck U, et al. Complications of pelvic lymphadenectomy in 1,380 patients undergoing radical retropubic prostatectomy between 1993 and 2006. J Urol 2008;179(3):923–8 [discussion: 928–9].

40. Loeb S, Partin AW, Schaeffer EM. Complications of pelvic lymphadenectomy: do the risks outweigh the benefits? Rev Urol 2010;12(1):20–4.

41. Gotto GT, Yunis LH, Guillonneau B, et al. Predictors of symptomatic lymphocele after radical prostatectomy and bilateral pelvic lymph node dissection. Int J Urol 2011 Feb 10. [Epub ahead of print].

42. Heinzer H, Hammerer P, Graefen M, et al. Thromboembolic complication rate after radical retropubic prostatectomy. Impact of routine ultrasonography for the detection of pelvic lymphoceles and hematomas. Eur Urol 1998;33(1):86–90.

43. Naselli A, Andreatta R, Introini C, et al. Predictors of symptomatic lymphocele after lymph node excision and radical prostatectomy. Urology 2010;75(3): 630–5.

44. Catalona WJ, Kadmon D, Crane DB. Effect of minidose heparin on lymphocele formation following extraperitoneal pelvic lymphadenectomy. J Urol 1980; 123(6):890–2.

45. Kropfl D, Krause R, Hartung R, et al. Subcutaneous heparin injection in the upper arm as a method of avoiding lymphoceles after lymphadenectomies in the lower part of the body. Urol Int 1987;42(6): 416–23.

46. Fallick ML, Long JP. Laparoscopic marsupialization of lymphocele after laparoscopic lymph node dissection. J Endourol 1996;10(6):533–4.

47. Kavoussi LR, Sosa E, Chandhoke P, et al. Complications of laparoscopic pelvic lymph node dissection. J Urol 1993;149(2):322–5.

48. Donohue JP, Zachary JM, Maynard BR. Distribution of nodal metastases in nonseminomatous testis cancer. J Urol 1982;128(2):315–20.

49. Donohue JP. Evolution of retroperitoneal lymphadenectomy (RPLND) in the management of nonseminomatous testicular cancer (NSGCT). Urol Oncol 2003;21(2):129–32.

50. Whitmore WF Jr. Surgical treatment of adult germinal testis tumors. Semin Oncol 1979;6(1):55–68.

51. Albers P, Siener R, Kliesch S, et al. Risk factors for relapse in clinical stage I nonseminomatous testicular germ cell tumors: results of the German Testicular Cancer Study Group Trial. J Clin Oncol 2003; 21(8):1505–12.

52. George DW, Foster RS, Hromas RA, et al. Update on late relapse of germ cell tumor: a clinical and molecular analysis. J Clin Oncol 2003;21(1):113–22.

53. Baniel J, Foster RS, Rowland RG, et al. Complications of post-chemotherapy retroperitoneal lymph node dissection. J Urol 1995;153(3 Pt 2):976–80.

54. Abouassaly R, Klein EA, Raghavan D. Complications of surgery and chemotherapy for testicular cancer. Urol Oncol 2005;23(6):447–55.

55. Christmas TJ, Smith GL, Kooner R. Vascular interventions during post-chemotherapy retroperitoneal lymph-node dissection for metastatic testis cancer. Eur J Surg Oncol 1998;24(4):292–7.

56. Albers P, Melchior D, Muller SC. Surgery in metastatic testicular cancer. Eur Urol 2003;44(2):233–44.

57. Baniel J, Sella A. Complications of retroperitoneal lymph node dissection in testicular cancer: primary and post-chemotherapy. Semin Surg Oncol 1999; 17(4):263–7.

58. Jewett MA, Kong YS, Goldberg SD, et al. Retroperitoneal lymphadenectomy for testis tumor with nerve sparing for ejaculation. J Urol 1988;139(6): 1220–4.

59. Sheinfeld J, Herr HW. Role of surgery in management of germ cell tumor. Semin Oncol 1998;25(2): 203–9.

60. Baniel J, Foster RS, Rowland RG, et al. Management of chylous ascites after retroperitoneal lymph node dissection for testicular cancer. J Urol 1993;150 (5 Pt 1):1422–4.

Index

Note: Page numbers of article titles are in **boldface** type.

Urol Clin N Am 38 (2011) 519–523
doi:10.1016/S0094-0143(11)00104-2
0094-0143/11/$ – see front matter © 2011 Elsevier Inc. All rights reserved.

urologic.theclinics.com

United States Postal Service

Statement of Ownership, Management, and Circulation
(All Periodicals Publications Except Requestor Publications)

1. Publication Title	2. Publication Number		3. Filing Date
Urologic Clinics of North America	0 0 0	- 7 1 1 1	9/15/11

4. Issue Frequency	5. Number of Issues Published Annually	6. Annual Subscription Price
Feb, May, Aug, Nov	4	$291.00

7. Complete Mailing Address of Known Office of Publication (Not printer) (Street, city, county, state, and ZIP+4®)	Contact Person
Elsevier Inc. 360 Park Avenue South New York, NY 10010-1710	Stephen Bushing
	Telephone (Include area code)
	215-239-3688

8. Complete Mailing Address of Headquarters or General Business Office of Publisher (Not printer)

Elsevier Inc., 360 Park Avenue South, New York, NY 10010-1710

9. Full Names and Complete Mailing Addresses of Publisher, Editor, and Managing Editor (Do not leave blank)

Publisher (Name and complete mailing address)

Kim Murphy, Elsevier, Inc., 1600 John F. Kennedy Blvd. Suite 1800, Philadelphia, PA 19103-2899

Editor (Name and complete mailing address)

Stephanie Donley, Elsevier, Inc., 1600 John F. Kennedy Blvd. Suite 1800, Philadelphia, PA 19103-2899

Managing Editor (Name and complete mailing address)

Barton Dudlick, Elsevier, Inc., 1600 John F. Kennedy Blvd. Suite 1800, Philadelphia, PA 19103-2899

10. Owner (Do not leave blank. If the publication is owned by a corporation, give the name and address of the corporation immediately followed by the names and addresses of all stockholders owning or holding 1 percent or more of the total amount of stock. If not owned by a corporation, give the names and addresses of the individual owners. If owned by a partnership or other unincorporated firm, give its name and address as well as those of each individual owner. If the publication is published by a nonprofit organization, give its name and address.)

Full Name	Complete Mailing Address
Wholly owned subsidiary of	4520 East-West Highway
Reed/Elsevier, US holdings	Bethesda, MD 20814

11. Known Bondholders, Mortgagees, and Other Security Holders Owning or Holding 1 Percent or More of Total Amount of Bonds, Mortgages, or Other Securities. If none, check box ☐ None

Full Name	Complete Mailing Address
N/A	

12. Tax Status (For completion by nonprofit organizations authorized to mail at nonprofit rates) (Check one)
The purpose, function, and nonprofit status of this organization and the exempt status for federal income tax purposes:
☐ Has Not Changed During Preceding 12 Months
☐ Has Changed During Preceding 12 Months (Publisher must submit explanation of change with this statement)

PS Form 3526, September 2007 (Page 1 of 3 (Instructions Page 3)) PSN 7530-01-000-9931 PRIVACY NOTICE: See our Privacy policy in www.usps.com

---

13. Publication Title	14. Issue Date for Circulation Data Below
Urologic Clinics of North America	August 2011

15. Extent and Nature of Circulation			Average No. Copies Each Issue During Preceding 12 Months	No. Copies of Single Issue Published Nearest to Filing Date
a. Total Number of Copies (Net press run)			2313	2000
b. Paid Circulation (By Mail and Outside the Mail)	(1)	Mailed Outside-County Paid Subscriptions Stated on PS Form 3541. (Include paid distribution above nominal rate, advertiser's proof copies, and exchange copies)	860	794
	(2)	Mailed In-County Paid Subscriptions Stated on PS Form 3541 (Include paid distribution above nominal rate, advertiser's proof copies, and exchange copies)		
	(3)	Paid Distribution Outside the Mails Including Sales Through Dealers and Carriers, Street Vendors, Counter Sales, and Other Paid Distribution Outside USPS®	614	639
	(4)	Paid Distribution by Other Classes Mailed Through the USPS (e.g. First-Class Mail®)		
c. Total Paid Distribution (Sum of 15b (1), (2), (3), and (4))		▶	1474	1433
d. Free or Nominal Rate Distribution (By Mail and Outside the Mail)	(1)	Free or Nominal Rate Outside-County Copies Included on PS Form 3541	97	78
	(2)	Free or Nominal Rate In-County Copies Included on PS Form 3541		
	(3)	Free or Nominal Rate Copies Mailed at Other Classes Through the USPS (e.g. First-Class Mail)		
	(4)	Free or Nominal Rate Distribution Outside the Mail (Carriers or other means)		
e. Total Free or Nominal Rate Distribution (Sum of 15d (1), (2), (3) and (4))		▶	97	78
f. Total Distribution (Sum of 15c and 15e)		▶	1571	1511
g. Copies not Distributed (See instructions to publishers #4 (page #3))		▶	742	489
h. Total (Sum of 15f and g)		▶	2313	2000
i. Percent Paid (15c divided by 15f times 100)			93.83%	94.84%

16. Publication of Statement of Ownership

☐ If the publication is a general publication, publication of this statement is required. Will be printed
in the November 2011 issue of this publication.

☐ Publication not required

17. Signature and Title of Editor, Publisher, Business Manager, or Owner	Date
Stephen R. Bushing – Fulfillment/Inventory Specialist	September 15, 2011

I certify that all information furnished on this form is true and complete. I understand that anyone who furnishes false or misleading information on this form or who omits material or information requested on the form may be subject to criminal sanctions (including fines and imprisonment) and/or civil sanctions (including civil penalties).

PS Form 3526, September 2007 (Page 2 of 3)

Moving?

Make sure your subscription moves with you!

To notify us of your new address, find your **Clinics Account Number** (located on your mailing label above your name), and contact customer service at:

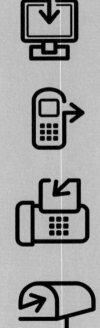

Email: journalscustomerservice-usa@elsevier.com

800-654-2452 (subscribers in the U.S. & Canada)
314-447-8871 (subscribers outside of the U.S. & Canada)

Fax number: 314-447-8029

Elsevier Health Sciences Division
Subscription Customer Service
3251 Riverport Lane
Maryland Heights, MO 63043

*To ensure uninterrupted delivery of your subscription, please notify us at least 4 weeks in advance of move.